Psychological Interventions in Childhood Chronic Illness

GRACE LIBRARY CARLOW UNIVERSITY
PITTSBURGH PA 15213

Psychological Interventions in Childhood Chronic Illness

DENNIS DROTAR

with

DAWN O. WITHERSPOON,

KATHY ZEBRACKI,

and

CATHERINE CANT PETERSON

RJ
380
D76
2006

American Psychological Association
Washington, DC

CATALOGUED

Copyright © 2006 by the American Psychological Association. All rights reserved. Except as permitted under the United States Copyright Act of 1976, no part of this publication may be reproduced or distributed in any form or by any means, including, but not limited to, the process of scanning and digitization, or stored in a database or retrieval system, without the prior written permission of the publisher.

Published by
American Psychological Association
750 First Street, NE
Washington, DC 20002
www.apa.org

To order
APA Order Department
P.O. Box 92984
Washington, DC 20090-2984
Tel: (800) 374-2721
Direct: (202) 336-5510
Fax: (202) 336-5502
TDD/TTY: (202) 336-6123
Online: www.apa.org/books/
E-mail: order@apa.org

In the U.K., Europe, Africa, and the Middle East, copies may be ordered from
American Psychological Association
3 Henrietta Street
Covent Garden, London
WC2E 8LU England

Typeset in Goudy by World Composition Services, Inc., Sterling, VA

Printer: Data Reproductions, Auburn Hills, MI
Cover Designer: Go! Creative, Kensington, MD
Technical/Production Editor: Harriet Kaplan

The opinions and statements published are the responsibility of the authors, and such opinions and statements do not necessarily represent the policies of the American Psychological Association.

Library of Congress Cataloging-in-Publication Data

Drotar, Dennis.
    Psychological interventions in childhood chronic illness / by Dennis Drotar ; with Dawn O. Witherspoon, Kathy Zebracki, and Catherine Cant Peterson.—1st ed.
        p. cm.
    Includes bibliographical references and index.
    ISBN 1-59147-330-6
    1. Chronic diseases in children—Psychological aspects. 2. Chronically ill children—Medical care. 3. Chronically ill children—Services for. I. American Psychological Association. II. Title. [DNLM: 1. Chronic Disease—psychology—Child. 2. Chronic Disease—psychology—Adolescent. 3. Mental Health Services—Child. 4. Mental Health Services—Adolescent. 5. Child Psychology. 6. Adolescent Psychology.

WS 200 D787p 2006] RJ380.D76 2006
618.92—dc22   2005025428

British Library Cataloguing-in-Publication Data
A CIP record is available from the British Library.

Printed in the United States of America
First Edition

RIT $49.95 11-25-08 GROONS

This book is dedicated to my wife, Peggy Crawford, who has taught me (and teaches me every day) about the compassion, commitment, and integrity that are ideally necessary to care for individuals affected with chronic illness and their families and about the meaning of love and long-term commitment.

CONTENTS

ACKNOWLEDGMENTS

The work reflected in this book represents the cumulative product of my many years of clinical experiences with children and families with chronic illnesses, who have taught me so much about human courage in the face of difficult odds; collaborations with physician colleagues, who have dedicated their lives to the care of children and adolescents with chronic illness; work with students and fellows, who have made an extraordinary commitment to research and clinical care for children and adolescents with chronic illness; and my colleagues in the field of pediatric psychology, who have provided wisdom, inspiration, and models of clinical care and research. Their support and influence is gratefully acknowledged. In addition, special acknowledgment is given to Susan Wood, who typed this book (which became a chronic condition in itself) with her usual extraordinary care and attention to quality.

Psychological Interventions in Childhood Chronic Illness

INTRODUCTION

The impetus for this book came from my years of clinical and research experience with children and adolescents with chronic illness and their families. As a practitioner, I have worked with children and adolescents with a range of conditions, such as cystic fibrosis, diabetes, asthma, and renal disease, who also presented with a range of psychological adjustment problems such as anxiety and depression. These experiences led me to wonder why it was that some children with very serious illnesses managed to cope very well with the rigors of a chronic condition whereas others with milder illnesses demonstrated significant psychological problems. The following questions fascinated me then and still do to this day: (a) What was it about these children and families that contributed to their resilience in the face of stress? (b) Alternatively, what heightened their risks for psychological problems? These questions became the focus of my initial research on pediatric chronic illness. Over the past 10 years, I have become interested in applying data from such descriptive studies to developing and testing interventions. The current focus of my research revolves around questions that concern the effects of psychological interventions delivered by psychologists and other professionals to children with chronic illness and families to improve their ability to adjust to and manage a serious chronic illness.

This book was written to summarize some of the lessons I have learned in the course of my experiences in clinical care and research, to provide a synthesis of current empirical knowledge concerning psychological interventions, and to consider recommendations to develop and evaluate psychological interventions that would be most helpful to children with chronic illness and their families. To accomplish this purpose, this book has the following specific aims: (a) to describe key research findings concerning strategies of interventions to promote illness management, reduce rates of nonadherence to medical treatment among children, and improve psychological adaptation of children and adolescents with chronic illness and their families; (b) to consider key methodological and measurement problems in psychological intervention research; (c) to describe short- and long-range implications of research priorities to advance scientific knowledge concerning psychological interventions to promote adherence to treatment and adaptation in pediatric chronic illness; and (d) to consider implications of research findings, clinical applications, and policies concerning psychological interventions for children and adolescents with chronic illness.

NEED FOR THE PRESENT VOLUME

Reviews of empirically supported interventions in psychological and health-related morbidity of childhood chronic illness have underscored the efficacy of various interventions to improve psychological adaptation (Bauman, Drotar, Leventhal, Perrin, & Pless, 1997; Kibby, Tyc, & Mulhern, 1998), ensure adherence to treatment (Lemanek, Kamps, & Chung, 2001), and reduce the impact of pain, both illness related (G. W. Walco, Sterling, Conte, & Engel, 1999) and procedure related (Kuppenheimer & Brown, 2002; Powers, 1999). Kibby et al. (1998) conducted what is to my knowledge the only meta-analysis of psychological interventions for children and adolescents with a broad group of chronic health conditions on 42 studies that focused on disease management (e.g., adherence to treatment), emotional–behavioral problems, and health promotion and prevention. Overall, psychological interventions were found to be effective with a large effect size of 1.12, based on J. Cohen (1988). Moreover, these intervention gains were maintained for at least 12 months posttreatment in some studies. Psychological interventions directed at emotional–behavioral problems were found to be effective. However, Kibby et al.'s (1998) analysis did not include a substantial body of recent intervention research. Moreover, they did not review the findings of psychological interventions that focused on enhancement of adherence to the medical treatment of pediatric chronic illness. In recent years, there has been significant progress in development of empirically supported psychological interventions in a range of pediatric chronic illnesses (Bauman et al., 1997; Kibby et al., 1998; Lemanek et al., 2001;

McQuaid & Nassau, 1999; Powers, 1999). However, this work has not been synthesized.

Despite considerable progress in recent years with interventions with various chronic illness populations, relatively few such interventions can be considered as well established on the basis of criteria for empirically supported interventions (Lemanek et al., 2001; McQuaid & Nassau, 1999; Powers, 1999). Moreover, substantial methodological problems in the design and evaluation of psychological interventions that relate to the inherent challenges of conducting intervention research in childhood chronic illness have limited scientific progress (Bauman et al., 1997; Drotar, 1997a, 1997b, 2002; Kibby et al., 1998; Lemanek et al., 2001; Powers, 1999; Rapoff, 1999). To my knowledge, these issues have not been well described. The present volume was designed to address these gaps in scientific understanding and clinical relevance by describing the state of the art in psychological intervention research, detailing relevant methodological and clinical challenges in conducting such research, and proposing recommendations to improve the science and practice of psychological interventions.

ORGANIZATION OF THE BOOK

The volume is organized in four parts: Part I presents an overview of research on psychological interventions; Part II describes pragmatic strategies in conducting intervention research; Part III details psychological interventions with representative chronic pediatric conditions, including research and clinical applications; and Part IV provides recommendations for research on psychological intervention, practice, and policy.

Part I: Overview of Research

Part I includes two chapters that provide an introduction and framework for the book. The first chapter of the book provides an overview of the incidence and prevalence of childhood chronic illness, including the psychological impact of chronic illness on children, adolescents, and their families, as well as targets for relevant interventions, developmental issues, and individual differences in patterns of psychological adjustment. Chapter 2 provides an overview and critique of theories that have guided psychological research on pediatric chronic illness and the implications for psychological intervention.

Part II: Pragmatic Strategies

The chapters in Part II describe the pragmatic issues involved in conducting intervention research with children and adolescents with chronic illness. Chapter 3 is devoted to research methods and covers such issues as design of interventions, sampling considerations, choice of target outcomes, options for study design, data analysis, sample attrition, and measurement issues. Chapter 4 describes the pragmatic issues that are involved in conducting psychological intervention research, such as developing collaborative resources to support research and a research team, sample recruitment and retention, and management of intervention studies. Chapter 5 considers relevant ethical issues in conducting research on pediatric chronic illness, including informed consent and assent with children and adolescents.

Part III: Psychological Interventions With Representative Pediatric Chronic Conditions

Part III (chaps. 6–10) synthesizes current research on psychological interventions with a range of pediatric chronic conditions, including asthma (chap. 6), diabetes (chap. 7), cancer (chap. 8), sickle cell disease and juvenile rheumatoid arthritis (chap. 9), and cystic fibrosis (chap. 10). These pediatric chronic conditions were chosen to reflect a broad spectrum in which psychological intervention research has been conducted. Choice of these chronic conditions also reflects my experience. Syntheses of research in chapters 6 and 7 include a detailed summary of published reviews of psychological interventions in asthma and diabetes, which represent conditions for which a critical mass of intervention research has been reviewed critically. In contrast, other chapters (8–10) focus on pediatric cancer, sickle cell disease, rheumatoid arthritis, and cystic fibrosis, all of which are chronic conditions for which empirically supported interventions have been published less frequently. Chapters devoted to each of these conditions include tables that summarize findings from intervention studies. Recommendations for future research and clinical applications, including comprehensive care, are described in each chapter.

Part IV: Summary and Conclusion

The final section includes a summary chapter (chap. 11) that provides recommendations to enhance psychological intervention science, clinical applications, dissemination of intervention science, developing the field of intervention research, and policy. This chapter describes a framework to consider the interrelationship among research, practice, training, policy, and the stages of intervention research. Finally, a detailed agenda for future work on psychological interventions is provided.

I

OVERVIEW OF RESEARCH

1

PSYCHOLOGICAL INTERVENTION RESEARCH: NEEDS AND CRITICAL ISSUES

This chapter presents an overview of issues that relate to the need for psychological interventions among children and adolescents with chronic illness. Each of the issues described in this chapter has relevance for the clinical significance, design, and implementation of psychological intervention research. These issues include (a) the prevalence of childhood chronic illness; (b) description of the multifaceted impact of pediatric chronic illness on children and families; (c) barriers to psychological intervention; (d) targets, methods, and outcomes of intervention, including examples of psychological interventions; and (e) individual differences.

PREVALENCE OF PEDIATRIC CHRONIC ILLNESS

For the purpose of this book, a chronic or ongoing health condition is defined as one that (a) lasts a year or longer; (b) requires specialized treatments or technologies; and (c) causes limitations in function, activities, or social roles in patients compared with physically healthy peers (R. E. K. Stein, Bauman, Westbrook, Coupey, & Ireys, 1993). The importance of psychological interventions for children with chronic physical illness relates to the prevalence and psychological impact of these conditions. Chronic pediatric illness affects large numbers of children, adolescents, and families. For example, a national survey estimated that the prevalence rate of children with chronic health conditions was 18% (Newacheck, McManus, Fox, Hung, & Halfon, 2000). Children from economically disadvantaged families have a higher risk of experiencing severe chronic conditions than children from higher income families (Newacheck, 1994).

It should be noted that the specific estimates of prevalence of pediatric illness will vary considerably depending on the method of sampling, the population that is sampled, and the specific measures and questions that are used to define chronic conditions. For this reason, investigators should carefully consider the sources from which data concerning the prevalence of pediatric chronic illness are drawn. National estimates of prevalence are important in defining the overall scope of the problem of pediatric chronic illness. However, national estimates are not necessarily useful to individual investigators and practitioners who will be most interested in the numbers of children and adolescents in the age range of interest who are affected with a specific chronic condition in a particular setting. The prevalence of specific chronic conditions varies from the relatively common pediatric asthma to rarer conditions such as cystic fibrosis (see chaps. 6–10).

The number of children and adolescents available to participate in a psychological intervention study will depend on the number being followed for medical care in a particular setting, which investigators can ascertain by reviewing patient rosters and databases (see chap. 3). In general, the number available to participate in a psychological intervention study at any particular site may be relatively small, unless the site is a major referral and clinical center for the region. For this reason, multisite studies involving different clinical settings in the same city or, depending on available resources, centers in different parts of the country may be needed (see chap. 3).

MULTIFACETED PSYCHOLOGICAL IMPACT OF PEDIATRIC CHRONIC ILLNESS

One of the most compelling aspects of childhood chronic illness is the multifaceted nature of the psychological impact of the illness on children and their families. As shown in Figure 1.1, a chronic illness can affect the individual child's psychological adjustment as well as his or her activities and level of functioning in a wide range of important settings, such as health care, school, and with peers. In addition, the impact of a pediatric chronic illness transcends the individual child and includes his or her family members.

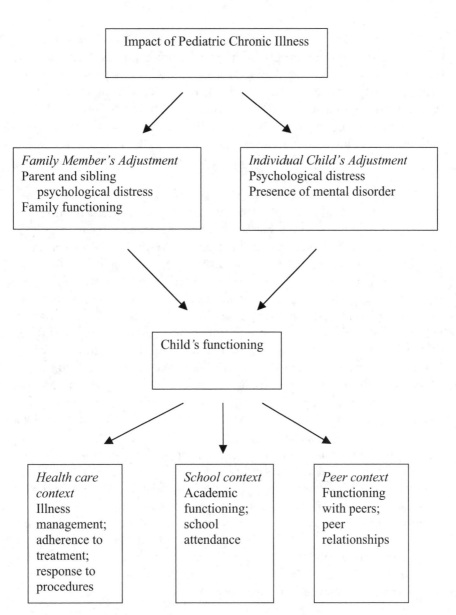

Figure 1.1. Description of the multifaceted psychological impact of pediatric chronic illness.

The multifaceted impact of pediatric chronic illness has a number of relevant implications for the design and implementation of psychological intervention research. First, to be most effective, interventions generally need to be focused on specific target problems that are interfering with the child's functioning (health or psychological adaptation) in specific settings

(Kazdin, 2000). Target problems should have a clinically significant impact on the current functioning of children or family members in at least one clinically relevant context (see Figure 1.1). In the case of preventive interventions, the focus is on the prevention of clinically significant target problems and enhancement of functioning. It should be noted that the specific intervention approach will generally vary as a function of the target problem. For example, different psychological intervention approaches may be required to manage target problems that interfere with school functioning versus illness management.

A second implication of the multifaceted impact of chronic illness is that children and adolescents with chronic illness and their families may experience other problems that affect their functioning (e.g., comorbid problems) that could affect the child or family's responsiveness to an intervention that is targeted to a specific problem. For example, children who are enrolled in an intervention designed to manage problems with adherence to treatment may also experience significant psychological problems that may interfere with their response to the intervention. Consequently, investigators will need to consider whether it is desirable or realistic to include children or their families who demonstrate problems in multiple domains of functioning in an intervention study. Such a decision may involve a difficult trade-off between the need to focus the intervention on target problems and the need to generalize the findings of the intervention to clinical care. The clinical examples in the next section illustrate potential targets of psychological intervention (see chap. 3).

A third implication concerns the prevalence of the psychological problems that are potential targets of intervention. The prevalence and functional impact of specific problems (e.g., psychological and adherence related) associated with various chronic conditions vary with the demands of the specific condition as well as associated risk factors that affect the child's adjustment (Drotar, 1981; see chaps. 6–10). Problems that are targeted for psychological intervention in research should be sufficiently prevalent in the sample that is being studied to facilitate the achievement of sufficient statistical power to detect intervention effects (see chap. 3).

Psychological Impact on the Child

This section considers specific clinical examples of the psychological impact of pediatric chronic illness on children and families and the prevalence of these problems.

Psychological Adjustment Problems

Consider the following example of an adolescent with chronic illness who is at psychological risk. Alice, a 14-year-old child with a 5-year history of cystic fibrosis, adjusted well to her condition when she was younger. However, as an adolescent she has become increasingly sensitive to and distressed about her illness and treatment. She now feels embarrassed and ashamed about her symptoms and has begun to avoid school and contact with friends. She believes that her illness is "impossible" and has also told her mother that she is not sure that she wants to "go on living" if she has to suffer so much. Her family has become increasingly concerned about Alice and has sought psychological help for her.

Alice's distress illustrates how a chronic physical illness can place significant physical and psychological burdens on children that can disrupt the quality of their lives, including their mental health. Epidemiological studies have consistently indicated that a higher than average risk for mental health disorders is associated with childhood chronic health conditions (e.g., Cadman, Boyle, Szatmari, & Offord, 1987; Gortmaker, Walker, Weitzman, & Sobol, 1990). The Ontario Child Health Survey, which included more than 3,000 children with chronic health conditions and physical disabilities, described a risk of developing a diagnosable psychiatric disorder 3 times greater (and in the absence of physical disability, a 2 times greater risk) compared with healthy children (Cadman et al., 1987). Gortmaker et al.'s (1990) study of a U.S. sample of nearly 12,000 children and adolescents found that the presence of a chronic physical condition was a risk factor for behavior problems.

Research reviews, including meta-analyses of studies of psychological adjustment of children and adolescents with a range of chronic illnesses, have also identified a relationship between childhood chronic illness and risk for psychological maladjustment. For example, Pless and Nolan's (1991) review concluded that children with chronic health conditions were twice as likely to demonstrate psychosocial maladjustment compared with physically healthy children. Lavigne and Faier-Routman's (1992) meta-analytic review of 87 studies found that children with chronic physical conditions were at an increased risk for internalizing and externalizing symptoms. Bennett's (1994) meta-analysis of 60 studies concluded that children with chronic health conditions were at higher risk for depressive symptomatology than physically healthy children. Finally, similar findings have been obtained from meta-analyses of the psychological adjustment of children with individual chronic conditions such as asthma (McQuaid, Kopel, & Nassau, 2001) and juvenile rheumatoid arthritis (JRA; LeBovidge, Lavigne, Donenberg, & Miller, 2003).

Taken together, these results underscore the salient risk of childhood chronic illness to children's mental health and the need to develop and evaluate interventions to reduce the negative impact on children's psychological adjustment. However, investigators need to recognize that these population-based data do not necessarily reflect the prevalence of children and adolescents with chronic conditions who demonstrate psychological adjustment problems in their settings. The prevalence of specific adjustment problems (e.g., depression) among children and adolescents with a specific chronic condition in any particular setting will vary as a function of the presence or absence of associated risk factors such as socioeconomic disadvantage and other factors. For this reason, it may be important for investigators to obtain information concerning the prevalence of target psychological adjustment problems among children and adolescents with the chronic condition of primary interest in their setting.

Distress Associated With Pain

Children and adolescents with chronic illness generally experience procedural pain that is associated with diagnostic and treatment procedures (Blount, Piira, & Cohen, 2003). Moreover, large numbers of children and adolescents with chronic illness experience acute or chronic pain associated with their illness (Dahlquist & Switkin, 2003; McGrath & Finley, 1999; for a review of the epidemiology of pain in children and adolescents, see Goodman & McGrath, 1991). Pain and psychological distress associated with medical procedures increase children's suffering and disrupt children's functioning in the health care context (Palermo, 2000). Consequently, they are important targets of psychological intervention for a range of chronic conditions (Kuppenheimer & Brown, 2002; Powers, 1999).

Consider Johnny, a 7-year-old with end-stage renal failure who reacted to the onset of dialysis with unmitigated panic and anger. His distress was so severe that it interfered with adherence to his dialysis treatment and was a source of great concern for his parents and physician. Johnny was given a pain management intervention involving imagery and distraction to help him manage his pain and was eventually able to cope with the dialysis procedures.

Children with chronic conditions such as Johnny's often have to endure painful diagnostic procedures that can range from injections to more invasive procedures, such as bone marrow aspirations (see chaps. 6–10; Powers, 1999). The psychological management of painful diagnostic treatment procedures is relevant for many chronic conditions (McGrath & Finley, 1999). In addition, pain is a hallmark characteristic of conditions such as cancer, sickle cell disease, and JRA (see chaps. 7–9; Kuppenheimer & Brown, 2002; Lemanek, Buckloh, Woods, & Butler, 1995; Rapoff, McGrath, & Lindsley, 2003; Wild & Espie, 2004).

Children with chronic illnesses demonstrate a wide range of patterns in adapting to acute and chronic pain. Some children cope very well with extraordinarily difficult procedures and high levels of pain, whereas others can become unduly distressed and experience problems in functioning in response to relatively minimal levels of pain. For this reason, a range of interventions have been designed and implemented to lessen the intensity of acute and recurrent pain (Walco, Sterling, Conte, & Engel, 1999; Wilson & Gil, 1996) and improve functioning in response to pain (Palermo, 2000; Palermo & Scher, 2001). The numbers of children and adolescents with chronic illness who are affected with acute or chronic pain will vary from condition to condition and from setting to setting. Moreover, the intensity and pattern of pain experienced by an individual child may vary over time. Also, children experience varying levels of dysfunction and activity limitations in response to pain (Palermo, 2000). For this reason, detailed assessments of pain and the functional consequences of pain are generally needed in the design and evaluation of intervention studies that are focused on these problems.

Illness Management and Nonadherence to Medical Treatment

The multidimensional tasks of chronic illness management include daily adherence to the prescribed treatment regimen as well as preventive management of a range of symptoms and their consequences, such as visits to the doctor or emergency room or hospitalization. Optimal illness management and adherence to medical treatment require a great deal of support from families, physicians, and comprehensive care teams and are important potential foci of preventive psychological interventions (Creer, 2000; Drotar, Crawford, & Bush, 1984).

Many children and families have difficulty coping with the complex tasks of chronic illness management and may need additional help to facilitate their management. Consider Alex, a 15-year-old who was admitted to the hospital for evaluation and treatment planning concerning control of his asthma. Poor control had been very problematic and had caused recurrent asthma attacks, which threatened his health and necessitated multiple hospitalizations. Family problems, including serious conflict with his parents about his asthma, had played a role in his problematic asthma management. Alex had also struggled with acceptance of his asthma and with adherence to his prescribed treatment. He and his family were referred for family-centered psychological intervention.

As shown in the case of Alex, problematic illness management can result in nonadherence to the prescribed treatment regimen (also termed *noncompliance*) and can have a significant impact on the child's health and health care utilization (Drotar, 2000c; La Greca & Bearman, 2003; La Greca & Schuman, 1995; Lemanek, Kamps, & Chung, 2001). Moreover, nonadherence to prescribed medical treatment for pediatric chronic illness is a prevalent problem: Rates of nonadherence of 50% or greater have been described across a range of chronic conditions (La Greca & Schuman, 1995).

However, as with psychological adjustment problems, investigators should not assume that the prevalence rates of nonadherence to medical treatment based on published research conducted in other settings will be equivalent to the rates that are demonstrated by children who are seen in their settings. For this reason, to design intervention studies that focus on nonadherence to treatment, investigators should gather information concerning the prevalence of nonadherence among children and adolescents with the target chronic illness of interest in their setting.

One reason that nonadherence to treatment is an important target of psychological intervention concerns its potential effects on children's current health and symptoms and, in some cases, on the long-term health outcomes. The precise nature of the relationship between nonadherence to prescribed medical treatment and children's short- and long-term health has yet to be documented for pediatric chronic conditions (Johnson, 1995). However, problematic adherence to treatment, especially if it continues across time, may result in clinically significant symptoms such as wheezing in asthma (see chap. 6) and high blood sugar in diabetes (see chap. 7). On the other hand, optimal illness management, which includes adherence to prescribed treatment, has been shown to reduce the rate of complications for chronic illnesses such as diabetes (Diabetes Control and Complications Trial Research Group, 1993). Moreover, clinical observations have indicated that serious problems with adherence to medical treatment can have a negative effect on the physical health of children and adolescents with chronic illnesses and the costs of their medical care (La Greca & Bearman, 2003).

Similar to mental health problems, the etiology of illness management and treatment adherence to problems are heterogeneous. A wide range of individual and family factors can influence adherence to medical treatment, which has important implications for targeting interventions (Rapoff, 1999). For example, Sally, a 17-year-old with a 7-year history of diabetes, had controlled her blood sugar within medically acceptable limits up until the past year, when she was diagnosed with depression. Since then, Sally has lost interest in keeping track of her blood sugar and managing her diet. As a consequence, her blood sugar has become increasingly less well controlled. Psychological intervention is indicated to help treat her depression and to evaluate whether pharmacological treatment is also needed.

A chronic physical illness can affect children's functioning in multiple life contexts, each of which may be the focus of potential psychological interventions. The two primary contexts in which problems may be experienced by children with chronic illness include peer relationships and school.

Peer relationships. Children and adolescents with chronic illness may experience social stigma (Westbrook, Bauman, & Shinnar, 1992) and missed opportunities for peer interaction owing to their illness and its treatment. Moreover, the experiences associated with chronic illness may lead to social withdrawal and peer-related stress (La Greca, 1990). However, it should be emphasized that the prevalence of peer relationship problems has not been well documented for many chronic conditions. Nevertheless, peer-related problems are experienced in children with chronic illness (see chaps. 6–10). For this reason, psychological interventions may be needed to enhance children's social skills and peer relationships (Varni, Katz, Colegrove, & Dolgin, 1993). For example, consider the social problems experienced by Adam, a 13-year-old with inflammatory bowel disease, who has been distressed about how his peers treat him. He is smaller than his peers and is not good at sports. He also has been absent from school multiple times because of hospitalizations, which has limited his participation in school activities and isolated him from his peers. Shy by temperament, he has few friends and feels very disengaged from his peers. He is in need of psychological intervention to facilitate his motivation to participate in peer activities and to enhance his social skills.

Functioning in school. Children and adolescents with chronic illness also can experience problems in school-related functioning. These problems may involve school absences because of hospitalizations as well as learning and academic difficulties, stemming from central nervous system disorders, that can be very stressful for children and families (R. T. Brown, 1999; Drotar, Palermo, & Barry, 2003). Moreover, as a result of advances in medical technology, large numbers of children (10%–15%) with chronic pediatric health conditions are attending school on a regular basis and may require accommodations in their curricula and academic programs, monitoring of their symptoms, or supervision or provision of medical treatment in the school setting (Clay, 2004). Although population-based estimates of the prevalence of school-related problems for children with chronic conditions are not available to my knowledge, such problems are frequently encountered in chronic conditions such as cancer and sickle cell disease (see chaps. 7 and 9).

For example, Joey, age 14, suffered a brain tumor that was treated with surgery and radiation, and he now experiences significant learning problems. His parents note that he has serious problems in organizing his behavior at home and at school and in processing academic information. These problems have affected his grades and caused a great deal of emotional distress. Problems such as Joey's may be helped by school-based interventions designed to integrate children with chronic illness who have experienced lengthy hospitalizations back into the school setting (Varni et al., 1993) and psychoeducational planning including specialized academic programs (R. T. Brown, 1999).

Psychological Impact of Pediatric Chronic Illness on Family Members

The impact of pediatric chronic illness is not restricted to the affected child but also involves the child's family. The powerful impact of pediatric chronic illness on family members can be illustrated by returning to Alice, the psychologically distressed adolescent with cystic fibrosis considered earlier in this chapter. Alice's psychological distress has had a significant impact on her family. Her parents have very different interpretations of her problems. Her mother feels responsible for Alice's distress and wonders how she failed her daughter. Alice's father believes that his daughter has been "babied" and wonders why Alice cannot accept her illness. The parents disagree about how to manage Alice's problems. Alice's younger sibling Lisa is worried about her sister but also resents the time and attention her sister receives from her parents because of her illness. Alice's family is in need of psychological intervention to address these family relationship issues.

The fact that the psychological impact of childhood chronic illness transcends the individual child and affects the entire family, including siblings and parents, has significant implications for the design and implementation of psychological intervention research. Cadman, Boyle, and Offord (1988) noted a twofold increase in risk for emotional disorders, especially depression and anxiety, among siblings of children with chronic illness. Sharpe and Rossiter's (2002) meta-analysis also identified a negative impact of chronic illness on siblings. In addition, researchers have consistently identified a high level of emotional distress among mothers of children with chronic illness, who shoulder much of the burden of the child's medical care and treatment as well as psychological management (e.g., supporting the child and family, providing information to the child and family members; Goldberg, Morris, Simmons, Fowler, & Levison, 1990; Hausenstein, 1990; Jessop, Riessman, & Stein, 1989). The impact of pediatric chronic illness on the entire family underscores the need to target interventions to reduce the level of distress on affected siblings and parents of children with chronic health conditions (Ireys, Sills, Kolodner, & Walsh, 1996; Jessop et al., 1989; R. E. K. Stein & Jessop, 1984, 1991) and to develop interventions that involve multiple family members, including parents and children (Lewis, Hatton, Salas, Leake, & Chiofalo, 1991) or siblings (Sharpe & Rossiter, 2002).

BARRIERS TO PSYCHOLOGICAL INTERVENTIONS

The need is considerable for interventions to address the wide range of adjustment and illness management problems experienced by children and adolescents with pediatric chronic illness and their families. Unfortunately, barriers to intervention and service delivery limit the numbers of children with chronic illness who receive psychological services, including those who have a clear need for them (Drotar, 1999; Sabbeth & Stein, 1990; Walders & Drotar, 1999). Cadman et al. (1987) found that among children with chronic physical illness who had a diagnosable mental health disorder, only one in four received mental health services and access to psychologists and others who deliver such services. A wide range of other barriers can also limit access to and participation in psychological intervention services in clinical settings. Some of these barriers can also interfere with child or family participation in psychological intervention research or their adherence to protocols for psychological intervention (see chap. 4). For example, the physical demands of caring for a child with a chronic physical illness can interfere with families' ability to participate in mental health services for their children with chronic health conditions. In addition, caring for a child with a chronic physical illness can generate intense emotions for parents that heighten their need to deny the magnitude and implications of the child's psychological problems (Sabbeth & Stein, 1990). For example, some parents may feel that the medical team will question the quality of their parenting if their child is identified as having a psychological problem. In addition, economic barriers that affect access to psychological intervention and cultural barriers such as mistrust may limit the ability of children with chronic illness and family members to participate in psychological services (R. T. Brown, Fuemmeller, & Forti, 2003; Maloney, Clay, & Robinson, 2005).

Reimbursement for psychological intervention under managed care is one critical barrier to such services among children with chronic illness. Although such barriers are by no means unique to children with chronic illness, these children have special problems accessing mental health services. An example is the separation of reimbursement for services for children's physical health and mental health that is inherent in the "carve out" of mental health services from a more comprehensive benefits package. This policy limits the integration of mental health services and pediatric specialty care, which can be an important component of comprehensive care for children with these conditions (Walders & Drotar, 1999).

It is important to recognize that the above barriers not only affect family participation in psychological services in clinical settings but can also limit their capacity to participate in research-based interventions. Family nonparticipation in or dropout from psychological intervention research is a significant problem that can threaten the validity and generalizability of findings (see chap. 3). For this reason, investigators need to consider methods of enhancing family members' participation in intervention research by reducing the burden of participation, enhancing family access to interventions, and increasing family members' trust of the intervention staff (see chap. 4).

A final set of barriers to psychological intervention research that are especially relevant to this book is posed by limitations in available data concerning the outcomes of intervention. Data are needed for *intervention efficacy*, which is defined as the demonstration of psychological intervention effects in randomized controlled trials (RCTs), as well as *effectiveness*, which is defined as the impact of psychological services as they are delivered to children with chronic illness and their families in clinical settings (Bauman, Drotar, Leventhal, Perrin, & Pless, 1997; Lemanek et al., 2001). In the absence of such data, it is difficult to know how best to allocate psychological services to children with specific chronic illnesses. For example, for which chronic-illness-related problems are psychological interventions most effective? What is the most efficient and cost-effective way of allocating such services? (See chap. 11.)

It is important to recognize that the data generated by psychological intervention research may eventually be useful in reducing barriers to psychological services for children and adolescents with chronic illness by influencing policy (see chap. 11). For example, research that demonstrates the efficacy of psychological intervention in reducing problems in functioning or adherence to treatment may be used to demonstrate the importance of providing reimbursement for such services. Data concerning the cost-effectiveness of outcomes of psychological interventions for children with chronic health conditions are of primary interest to hospital administrators and managed-care companies that make decisions concerning the funding of psychological services. Demonstration of cost-effective psychological services may help to create changes in reimbursement policies. These practical considerations underscore the importance of conducting research on psychological interventions that can be generalized beyond local clinical experience (see chap. 11).

Finally, intervention research may also increase the access of children with chronic illness and their families to psychological services in selected circumstances. For example, psychological intervention research is generally free to participants. In contrast, access to preventive psychological interventions, which may be offered to children and adolescents with pediatric chronic illness in research studies, is very limited in current patterns of reimbursement, at least up until the recent advent of the Health and Behavior Codes (Noll & Fischer, 2004; see chaps. 3 and 6–10).

TARGETS, METHODS, AND OUTCOMES OF INTERVENTION

A wide range of interventions have been designed and delivered to children with chronic illnesses and their families and reported in the peer-reviewed literature (Bauman et al., 1997, Kibby, Tyc, & Mulhern, 1998).

TABLE 1.1
Examples of Intervention Targets in Childhood Chronic Illness

Target of potential intervention	Method of potential intervention	Potential outcome
Primary caregiver	Social support, stress management education	Improved mental health and social support; lower distress among caregivers
Family	Psychological support, education, stress management, problem solving	Improved psychological adjustment, adherence to treatment for children and adolescents, adjustment for siblings
School environment	Education, anticipatory guidance, individualized educational plans	Improved psychological adjustment, school performance and attendance, social support, social skills, illness management
Peer relationships	Social support, problem solving, social skill enhancement	Improved social support, social skills, illness management
Child	Cognitive–behavioral intervention, coping, problem-solving skills	Lower frequency and intensity of pain and psychological distress; improved adherence to treatment

Such interventions have been designed to focus on specific problems that are demonstrated by children with chronic illness in multiple domains of functioning. As shown in Table 1.1, research on childhood chronic illness has considered a number of potential targets for intervention methods and outcomes (Bauman et al., 1997; Eiser, 1990; Garrison & McQuiston, 1989; Kibby et al., 1998; Hobbs & Perrin, 1985; Pless & Pinkerton, 1975; R. J. Thompson & Gustafson, 1996). Table 1.1 describes the range of models of psychological intervention that have been used, organized by target of intervention, method of intervention, and outcome. This table illustrates the range of psychological interventions that have been conducted to manage the spectrum of psychological problems experienced by children with chronic illness and their families. Examples of such interventions that have been conducted in the context of research are described in this section. It is useful to consider the variety in models of intervention that have been used to manage target problems associated with pediatric chronic illness. The variety of interventions, though a tribute to the ingenuity of individual investigators, makes it difficult to generalize conclusions about specific intervention models across different chronic conditions.

One issue that should be considered in reviewing the results of different models of intervention (e.g., cognitive–behavioral) is that the same model of intervention that is applied to different targets in different chronic illnesses may necessitate somewhat different strategies (see chaps. 6–10). For example, a cognitive–behavioral intervention in pediatric asthma may focus on anxiety reduction to enhance the management of asthma symptoms, whereas a cognitive–behavioral intervention in sickle cell disease may focus on enhancing coping skills to improve pain management (see chap. 10).

Primary Caregiver–Centered Models

A number of interventions have focused on enhancing support for mothers or primary caregivers of children with chronic illness. One of these is the Pediatric Ambulatory Care Treatments (PACT) program, which evaluated the impact of a program that was designed to provide integrated biomedical and psychosocial care to children with a wide range of different chronic illnesses (R. E. K. Stein & Jessop, 1984, 1991). In addition to comprehensive medical care, PACT provided coordination of health services and social and community resources, education, and training in self-care skills. The intervention model included an initial home visit by a pediatric nurse practitioner and general pediatrician and at least one contact a month thereafter in person or by telephone for a period of at least 6 months (R. E. K. Stein & Jessop, 1984). At 6- to 12-month follow-up, children who received the comprehensive care program had better psychological adjustment than did children who received medical standard care (R. E. K. Stein & Jessop, 1984). Mothers who received the comprehensive care program also had fewer psychiatric symptoms and greater satisfaction with care. These findings were sustained on a 5-year follow-up (R. E. K. Stein & Jessop, 1991). However, these interventions did not affect the impact of the illness on other family members.

Ireys et al. (1996) evaluated the efficacy of a comprehensive social support intervention, including informational support (e.g., sharing information), affirmational support (e.g., identification of competency and giving positive feedback), and emotional support (e.g., listening to concerns) that was provided by mentors. These mentors were the mothers of adults who had had JRA since childhood. Mothers who received the intervention demonstrated greater improvement on several measures of social support compared with controls.

Family-Centered Models

A range of family-centered intervention models have been shown to enhance child and maternal adjustment. For example, Pless et al. (1994) tested the efficacy of a family-centered nursing intervention that focused on helping families manage the impact of the chronic illness on the family, address parental concerns related to their children's behavior and school performance, resolve parenting issues, improve their problem solving, enhance emotional support, and obtain resources and services. Intervention was associated with less anxiety and depression, greater scholastic confidence, and higher global self-worth among children with different chronic conditions.

Lobato and Kao (2002) evaluated an integrated group intervention for siblings and parents that was designed to increase sibling understanding of and adjustment to chronic illness and developmental disability. The intervention was associated with improved and reduced sibling and parental reports of negative adjustment to the disorder, regardless of the type of diagnostic condition, that were maintained at 3-month follow-up.

Family-centered intervention models have also been targeted to improve adherence to treatment among children and adolescents with chronic illness. Greineider, Loane, and Parks (1995) tested the efficacy of an individualized outreach treatment program that included instruction in asthma management medications, triggers, and use of inhalers and peak flow meters. Personal telephone contact was maintained with families to enhance adherence. The intervention was associated with significant reductions in rates of emergency room visits and hospital admissions in a group of predominantly African American children and adolescents drawn from an inner-city population.

Wysocki, Greco, Harris, and White (2000) tested the effects of behavioral family systems therapy (BFST), which involves a combination of problem-solving training, communication skills training, cognitive restructuring, and family therapy interventions applied to parent–adolescent conflict, treatment adherence, psychological adjustment to diabetes, and diabetes control at 6- and 12-month follow-up. Compared with education and support or current therapy, the BFST group demonstrated improvement in parent–child relations and diabetes-specific conflict between parents and adolescents. On the other hand, there were no effects on treatment adherence. Moreover, the effects on psychological adjustment to diabetes and diabetes control depended on age and gender: Younger girls showed the most improvement in diabetes control, whereas older boys were the most improved on diabetes-related adjustment.

School-Based Models

Katz, Varni, Rubenstein, Blew, and Hubert (1992) evaluated a program designed to help children newly diagnosed with cancer return to school as quickly as possible. The program included arranging conferences with school personnel to help them understand basic facts about the child's illness and medical treatment, planning for absences, anticipating peers' reactions to the child, and formulating an individualized educational plan. Classroom presentations provided peers with information about their illness, medical procedures, and common side effects such as hair loss. Compared with pretest measures, children who received the intervention reported fewer internalizing and behavioral problems, more social confidence, fewer self-reported depressive symptoms, greater perceived social confidence, and better adjustment to school as rated by their teachers.

Peer-Centered Models

Greco, Shroff-Pendley, McDonell, and Reeves (2001) devised a peer-group intervention designed to increase diabetes knowledge and social support of diabetes care. Following the intervention, adolescents and their friends demonstrated higher levels of knowledge about diabetes and support as well as a higher ratio of peer-to-family support, and friends demonstrated improved self-esteem.

Barakat et al. (2003) evaluated the effectiveness of a manual-based, social skills training group intervention to improve social skills and social functioning of children treated for brain tumors. Social skills and social functioning changed in the direction of improved functioning, with several scores showing significant improvement from baseline to the follow-up assessment.

Peer-group interventions have also been designed to improve illness management by enhancing problem solving and self-monitoring of blood glucose (B. J. Anderson, Wolf, Burkhart, Cornell, & Bacon, 1989) and social skills related to peer influences on illness management (Kaplan, Chadwick, & Schimmel, 1985). B. J. Anderson et al. (1989) found that adolescents who received the problem-solving intervention demonstrated better metabolic control and increased use of self-monitoring of blood glucose levels than adolescents who received standard diabetes education and care.

Child-Centered Models

Child-centered models of psychological intervention have been used to address a range of outcomes, including psychological distress and adherence to treatment. Some of these interventions have been designed to reduce distress associated with pain, including procedure-related pain (Powers, 1999), or to reduce acute and chronic pain associated with chronic illness (Walco et al., 1999). Varni, Blount, Waldron, and Smith (1995) grouped the content of pain-related interventions into three categories: (a) pain perception regulation focused on reducing subjective experiences of discomfort; (b) increasing mastery over the pain using techniques such as progressive muscle relaxation, meditative breathing, guided imagery, and self-hypnosis; and (c) behavioral reinforcement designed to decrease pain-related behaviors. In addition, Blount et al. (2003) described an interesting model that groups medical and coping interventions by phase of medical procedure (e.g., approach, preprocedure, procedure, postprocedure) and by specific goals and interventions for each phase for parents, children, and staff in three broad areas of content. These three areas include information provision and distraction, coping, and medical factors.

A range of cognitive–behavioral interventions has been tested to enhance pain management. For example, Lavigne, Ross, Berry, Hayford, and Pachman (1992) evaluated the effects of psychological treatment for children with JRA who were experiencing moderate to high levels of pain. Six sessions completed over a 3-month period involved both parent and child in progressive muscle relaxation, electromyogram feedback, and operant pain management. A significant 25% reduction in mean pain scores based on child and maternal report was found from baseline to 3-month follow-up.

Jay, Elliott, Ozolins, Olson, and Pruitt (1985) reported one of the first studies that tested the effects of cognitive–behavioral treatment to reduce pain and distress for children with cancer who underwent bone marrow aspiration and lumbar puncture. Intervention components included breathing exercises; imagery; filmed modeling coping, which depicted a child showing some signs of distress but coping well; reinforcement and incentive for lying still and using breathing skills; and behavioral rehearsal, in which the child pretended to do a medical procedure on a doll and then on a psychologist who modeled breathing skills, and then the child practiced lying still and using deep breathing skills. Such interventions have been demonstrated to be superior to baseline conditions (Jay et al., 1985) and to medication and a minimal treatment–attentional control (Jay, Elliott, Katz, & Siegel, 1987).

Rapoff et al. (2002) conducted an RCT that evaluated a clinic-based, nurse-administered educational and behavioral intervention to prevent the reduction in adherence to nonsteroidal medications in newly diagnosed children and adolescents with JRA. Behavioral interventions included contingency management, monitoring, and positive reinforcement. The intervention was associated with significant differences in adherence to treatment as assessed via electronic monitoring over a 13-month follow-up. The educational intervention included information about the types of JRA, signs and symptoms, and medical treatments.

Some child-centered interventions have used computer and telecommunication technology-based approaches. For example, Erickson, Ascione, Kirking, and Johnson (1998) provided individuals with asthma message–

based pagers that were programmed for multiple daily reminders to take the medication as well as specific directions about which medicines to take and subdirectories with administration steps or techniques (e.g., proper inhaler technique, what to do if having an asthma attack). Preliminary data for this intervention have suggested that this can be a viable and cost-effective means to improve adherence behaviors.

INDIVIDUAL DIFFERENCES: IMPLICATIONS FOR DATA GATHERING AND TARGETING INTERVENTIONS

The previous section described examples of a number of psychological interventions that have been developed to address problems that are manifest in various domains of child, parent, or family functioning. Individual differences in clinically relevant characteristics affect the way children and families respond to interventions and hence the efficacy of interventions. It is doubtful that any single model of psychological intervention will be equally effective with each and every child, adolescent, or family member. Consequently, to develop powerful interventions, investigators will need to consider and evaluate the degree to which relevant individual difference characteristics affect or moderate the child and family response to intervention (see chap. 3). Such data are necessary to determine whether psychological interventions are most effective for subgroups of children or families. As shown in Figure 1.2, three dimensions of individual differences are most relevant to the design and implementation of psychological interventions in pediatric chronic illness: (a) type, severity, and stage of target psychological problem; (b) nature and stage of chronic illness; and (c) child's developmental stage.

These dimensions need to be considered in describing samples of children and families who participate in interventions. Individual samples of children and adolescents with chronic illness at individual sites may vary significantly from children at other sites on these characteristics. Consequently, it may be difficult for investigators to compare the results of interventions that are conducted at different sites. For this reason, depending on the purpose of the study and availability of data, information concerning individual differences in relevant characteristics such as severity and stage of problem, developmental stage of illness, and age should be included in the description of participants in intervention studies (see chap. 3). This will help other investigators understand the potential generalizability of intervention findings that are conducted at a particular site or sites to their patient populations.

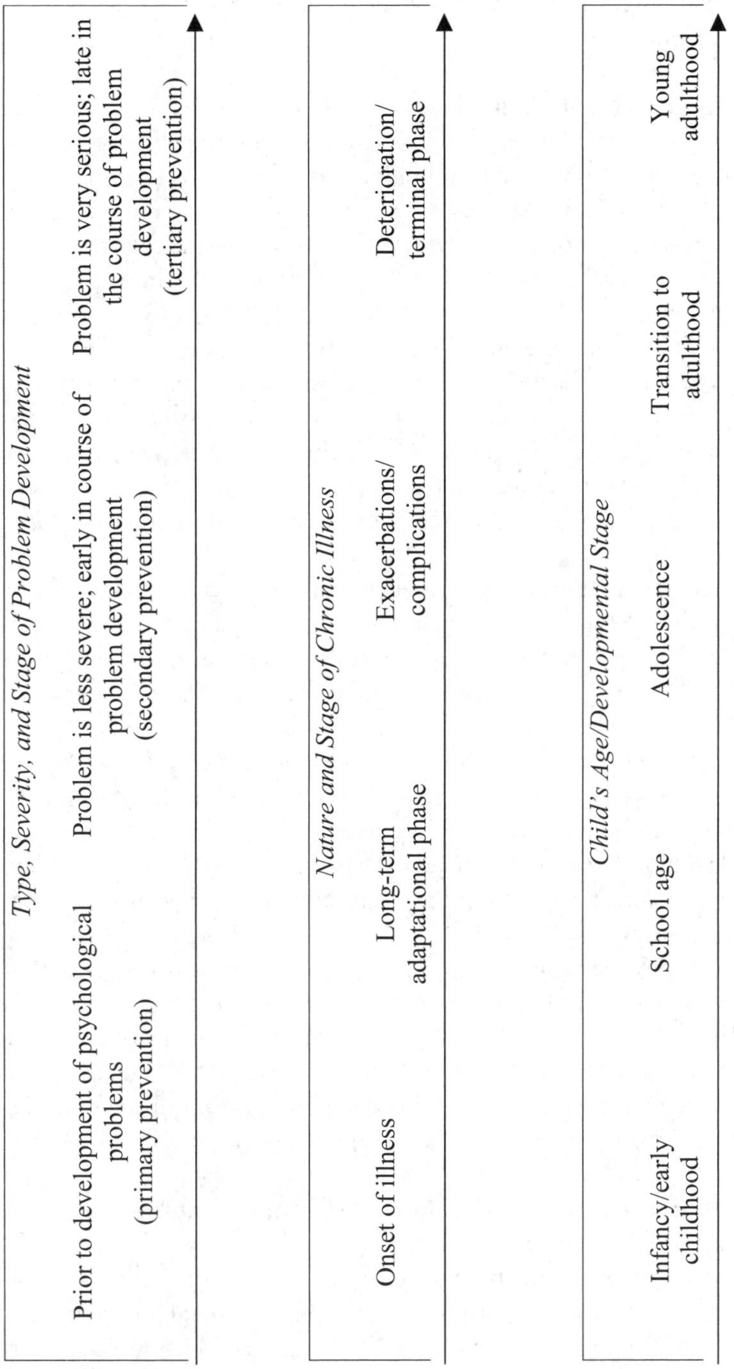

Type, Severity, and Stage of Problem Development

Prior to development of psychological problems (primary prevention) → Problem is less severe; early in course of problem development (secondary prevention) → Problem is very serious; late in the course of problem development (tertiary prevention)

Nature and Stage of Chronic Illness

Onset of illness → Long-term adaptational phase → Exacerbations/complications → Deterioration/terminal phase

Child's Age/Developmental Stage

Infancy/early childhood → School age → Adolescence → Transition to adulthood → Young adulthood

Figure 1.2. Individual difference characteristics that are relevant to intervention.

Individual Differences in the Type, Severity, and Stage of Target Problem

There is extraordinary individual variation in the type and severity of individual children's psychological adjustment problems to pediatric chronic illness that need to be considered in designing interventions (Drotar, 1981; Drotar & Bush, 1985; R. J. Thompson & Gustafson, 1996). Some children with chronic illness demonstrate remarkable psychological resilience and may not need any psychological interventions other than those provided in the context of comprehensive care (Gerhardt, Walders, Rosenthal, & Drotar, 2003). Other children and adolescents may demonstrate more serious psychological problems that are potentially classifiable as mental disorders by the *Diagnostic and Statistical Manual of Mental Disorders* (4th ed., *DSM–IV*; American Psychiatric Association, 1994). A third group may demonstrate problems that significantly interfere with their functioning (e.g., treatment nonadherence, psychological distress) yet not meet the threshold for a *DSM–IV* diagnosis.

The heterogeneity in the psychological problems associated with childhood chronic illness has significant implications for planning and implementing research on psychological interventions. For example, investigators need to think carefully and critically about the nature and prevalence of specific problems to which the intervention will be targeted (see chap. 3). Moreover, to be acceptable to the consumers of services, psychological interventions need to be targeted to problems that are considered problematic by children or their parents or physicians.

Individual differences in the stage of development of the target problem also have implications for the targeting of interventions. For example, nascent problems or signs of psychological distress that signal risk for the development of disorders may benefit from preventive interventions that can be delivered in conjunction with medical care (Drotar, Crawford, & Ganofsky, 1984; Kazak, 2005; Rapoff, 2000). On the other hand, problems that are more severe (e.g., psychological disturbance) and problematic (e.g., adherence to medical treatment) generally require more intensive psychological interventions (Ellis, Frey, et al., 2005; Ellis, Naar-King, et al., 2005).

Heterogeneity in the Nature and Course of Chronic Illnesses

Individual differences in the course of different chronic illnesses also have implications for the targeting and design of psychological interventions. By definition, all pediatric chronic illnesses have a long duration. However, there is substantial variation in the age of onset, course, and progression of different chronic conditions. Some conditions, such as cystic fibrosis, are generally diagnosed in infancy, whereas others, such as diabetes, may be diagnosed at various ages from preschool through adolescence. Moreover, children and adolescents with the same chronic condition may also experience substantial differences in the course and severity of their condition (Rolland, 1987).

How illness-related demands affect children and families depends on the specific condition, the nature of medical treatment (Quittner et al., 1996), and the stage of the child's illness (Rolland, 1987). For example, the physical and psychological stressors that are associated with an illness such as diabetes (Johnson, 1995) are very different from those that are involved in cancer (Wolznick & Goodheart, 2002). These condition-specific differences need to be considered in targeting psychological interventions (see chaps. 6–10 for examples). Moreover, different stressors and burdens are also associated with a recent diagnosis of a chronic illness, the long-term adaptational phase, the terminal phase (Rolland, 1987) in the case of cancer, or transition from treatment to survivorship (see chap. 7). Such stage-specific stressors and burdens may need to be carefully considered in designing and implementing psychological interventions. Clinical experience and theories of stress and coping (Hobfoll, 1988, 1989) suggest that psychological interventions that coincide with periods of greatest psychological stress may be most accepted by families. Predictable stress points for children with chronic illness and their families include the diagnosis of a chronic condition, changes in the children's illness status requiring hospitalization or extraordinary treatments, or deteriorations in conditions resulting in a loss of functional independence (Rolland, 1987) and, for conditions such as cancer, the end of treatment (Koocher & O'Malley, 1981; Noll & Kazak, 2004). Each of these stress points can engender specific psychological threats. Moreover, the different phases of a chronic illness and associated medical treatment require family members to learn specific responsibilities for the child's care that are appropriate to that phase.

For the most part, psychological interventions have not focused specifically on the stage of a chronic illness. One exception is Delamater et al.'s (1990) study of family-based self-management training for children with diabetes, which is an interesting example of an intervention that was targeted to children with a recent onset of a chronic condition, in this case Type 1 diabetes (DM1). Following standard in-hospital diabetes education, children who were newly diagnosed with DM1 were randomized to conventional follow-up, supportive counseling, or self-management training that focused primarily on enhancing utilization of data obtained from self-monitoring of blood glucose. All interventions took place during the first 4 months following diagnosis, with booster sessions at 6 and 12 months. Self-management training was associated with better metabolic control 1 and 2 years later but did not affect family adaptation.

In addition to the stage of a chronic condition illness course, exacerbations of symptoms or the onset of illness-related complications may be a source of distress and burden and may be the focus of psychological intervention. For example, illnesses such as Crohn's disease have an unpredictable course in which symptom-free periods are followed by flare-ups of symptoms, which engender distress. Other chronic conditions, such as cystic fibrosis, have a deteriorating course that may require painful adjustments in school, work-related activities, or life goals, which can result in psychological distress needing intervention (Drotar, 1978). Despite the stressors associated with exacerbations in illness-related symptoms and complications, to my knowledge they have not been the focus of psychological intervention research. One reason is that changes in illness course are unpredictable, and it may be difficult to identify sufficient numbers of children and adolescents with these stressors and recruit them in a realistic time frame.

Individual Differences in Age, Developmental Stage, or Transition

Individual differences in the child's age and developmental stage also have important implications for the design of psychological intervention research as well as for data analysis of such studies (Garrison & McGuiston, 1989). For the most part, the child's age is a useful indicator of his or her developmental level or stage, but children of the same chronological age may differ substantially in cognitive and physical maturity (Williams, Holmbeck, & Greenley, 2002; Wysocki, Hough, Ward, & Green, 1992). Such differences may have implications for interventions in that they can affect individual psychological resources as well as family conflict. Consequently, depending on the design and focus of the intervention study, cognitive and physical maturity may need to be considered in describing the sample of participants in targeting interventions and in evaluating moderators of psychological intervention (see chaps. 3 and 11).

Developmental transitions (e.g., the beginning of school, onset of adolescence) may also pose salient stresses to children with chronic illness. Psychological intervention may be needed to manage the socialization as well as illness-related demands of a new developmental phase, which may also involve increased responsibilities for illness management (Whitt, 1984). Such developmental transitions also have important influences on the development of coping skills, competencies, and goals (L. Schwartz & Drotar, 2005) that may affect children's response to, the need for, and the focus of psychological interventions (Williams et al., 2002). For example, the development of psychological autonomy during adolescence may facilitate self-management of a chronic illness but only if it is supported by parents (B. J. Anderson, Ho, Brackett, Finkelstein, & Laffel, 1997; Wysocki, Hough, Ward, & Green, 1992). On the other hand, parents' and physicians' expectations for the management of a chronic illness such as diabetes may exceed some adolescents' levels of maturity and their families' capacities for support, thus creating a need for intervention. For example, excessive independence in managing diabetes coupled with the relative absence of parental involvement and monitoring has been associated with problematic treatment adherence in DM1 (Wysocki, Hough, Ward, Allen, & Murgai, 1992).

It should be noted that with some chronic conditions, developmental transitions may coincide with transitions in the stage of treatment or course of a chronic illness in ways that pose special psychological challenges and targets for psychological intervention research. For example, adolescents and young adults who have been cured of cancer and now face the transition from patient to survivor are also called on to manage the critical developmental transition to adolescence and young adulthood at the same time (see chap. 7).

Another example is that young adults with cystic fibrosis can face extraordinary stressors associated with progressive deterioration of their chronic condition at a point in their psychological development when they also face transitions to adulthood and family formation (Stark, Mackner, Patton, & Acton, 2003; see chap. 10). The burdens created by the combination of developmental and illness-related transitions can afford special opportunities for psychological intervention. A related point is that some important outcomes of pediatric chronic illness only become apparent at specific ages or developmental transitions. For example, the late effects of pediatric cancer become most apparent in late adolescence and adulthood (see chap. 8).

For the most part, research on psychological interventions in childhood chronic illness has not focused on developmental transitions, primarily because it is difficult to obtain sufficient numbers of participants at one age or developmental stage at a single center. Nevertheless, one example of a developmentally focused intervention is Satin, La Greca, Zigo, and Skyler's (1989) multifactorial intervention that focused on helping adolescents with juvenile diabetes express feelings about their illness and enhance communication about the management of this condition, especially assertive diabetes-related communication. One interesting component of this particular intervention model was an exercise in which adolescents taught their parents how to manage diabetes by reviewing management skills and serving as instructors while their parents actually carried out aspects of the regimen. Adolescents who participated in their family group demonstrated clinically significant improvements in metabolic control that were maintained at 6-month follow-up (Satin et al., 1989).

CONCLUSION

The complexity of psychological intervention research raises considerable challenges that have been examined in this introductory chapter and will be addressed throughout this volume. The primary issues that have been raised here concerning prevalence and impact of a chronic illness; targets, methods, and outcomes of interventions; barriers to psychological intervention; and intervention in reference to target problem severity and development, nature and stage of chronic illness, and age and developmental stage are explored throughout this volume. As you read subsequent chapters on theory, research design, and implementation (chaps. 2–4) and the chapters on individual chronic conditions (chaps. 6–10), consider how the above issues were evaluated in study designs, in the presentation, and in the critique of findings. In reading the information that is contained in chapters 6–10, which focus on interventions for specific chronic conditions, readers should consider how the individual differences in illness characteristics influenced the target and focus of the intervention and relevant outcomes.

2

THEORETICAL MODELS AND FRAMEWORKS FOR PSYCHOLOGICAL INTERVENTION

Theoretical models and frameworks that describe risk factors for problematic psychological adjustment and medical treatment adherence in childhood chronic illness can provide a foundation for developing psychological interventions (Drotar, 1992, 1999; R. J. Thompson & Gustafson, 1996; Wallander et al., 1989). In addition, models and frameworks can also be used to evaluate the key processes that mediate changes in critical outcomes that occur in response to psychological interventions (Drotar, 2002). Despite these salient advantages, theoretically guided psychological interventions have been more the exception than the rule in the field of pediatric chronic illness. To address this need, this chapter considers applications of theoretical models and frameworks to psychological intervention research in pediatric chronic illness, including (a) specific theoretical models that have been proposed to account for relevant empirical evidence and (b) relevant implications for the development of psychological interventions.

APPLICATIONS OF THEORETICAL MODELS AND FRAMEWORKS FOR INTERVENTION RESEARCH

Theoretical models and frameworks can facilitate practitioners' and researchers' decision making concerning designing and delivering psychological interventions with children with chronic illness. For example, consider Lisa, who is an adolescent with diabetes who presents with symptoms of depression and nonadherence to treatment. Lisa's symptoms have interfered with both her day-to-day functioning and her capacity to manage her illness and have been distressing to her mother and younger siblings. In developing a treatment plan to manage Lisa's symptoms in clinical care or a psychological intervention study, one may need to consider the following issues: (a) the factors that triggered Lisa's depressive symptoms and problems in treatment adherence, (b) the factors that are maintaining them, and (c) the most effective way to involve the child and family to facilitate change in the target areas. To accomplish these tasks, practitioners and intervention researchers would benefit from a working knowledge of theories that first identify key factors in the etiology of risk for Lisa's depression and treatment adherence problems and, second, describe effective strategies and processes that will reduce Lisa's depression and its impact on her adjustment to her illness, family, and peers. Some of the theories and models that are considered in this chapter are applicable to Lisa's treatment plan.

Models and frameworks can also inform and facilitate the development of intervention programs for children with chronic illness and their families. Consider the following example: A new program is being developed to provide intervention at the point of diagnosis of pediatric cancer to prevent psychological distress in children and families. The program developer wants to identify the following information: (a) the most relevant targets of psychological intervention (e.g., psychological distress in children, parents, or both), (b) potential risk factors (e.g., family dysfunction) that may be reduced by the intervention, and (c) resilience factors or competencies (e.g., parent and child problem solving and adaptive coping) that can be enhanced by the intervention. The theories and models described in this chapter can inform the design of new programs that need to be developed.

Theoretical models can facilitate the development of study design, data analysis, and interpretation of findings in psychological intervention research (Drotar, 2002). For example, theory can facilitate the investigators' decisions concerning the focus of psychological interventions for children with chronic illness, including the specific individuals and psychological processes that need to be targeted to create change (see chap. 3). In addition, theory can help develop and test an intervention model by specifying how and why the intervention is expected to change a target behavior or outcome. This is important for the following reason: If a specific intervention model (e.g., cognitive–behavioral) is found to be effective in relieving psychological distress, but the theory that guided the intervention model is not clearly specified, it will be very difficult to identify the processes by which the effect was achieved. This intervention may have achieved change by application of cognitive–behavioral principles. Alternatively, the intervention may have achieved its effect solely by providing more support to the child and parents. Unless the mechanism of change that underlies the intervention is specified, it will be difficult to decide between these different explanations. On the other hand, if a theory concerning predicted intervention-related change is proposed, and the hypothesized change is demonstrated by the intervention, it can enhance the validity of the theory and the generalizability of findings because the processes of intervention change are specified (Drotar, 2002).

Designing an intervention study to test competing conceptual models of intervention effects is an especially powerful application of theory. For example, consider a study of intervention that is designed to promote adaptive functioning in response to chronic pain in children. Model A proposes that changing maladaptive patterns of parent–child communication concerning pain is the key ingredient in promoting positive adaptation to pediatric pain. In contrast, Model B suggests that it will not be sufficient to change parent–child communication to improve functioning and that changing the patterns of direct reinforcement for maladaptive functioning in response to pain is hypothesized to be a necessary ingredient for positive change. Such competing theoretical models can be tested by comparing the efficacy of alternative interventions, which have been designed to change processes specified by theories as critical for promoting adaptive functioning in response to chronic pain. Documenting the efficacy of one intervention model over the alternative model on the basis of measures of parent–child communication and reinforcement for maladaptive functioning in response to pain would provide empirical support for that theory.

Theories can also be useful in identifying and testing hypothesized mediators of intervention change that are potentially important in understanding underlying mechanisms of change and developing more powerful interventions. For example, suppose a theory predicts that improvement in parent–adolescent communication concerning illness management is the critical process in enhancing adherence to medical treatment for diabetes. If the intervention is found to be effective, an analysis of mediation can be conducted to determine whether parent–adolescent communication influenced adherence to treatment (Holmbeck, 1997). (See chap. 11 for additional discussion.)

SURVEY OF MODELS AND FRAMEWORKS THAT APPLY TO INTERVENTION RESEARCH

A number of theoretical models have potential application to interventions designed to enhance psychological adaptation and adherence to medical treatment in pediatric chronic illness. These theoretical perspectives can be categorized into the following broad content areas: (a) individual and family resource and risk factor models, (b) family systems models, (c) cognitive–behavioral models, (d) social–cognitive models, (e) states-of-change models, and (f) comprehensive models. Each of these models is discussed along with potential implications for interventions designed to promote psychological adaptation or adherence to medical treatment for chronic illness.

Individual and Family Resource and Risk Factor Models

Several theories have emphasized individual and family risks and resources as primary influences on the psychological adjustment of children with chronic illness. These include the disability, stress, and coping model (Varni & Wallander, 1988); the transactional stress and coping model (R. J. Thompson & Gustafson, 1996); and the family adjustment and adaptation response model (McCubbin & Patterson, 1982).

Disability, Stress, and Coping Model

Varni and Wallander's (1988) influential disability, stress, and coping model of psychological adjustment to chronic illness integrates several models of stress and coping (Lazarus & Folkman, 1984; Pless & Pinkerton, 1975). Varni and Wallander differentiated between risk factors that are hypothesized to increase the likelihood of adjustment problems in children with chronic illness and resistance or protective factors that are expected to decrease the probability of psychological disturbance. Relevant risk factors defined in this model include (a) disease or disability parameters (e.g., severity of disability, presence of medical problems, central nervous system involvement, and visibility of disability), (b) the child's functional independence, and (c) psychosocial stressors that encompass several domains such as disability-related problems, major life events, and daily hassles.

In this model, the impact of the above psychological risk factors is assumed to be moderated by three categories of resistance or coping resource factors. These include (a) stable individual factors (e.g., adaptive temperament and perceived competence), (b) stress-processing or coping ability factors (e.g., cognitive appraisal and coping behaviors), and (c) social–ecological influences such as the quality of family relationships.

Partial empirical support for this model, especially for the predictive power of family resources, has been obtained in a series of studies conducted over many years (Wallander, Thompson, & Alriksson-Schmidt, 2003). For example, Wallander et al. (1989) found that the combination of utilitarian and psychological family resources accounted for significant variance in children's psychological adjustment, but less so for behavioral problems than for social competence. Empirical tests of this model with children with various chronic conditions have found at least partial support in most studies, with different levels of empirical support for different risk and resilience factors. For the most part, condition type and severity have been found to have little impact on psychological adjustment. In contrast, child temperament, socioeconomic status, parent coping, and various aspects of family functioning (e.g., family cohesion) have been shown to influence psychological adjustment and social functioning of children with physical conditions (Wallander, Varni, Babani, Banis, & Wilcox, 1988).

Transactional Stress and Coping Model

In the transactional stress and coping model of adjustment to chronic illness, R. J. Thompson and colleagues (R. J. Thompson, Gil, Burbach, Keith, & Kinney, 1993; R. J. Thompson, Gustafson, Hamlett, & Spock, 1992) hypothesized that the psychological outcomes of children with chronic illness reflect the cumulative product of transactions among biomedical, developmental, and psychosocial processes, including the levels of stress and symptoms experienced by other family members. In this model, three types of psychosocial mediational processes are identified as influences on the psychological adjustment of children with chronic illness and their mothers: (a) cognitive processes, including stress appraisals (Lazarus & Folkman, 1984), expectations of locus of control, and self-efficacy (Bandura, 1997); (b) coping methods or strategies (Lazarus & Folkman, 1984); and (c) quality of family functioning (Moos & Moos, 1981). Several cross-sectional and longitudinal studies have supported the hypothesized role of maternal and child adaptational processes in both maternal and child psychological adjustment to a range of chronic illnesses, including cystic fibrosis, sickle cell disease, and spina bifida (R. J. Thompson & Gustafson, 1996; Wallander et al., 2003).

Family Adjustment and Adaptation Response Model

The family adjustment and adaptation response (FAAR) model differs from the family resource and resistance and the transactional stress and coping models in its focus on family level stress and burden as a primary risk or protective factor. The initial "ABCX" family crisis model (Hill, 1958) hypothesized that A (the stressor event) interacted with B (the family's crisis-meeting resources) and C (the family's definition of the event) to produce X (the crisis). In addition, McCubbin and Patterson's (1982) double ABCX model of family behavior, which identified processes by which families achieve precrisis adjustment and postcrisis adaptation, is potentially applicable to understanding psychological adaptation as well as adherence to treatment in pediatric chronic illness. Salient features of this model include the concept of pileup of demands on family resources and the identification of coping strategies used by the family, especially the need for family members to modify perceptions of their situation to adjust and adapt to a crisis. The most recent extension of the double ABCX model, the FAAR model (Patterson, 1988), emphasizes the importance of the personal meaning that family members attribute to stressors and level of resources for balanced family functioning.

In times of crisis, such as at the diagnosis of childhood chronic illness, stressors or demands on family members may exceed their capabilities. In such situations, family members may attempt to restore equilibrium by (a) acquiring new adaptive resources or coping behaviors, (b) reducing the pileup of multiple demands or stressors, or (c) changing the way they perceive their situation. According to the FAAR model, families can use many resources and capabilities for meeting these demands, including financial resources, personal resources (e.g., self-esteem, knowledge, and skills), systems resources (e.g., cohesion, organization, and communication skills), and community resources (e.g., schools, churches, medical care, and social support). *Coping behavior*, which is a major family resource in the FAAR model, is defined as action to either reduce demands or acquire resources, or changing the meaning of a situation to make it more manageable. The FAAR model assumes that some families are much more vulnerable than others to crises. For example, specific family resource problems, such as conflicted patterns of interaction, may develop into chronic strains that can trigger a crisis. On the other hand, families with very high resources are assumed to be resilient to most stresses.

The FAAR model generates predictions concerning the psychological adaptation of families to pediatric chronic illness as well as family adherence to the child's treatment regimen. In what is to my knowledge the only test of the FAAR model in pediatric chronic illness, Patterson (1985) tested the following hypotheses: (a) the level of family adherence to medical treatment for the child's cystic fibrosis would be negatively associated with the pileup of family demands in the past year, and (b) the family's subjective appraisal of the difficulty of demands would be positively associated with both family systems resources (e.g., cohesion and expressiveness) and personal resources (parental time, education, and coping efforts). Partial empirical support was obtained for this model: Contrary to prediction, neither the frequency of intrafamilial strains nor the total pileup of demands related to family compliance. On the other hand, the family resource of expressiveness correlated positively with adherence to treatment, whereas active recreation orientation correlated negatively (Patterson, 1985).

Implications for Intervention

Taken together, the individual and family resource and risk factor models have several implications for the targeting of psychological interventions in pediatric chronic illness. Risk factors such as illness-related psychological stressors and severity of disability are assumed to be fixed and hence not amenable to psychological intervention. On the other hand, resources (e.g., social support and coping strategies, appraisals, and some cognitive processes) are potentially modifiable targets of psychological intervention that can be the focus of intervention efforts. In the FAAR model, psychological intervention can be conceptualized as an added resource or support, along with information about the child's condition or generalized support and advocacy.

At the family level, the FAAR and individual and family resource and risk models also have implications for tailoring psychological interventions to families of children with chronic illness. For example, interventions can also be directed toward reducing the multiple demands on family members by modifying coping strategies or changing the way the demands are perceived. Moreover, psychological interventions may be targeted to families who are most vulnerable to recurrent crises or pileup of multiple demands owing to risk factors such as preexisting family conflict.

Family Systems Models

Family systems models, which describe how family processes (e.g., communication, quality of family relationships) can influence the chronic illness-related symptoms, have potential implications for psychological interventions (Fritz & McQuaid, 2000). Relevant family systems models include the psychosomatic family model, the family-centered biobehavioral model, and the miscarried helping model.

Psychosomatic Family Model

One example of the family systems model is Minuchin et al.'s (1975) psychosomatic family model, which hypothesizes that psychophysiological vulnerability to illness and family organization that potentiates this vulnerability influence the expression of children's chronic illness–related symptoms and illness behaviors. Unfortunately, the influence of Minuchin et al.'s innovative model has been limited by the lack of empirical support (Coyne & Anderson, 1988, 1989; Wood, 1993).

Family-Centered Biobehavioral Model

Wood's (1993) family-centered biobehavioral model describes the importance of reciprocal interactions among biological, psychological, and social processes in understanding psychological processes that can influence the activation of symptoms associated with chronic illnesses such as asthma. *Responsivity*, defined as (a) the strength with which an individual responds to physiological stimuli and (b) the intensity with which family members respond to one another, is a central construct of this model. Wood hypothesized that properties of family structure, such as generational hierarchy, parental relationships, and interpersonal responsivity, may interact with children's biobehavioral reactivity in ways that either buffer or activate psychological processes that can potentiate symptoms of chronic illness.

The model includes three levels: (a) a biologic level that corresponds to the child's disease process, (b) a psychological level that corresponds to the child's biobehavioral reactivity, and (c) a social level that corresponds to family patterns of interaction. Empirical support for this model includes the following. Family conflict has been linked with elevated stress levels in children (Gottman & Fainsilber-Katz, 1989). In addition, research with pediatric asthma has found that high levels of expressed emotion correlate with the frequency of asthma attacks (Hermanns, Florin, Dietrich, Rieger, & Hahlweg, 1989) and that specific emotional states correlate with autonomic reactivity (B. D. Miller & Wood, 1997). However, consistent demonstration that specific patterns of family members' interpersonal sensitivities influence disease activity through the specific activation of psychophysiological processes is needed to support the development of psychological interventions based on the biobehavioral model.

Miscarried Helping Model

B. J. Anderson and Coyne (1991) developed the family relationship construct of *miscarried helping*, which is defined as a process by which parental investment in achieving a positive health outcome for their children may trigger family interactions that ultimately constrain or disrupt the child's development. In their rationale for this model, Anderson and Coyne observed that many parents of children with chronic illnesses need to achieve a higher than normative level of vigilance and involvement in their children's lives to monitor their health status and facilitate their adherence to medical treatment. However, such parental investment and monitoring can conflict with the parents' focus on helping their children develop competencies and psychological autonomy. Even though parents' frequent monitoring may be well intentioned, it may be perceived as an unreasonable demand by children or adolescents who may resist the parents' interference. These interactions may potentiate a vicious cycle of family conflict that can disrupt children's illness management and psychological adaptation. Empirical data that have consistently shown a link between family conflict and psychological outcomes (Drotar, 1997b) as well as adherence to treatment (La Greca & Bearman, 2003) provide support for the Anderson and Coyne model.

Implications for Intervention

Family systems models have a number of potential implications for the development of psychological interventions. For example, psychosomatic and family-centered models have identified problematic family structure and relationships as potential targets of psychological interventions that will reduce family stress and potentially ameliorate illness-related symptoms. The miscarried helping model has several implications for preventive psychological interventions with families, some of which have been incorporated into psychological interventions for children with chronic conditions such as diabetes (B. J. Anderson, Brackett, Ho, & Laffel, 2000). For example, parents of children with chronic illness can be helped to anticipate that their emotional involvement (even if it is well meaning) may be disruptive to their children's psychological development, especially if it is interpreted as burdensome by the child. Moreover, parents, children, and adolescents can be taught communication skills to negotiate problem solving in their specific roles and responsibilities to reduce conflict (B. J. Anderson et al., 2000).

Cognitive–Behavioral Theories

Cognitive–behavioral theories have a number of important applications to research on psychological interventions in pediatric chronic illness. Relevant cognitive–behavioral theories include anxiety and pain reduction models and problem-solving theory.

Anxiety and Pain Reduction Models

Cognitive–behavioral models conceptualize anxiety and pain as having cognitive, behavioral, and physiologic features (Kendall, 1993). For example, anxious affect is hypothesized to be associated with physiologic arousal. Reinforcement contingencies in the child's environment and the child's information processing and beliefs are also emphasized. Cognitive–behavioral intervention also emphasizes performance-based procedures as well as a focus on cognitive and affective interventions to change thoughts, feelings, and behavior (Kendall, 1993). In this model, interventions are designed to teach the child to identify physiologic responses and use relaxation strategies in response to physiologic stimuli. Children are also given opportunities to reconsider interpretations of situations and to develop or learn new coping thoughts and actions to manage anxiety or pain through opportunities for exposure to the feared situation (Kendall, 1993). Strong empirical support has been generated for cognitive–behavioral anxiety and pain reduction models in a range of populations (Kendall, 1993; Kupperheimer & Brown, 2000; Powers, 1999).

Problem-Solving Theory

Problem-solving theory (Nezu, Nezu, & Perri, 1989) describes two core constructs that are relevant to psychological interventions with a range of populations including children with chronic illness and their families. These are (a) problem-solving skill or process, including problem definition, generation of alternatives, implementation, and evaluation; and (b) problem-solving orientation, including interpersonal motivational factors, attitudes, and belief systems. Problem-solving theory predicts that effective illness-related problem solving results from experience and practice in a positive problem-solving orientation and skills that include transfer of knowledge and experience to new illness-related problem situations (Hill-Briggs, 2003).

Considerable empirical support has been generated in research with adults with chronic illnesses for various components of the problem-solving model. For example, among adults with diabetes, decision-making processes such as problem symptom detection, appraisal or analysis, and evaluation have been described for responses to unanticipated blood glucose levels (Paterson & Thorne, 2000) and for decisions concerning action to take in response to hypoglycemia (Kovatchev, Cox, Gonder-Frederick, Schlundt, & Clarke, 1998).

Implications for Intervention

Cognitive–behavioral theoretical models have clear implications for the design of psychological intervention research. For example, interventions (e.g., relaxation and coping skills) that are derived from cognitive–behavioral models have been used effectively in the management of pain and psychological distress (Gil, Carson, et al., 2000; Gil, Porter, et al., 2000; Powers, 1999).

Problem-solving theory has stimulated the development of intervention models that have been shown to be acceptable to children, adolescents, and families. In addition, these models have been successful in promoting parental adjustment to their children's cancer (Sahler et al., 2002) as well as adherence to treatment in diabetes (Wysocki, Harris, et al., 2000) and cystic fibrosis (Quittner et al., 2000). These intervention models target problems that have been identified by children and parents and involve them in the process of devising and implementing solutions to manage the problems more effectively.

Social–Cognitive Models

Although social–cognitive models have been developed for the most part on the basis of research with adults, they are applicable to psychological interventions to enhance adherence to medical treatment in pediatric chronic illnesses. Relevant social–cognitive models include the following: the health belief model (Janz & Becker, 1984) and two related theories, the protection motivation theory (Boer & Seydel, 1996) and theory of planned behavior and reasoned action (Maddux & DuCharme, 1997); the self-efficacy theory (Bandura, 1997; Janz & Becker, 1984; Maddux & Du-Charme, 1997); the illness uncertainty theory (Bauman, 2000); and personal meaning models (Conrad, 1985).

Health Belief Model and Related Models

The health belief model postulates that people are more likely to act on advice to initiate preventive health practices if they understand that (a) they are at risk (i.e., that there is a threat or susceptibility of illness and consequences of that threat are serious), (b) there is an effective action that can be initiated (i.e., the intervention suggested will reduce the risk or severity of the consequences), and (c) the barriers or "costs" of adopting the preventive practice or behavior are less than the benefits.

Other social–cognitive models have also noted that the perceived threat of the chronic health condition and expectancies regarding the consequences of performing adherence behaviors are important in predicting adherence to treatment. However, these models use different names and definitions of these constructs (Norman & Conner, 1996). For example, *outcome expectancies* are defined as perceived benefits and barriers in the health belief model; as response efficacy and self-efficacy in the protection motivation theory; and as attitudes, subjective norms, and perceived behavioral control in the theory of planned behavior and reasoned action (Riekert & Drotar, 2000).

For the most part, research, including studies with pediatric populations, has generated at least partial empirical support for the health belief and related models. For example, severity of illness, defined as maternal and child perceptions of the seriousness of the child's chronic health condition if left untreated, has been shown to relate to treatment adherence (Brownlee-Duffeck et al., 1987). Moreover, maternal perceptions of illness-related susceptibility (e.g., the perception of risks related to health problems or complications that arise if the treatment regimen is not followed) correlated positively with treatment adherence (N. A. Smith, Ley, Seale, & Shaw, 1987).

Outcome expectancies are another key set of variables in the health belief and related models. These have been used in studies of the prediction of adherence to medical treatment but have broader applicability to a range of outcomes for the most part. Outcome expectancies include (a) *perceived benefits*, which are defined as one's judgment of the benefits of following the recommended treatment regimen, and (b) *perceived barriers* or costs of following a treatment regimen. Outcome expectancies such as perceived benefits have been found to relate to better treatment adherence in children with a range of chronic illnesses (Brownlee-Duffeck et al., 1987; Charron-Prochownik, Becker, Brown, Liang, & Bennett, 1993).

Self-Efficacy Theory

Self-efficacy theory (Bandura, 1997) has also been supported in previous research with children and adolescents with chronic illness. For example, several studies have found that adolescents who demonstrate higher self-efficacy for completing a treatment regimen (e.g., as measured by beliefs that they are capable of completing their treatment) are more adherent to such treatments (Clark et al., 1988; Czajkowski & Koocher, 1987; Littlefield et al., 1992). On the other hand, the variables (e.g., attitudes or beliefs) that are measured in studies of social–cognitive models, including self-efficacy theory, typically account for only a small proportion of variance in adherence behaviors (Rapoff, 1999).

Illness Uncertainty Theory

Uncertainty, which is defined in this context as the inability to determine the meaning of illness-related events (Mishel, 1988), is a cognitive state that is created when a child or parent cannot adequately understand or categorize an event or predict outcomes. Given the extraordinary individual differences in prognosis, course, and treatment of pediatric chronic illness, uncertainty in providers', parents', and patients' perspectives is ubiquitous. Uncertainty can result from any or all of the following factors: (a) ambiguity concerning illness status, (b) complexity of the treatments and systems of care for chronic illness, (c) lack of information about the diagnosis and severity of chronic illness, and (d) lack of information about the course and prognosis of a chronic illness. Perceived illness-related uncertainty can result in psychological distress and, in some instances, psychological symptoms (e.g., depression and anxiety; Stewart & Mishel, 2000). On the other hand, depending on the nature of a child or family member's individual interpretation of illness uncertainty, coping style, and pattern of coping with adversity, perceived uncertainty may not always have a negative psychological outcome. For example, to the extent that uncertainty is perceived as a challenge or opportunity rather than a threat, it may enhance psychological adjustment.

The frequency and pattern of chronic illness-related symptoms (e.g., the number, intensity, frequency, duration, and location of symptoms compared with parent–child expectations of symptoms) can relate to the degree of perceived uncertainty experienced by children and parents (Mishel, 1988).

Event congruence refers to the consistency between what is expected by children and parents versus what is experienced in illness-related events. Inconsistent or rapid changes in symptom patterns that are characterized by remissions and exacerbations or ambiguous symptoms may generate uncertainty. Lack of expected treatment-related change and novel illness and treatment-related events such as hospitalizations may also trigger perceptions of uncertainty. Stewart and Mishel's (2000) review found empirical support for the relationship of perceived uncertainty and psychological distress among parents of children with chronic illness.

Personal Meaning Models

Models that consider personal meaning of a chronic illness may have relevance for adherence to treatment. For example, adherence to some medical treatment regimens may be perceived by children, and especially adolescents, as a sign of unwanted dependence on family and doctors (Bauman, 2000; Conrad, 1985). Consequently, some children and adolescents with chronic conditions may decide to refuse treatment to reduce their dependence on their parents (M. T. Stein, 1999). Taking medications and following prescribed treatment for chronic illness can be perceived as acknowledging one's difference from peers. Consequently, some children and adolescents with chronic illnesses may try to reduce the stigma of their conditions by avoiding taking their medication in front of others or sometimes eliminating treatments entirely (Conrad, 1985; see also La Greca, 1990). Finally, parents and children may have very different personal beliefs about a chronic illness, the impact of the treatment, and treatment-related responsibilities that may engender conflict and can disrupt treatment adherence. For example, parents are much more interested in promoting their children's health by encouraging adherence to treatment as they are focused on their children's future. In contrast, on the basis of their personal goals that fit with their stage of development, children and adolescents are much more concerned about short-term consequences such as the burdens or side effects of treatment.

Implications for Intervention

Taken together, the social–cognitive models have several potential implications for psychological interventions. Parent and child beliefs about illness and treatment are important to consider in developing psychological interventions, especially in adherence promotion. Not surprisingly, differences between parents' and children's beliefs about chronic illness and its treatment may be a significant barrier to adherence to medical treatment that may be a relevant target of psychological intervention. For example, parent and child beliefs about the illness (e.g., the illness cannot be managed effectively with treatment) or treatment (e.g., the treatment will cause more harm than good) can be potential barriers to adherence to medical treatment. For this reason, they are a logical focus of psychological interventions. In addition, cognitive–behavioral interventions that elicit and challenge such beliefs may be useful in promoting psychological adjustment to pediatric chronic illness (Kazak et al., 2004). For example, family members may have competing beliefs and expectancies about the nature of an illness and its treatment. Psychological interventions that are designed to facilitate family communication about beliefs about impact of illness and treatment and limit their negative impact on family relations and adherence to treatment need to be evaluated in future research.

Uncertainty theory focuses on the need to develop psychological interventions to reduce the uncertainty experienced by children and families as a consequence of the child's chronic illness and its treatment. For example, children and parents can be informed concerning the potential sources of perceived uncertainty with respect to a chronic illness, their child's treatment, and the roles of the professional team. Psychological interventions can also help children and parents cope with or manage feelings of uncertainty and to reduce the level of uncertainty by asking questions of providers and developing problem-solving strategies to reduce uncertainty and its psychological impact. In this regard, Hoff (2003) found that an intervention based on these principles reduced parental distress in a sample of children and adolescents with diabetes.

Personal meaning models have applicability to the development of psychological interventions to promote adherence to medical treatment and to reduce the perceived psychological burdens that are associated with a chronic illness. For example, the identification and management of the perceived barriers that are associated with medical treatment of pediatric chronic illness may be an important component of psychological interventions designed to improve treatment adherence in pediatric chronic conditions such as asthma (Mansour, Lanphear, & DeWitt, 2000).

Stages-of-Change Models

Stages-of-change models consider how expectations for treatment adherence and psychological adjustment to a chronic illness vary as a function of the stage of the child's or family's psychological adaptation to the child's illness. For example, a child who is newly diagnosed with a chronic illness such as diabetes cannot be expected to adhere faithfully to a treatment regimen that involves an unfamiliar and personally demanding set of skills. It takes time to understand and accept the need for the treatment regimen. Moreover, the child's acceptance of the psychological and adherence-related demands of a chronic physical illness is not static and may be affected by his or her developmental phase. For example, increases in autonomy during adolescence may disrupt the child's acceptance of his or her treatment regimen (Koocher, McGrath, & Gudas, 1990). For this reason, conceptual models of treatment adherence that focus explicitly on the stages of acquisition and change of adherence behaviors are potentially applicable to children and adolescents.

Transtheoretical Model

The primary example of a stages-of-change model is the transtheoretical model, which postulates five stages of change in the acquisition of health-enhancing behaviors (Prochaska & DiClemente, 1984; Ruggiero & Prochaska, 1993): (a) precontemplation (i.e., not considering a change in behavior in the immediate future), (b) contemplation (i.e., considering change in behavior in the future), (c) preparation (i.e., considering change in behavior in the near future), (d) action (i.e., the process of changing behavior such as adherence-related behavior), and (e) maintenance (i.e., continued change over time). In this model, progression through these stages of change is not always linear. Individuals may relapse back through various stages. Moreover, individuals and families may be at different stages of change for the various specific components of adherence-related tasks (e.g., medication vs. diet; La Greca & Schuman, 1995). The transtheoretical model has conceptual appeal. However, pediatric application is limited by the absence of empirical data to support its validity or clinical utility in populations of children with chronic health conditions and the difficulty of categorizing children's and adolescents' behaviors into specific stages of change (Rapoff, 1999).

Implications for Intervention

Despite these limitations, stages-of-change models have potential clinical implications. For example, some children and parents who demonstrate significant difficulties in treatment adherence or serious psychological dysfunction (e.g., depression) do not acknowledge or accept that this is a problem that needs intervention. For such children and families, an initial step would be to educate and support them concerning the prevalence and clinical significance of nonadherence on psychological adjustment, which may serve to help them consider the need to make a change in their behavior (and hence to change from precontemplation to action). In addition, interventions that are based on motivational interviewing, which is a method designed to enhance motivation for change (W. R. Miller & Rollnick, 2002) that has been used increasingly in pediatric populations to enhance adherence to treatment recommendations (Sindelar, Abrantes, Hart, Lewander, & Spirito, 2004), is relevant to stages-of-change theory.

Motivational interviewing is based on the importance of understanding readiness to change and the personal importance or meaning of change to the individual and family.

Comprehensive Models

A number of comprehensive models of influence on adherence to treatment, illness management, and psychological adaptation have been developed. Each of these models integrates aspects of various models that have been described. One of these is Hanson's (1992) model of psychosocial factors of health outcomes, adherence, and metabolic control in youths with insulin-dependent diabetes mellitus. In Hanson's model, family factors such as cohesion and parental support of treatment are identified as salient influences on children's coping strategies and level of psychological stress, which, in turn, are hypothesized to influence treatment adherence and blood sugar control. Other hypothesized factors in this model include knowledge and family attitudes toward the health care system, peer pressure to engage in normal activities, and salient developmental variables (e.g., the child's age; Hanson, 1992). In support of the model, Hanson, Henggeler, and Burghen (1987a) found that older adolescents had less positive family relations than younger adolescents, which in turn was associated with poorer adherence to treatment. As adolescents became older and more independent, the decisions that they made regarding their behaviors were less likely to be based on health reasons and more on personal and social factors (Hanson et al., 1987a).

Kazak (1989) described a systems and social–ecological model of adaptation and challenge that integrates a broad range of concepts including (among others) child development, research, and theory (Garmezy, Masten, & Tellegen, 1984); the ABCX family crisis model (Hill, 1958); and Bronfenbrenner's (1979) social ecological model. This framework served to guide the systematic intervention program of Kazak and her colleagues in pediatric cancer (Kazak, 2001; see chap. 8). The model provides an important guide for intervention researchers to target relevant family processes.

De Civita and Dobkin (2004) recently proposed a new model of adherence to treatment in pediatric chronic illness that defines three central characteristics of treatment adherence: (a) multidimensional, emphasizing the multiple components of treatment plans and their potential interrelatedness; (b) triadic partnership, including mutually influential exchanges among the caregiver medical team (child–medical team and caregiver–child); and (c) dynamic, in relation to changes in developmental adaptive capacity (adaptive vs. maladaptive), contextual characteristics (favorable to unfavorable), and disease course (favorable to unfavorable). De Civita and Dobkin emphasized the necessity for research to test this new model, especially in prospective assessment and analysis of trajectories of treatment-related behaviors, adaptive capacities, contextual influences, and disease course.

For the most part, theoretical models have focused on either psychological adjustment or adherence to treatment and have not integrated these outcomes into one model. One exception is Varni, Jacobs, and Seid's (2000) integrated model of treatment adherence and health-related quality of life. Factors that are hypothesized to influence adherence to treatment include demographic (e.g., age, gender, socioeconomic status), disease (e.g., diagnosis, severity, time since diagnosis, symptoms), and health-related knowledge (e.g., attitudes and skills, problem solving, and coping). Treatment adherence is hypothesized to influence specific disease-related symptoms, which in turn is hypothesized to influence health-related quality of life, patient satisfaction, and health care utilization. Although there is supportive evidence for the components of this model (Varni et al., 2000), to my knowledge it has not been tested directly nor utilized to develop psychological interventions for children with chronic illness.

In general, comprehensive models have the advantage of integrating diverse perspectives to develop an intervention approach. In addition, comprehensive models promote flexibility and an individualized approach, which are often needed for psychological interventions. For example, the triadic partnerships model (De Civita & Dobkin, 2004) suggests interventions targeted toward enhancing family–physician communication (S. Y. Cohen & Wamboldt, 2000) to resolve discrepancies in prescribed medical treatment versus what is actually understood by children, adolescents, and family members. Finally, comprehensive models can incorporate multiple outcomes and specify the relationships among outcomes, which is an advantage in understanding mediators of intervention change.

FUTURE DIRECTIONS IN THE APPLICATION OF THEORY TO INTERVENTION RESEARCH

A wide range of theoretical models and frameworks have been proposed that are potentially relevant to psychological interventions for children and adolescents with chronic illness and their families. Broad, multifaceted frameworks that have been described provide important resources for researchers to use in developing interventions. Moreover, the key issues that are relevant to psychological interventions with pediatric chronic illness are already represented in available theories. Consequently, new theories are not needed. But a great deal of work is needed in refining and integrating current models. Progress in theory refinement would be achieved by the following agenda: (a) enhance specificity of theories, models, and frameworks for pediatric chronic illness; (b) articulate the role of family process in theory; (c) specify the critical processes in intervention change; (d) specify moderators of intervention change; and (e) refine and integrate theoretical models on the basis of data and practice.

Enhance Specificity of Models and Frameworks of Pediatric Chronic Illness Research

One important area for future development involves enhancing the specificity of theories and their application to research concerning psychological intervention with children with chronic illness. Although some theories, such as the individual and family resource and risk factor models (R. J. Thompson & Gustafson, 1996; Varni & Wallander, 1988), have been developed from research on pediatric chronic illness, others, such as the health belief model, have not. For this reason, the specific application and relevance to pediatric chronic illness need to be developed. In addition, specificity of the theories with respect to intervention change needs to be articulated (e.g., identification of key processes that are targets of intervention and mechanisms of change).

Nonspecific theories are difficult to operationalize in interventions. For example, family conflict, which is an important construct in risk and resilience models (R. J. Thompson & Gustafson, 1996; Wallander et al., 2003), is a broad dimension that may involve different domains and be operationalized in very different ways. To optimize the effectiveness of psychological interventions in promoting children's psychological adjustment or adherence to treatment, it is useful to specify the following: (a) nature of such conflict (e.g., is it illness specific or general conflict?), (b) the way family conflict is interfering with the target problem of interest (e.g., how specifically is conflict affecting children's psychological adjustment or adherence to treatment?), and (c) how family conflict might be changed by the intervention (e.g., by enhancing quality of family communication).

Another area in which greater theoretical specificity is needed is in the targeting of individuals and families and outcomes to be the focus of intervention efforts. It is useful to note that different theories may be applicable to different types of interventions and target outcomes. For example, individual and family resource and risk factors may be useful in targeting individuals and families who are at special risk for psychological problems and also identifying risk factors (e.g., family conflict) that relate to psychological distress among children with chronic illness and are potentially modifiable by psychological intervention. In contrast, social–cognitive models, such as health beliefs and personal meaning models, may be most relevant to identifying specific beliefs and concerns that affect children's psychological adjustment or adherence to treatment and may need to be modified in intervention. To enhance the applications of theory to psychological intervention research, researchers should describe how a specific theory or theories informed the design and implementation of their intervention (e.g., targets of intervention, intervention strategies).

In considering the potential applicability of theories to psychological intervention research, one should distinguish between modifiable risk factors or processes (e.g., coping strategies, reinforcement practices) and those that are more stable and less amenable to change (e.g., economic level, temperament). Individual and family risk and resource models (Patterson, 1988; R. J. Thompson & Gustafson, 1996; Varni & Wallander, 1988) have specified potentially modifiable versus stable factors. However, it is not clear whether and to what extent key variables in social–cognitive theories such as health or illness uncertainty beliefs are potentially modifiable, and if so, how this would affect children's psychological adjustment to chronic illness. Interventions need to focus on potentially changeable patterns of behavior and also consider how less modifiable factors may influence a family's response to a psychological intervention. For example, in working with the family of a child with asthma, one could help the child and parent develop a greater repertoire of adaptive behaviors in managing the treatment regimen and also consider how factors such as family economic resources might limit their participation in a specific intervention model.

Articulate the Role of Family Processes in Theory

Most theories and frameworks (e.g., risk and resource models, social–cognitive theories) have focused on individual psychological processes and factors rather than family processes. Individual psychological processes are clearly important. However, family processes are also critical to the development of children's patterns of psychological adjustment and adherence to medical treatment as well as the process of changing these patterns. For example, to accomplish change in maladaptive patterns of children's adaptation to chronic illness, psychological interventions need to engage both children and their parents in intervention. For this reason, family processes need to be emphasized and articulated in theories more than they have been. For example, greater attention to theoretical work that describes the influence of family-specific beliefs, perceptions, and behaviors on psychological adaptation and adherence to treatment in pediatric chronic illness is also necessary for several reasons (Kazak et al., 2004). Beliefs and behaviors are often the targets of psychological intervention because they can be modified. Moreover, changes in key behaviors and beliefs are likely to be mediators of intervention change. Other examples of behaviors and variables that have not received sufficient attention in models of intervention are specific child and family health behaviors such as feeding and diet (Mackner, McGrath, & Stark, 2001; Stark, 2000); the goals of children, adolescents, and parents for their chronic illness treatment; and quality of life in relation to personal goals (L. Schwartz, 2004; L. Schwartz & Drotar, 2005; Sheldon & Elliot, 1999).

Family-based theories, including the FAAR model and family systems models, have identified the family processes (e.g., family communications and relationships) that are important influences on clinically relevant chronic-illness-related outcomes such as adherence to treatment, illness management, and psychological functioning (e.g., see Blechman & Delamater, 1993; Fiese, Wilder, & Bickham, 2000). Psychological interventions need to target the critical family behaviors and reinforcers that support the child's optimal functioning in families, in school, and in response to chronic illness symptoms (e.g., pain) and illness management. The miscarried helping model (B. J. Anderson & Coyne, 1991) is one example of the level of specificity that will be needed to describe family processes that can result in problematic psychological outcomes and need to be targeted in psychological intervention research.

Family models also need to be developed to describe the way in which family interactions affect self-management of pediatric chronic illness. In this regard, Creer's (2000) theoretical work on the psychological components of chronic illness self-management for children and adolescents and their families provide a significant conceptual advance that should be incorporated in the development of intervention theory (see chap. 6). For example, Creer identified critical self-management behaviors (e.g., goal selection, information collection, decision making) that are learned in the family context, are critical to successful illness management, and hence are logical targets for change in families in which illness management is problematic.

Specify the Mediators of Intervention Change

Another area that theoretical models and frameworks should address is the process of change in response to psychological interventions (see chap. 11). Most theories have been developed to account for or understand the factors that have contributed to the development of psychological adjustment patterns associated with pediatric chronic illness as opposed to factors that influence change in these patterns. Rutter (2000) underscored the need to distinguish among factors, processes of risk, and resilience in understanding the causal mechanisms that underlie psychological outcomes. According to Rutter, the power of a theory or explanatory model relates to the specification of the dynamic process by which an outcome (e.g., adherence to treatment) develops and becomes resistant to change.

In general, available frameworks and models have focused on how problems with psychological adaptation to chronic illness or adherence to treatment may develop. However, processes of change that are needed to modify clinically significant problems once they develop are critical to interventions. The risk factors and processes that trigger the development of clinically significant problems such as serious adherence to treatment and psychological distress are related to but are not the same as those that maintain these problems (see chap. 1). For this reason, theoretical models need to consider and articulate these contrasting processes so that they can inform the development and evaluation of interventions. Another example is that the processes necessary for successful prevention of psychological problems may be very different from those that are needed to manage the negative impact of serious chronic and individual and/or family dysfunction (Kazak, 2001). Consequently, theories need to specify the processes by which problems develop so that interventions can address these processes.

A number of available theories are relevant to identifying and managing processes that are involved in positive change as a function of psychological intervention. For example, cognitive–behavioral theories have also specified some of the factors (e.g., avoidance) that are maintaining problematic patterns of psychological adjustment and would need to be targeted to create positive change. In addition, the transtheoretical model (Prochaska & DiClemente, 1984) is also relevant to understanding the various processes needed to occur to facilitate acceptance of and motivation for change (W. R. Miller & Rollnick, 2002). For this reason, this theory might be developed and operationalized with respect to specific targets of psychological intervention (e.g., psychological maladjustment or problematic adherence to treatment) that are applicable to children and adolescents. For example, stages-of-change models might be integrated with health belief models to consider how children and family members perceive the nature of their problems and address the following questions: Do they perceive the potential targets of intervention as a problem or not? If so, in what way? Do parents and children perceive the problem in similar or different ways? How do these perceptions affect their response to interventions?

Specify Moderators of Intervention Change

The extraordinary heterogeneity (e.g., type and severity) of adherence and psychological adjustment problems experienced by children and adolescents with chronic conditions poses significant challenges to theoretical models. One such challenge concerns the need to specify the critical individual and family factors that moderate the effects of psychological interventions and may need to be considered in tailoring psychological interventions. Greater theoretical emphasis on describing the relevance of individual difference factors that need to be addressed in individualizing psychological interventions would enhance the clinical relevance of theories and the power of interventions (see chap. 11). Theories such as individual and family risk and resource factor models (Patterson, 1988; R. J. Thompson & Gustafson, 1996; Varni & Wallander, 1988) are applicable to understanding potential moderators of intervention. For example, a psychological intervention may have different effects on families who present with different patterns of psychological risk versus resilience (i.e., some interventions would be expected to be more effective for families who demonstrate higher levels of resilience such as family cohesion and support).

Refine and Develop Theories

One of the important functions of intervention research in any field is to modify theory on the basis of data that are gathered (H. T. Chen, 1990). Research on psychological interventions in pediatric chronic illness is no exception. Unfortunately, many of the theoretical models described in this chapter have not been reevaluated or refined on the basis of research, especially intervention research. To address this need, specific theory-guided psychological interventions and data analyses will be necessary to develop intervention science in the field of pediatric chronic illness. Moreover, tests of alternative models of psychological intervention that are derived from competing theories provide another important but as yet little-used option for investigators. Syntheses of theory and intervention research findings in critical research reviews designed to enhance the development of theory to inform psychological intervention research are also very much needed.

Research on the description of change in clinically relevant outcomes, such as psychological adaptation and adherence to treatment in pediatric chronic illness, is highly relevant to theory development. The fact that psychological intervention research is prospective affords an important opportunity for researchers to develop theories and design research studies that generate knowledge about changes in the developmental trajectories of key outcomes (e.g., psychological adaptation and adherence to treatment) in response to intervention. Unfortunately, prospective research has been much more the exception than the norm in research on pediatric chronic illness, with notable exceptions (Coakley, Holmbeck, Friedman, Greenley, & Thill, 2002; Hauser et al., 1990; R. J. Thompson, Gustafson, Gil, Kinney, & Spock, 1999).

FUTURE DIRECTIONS: TOWARD AN INFORMED INTEGRATION OF THEORY, RESEARCH, AND PRACTICE

It is unlikely that any single theoretical model will be applicable to the broad range of processes and outcomes in psychological intervention research with children with chronic illness. For this reason, the most powerful theoretical models are likely to be comprehensive (i.e., those that facilitate the integration of different theories as they pertain to processes and outcomes that are relevant to multiple intervention targets across different clinic conditions). For example, with respect to interventions to promoting adherence to treatment, cognitive–behavioral models that enhance specific behaviors, health belief models that encourage change or reframing of beliefs about medications and their management, and problem-solving models that focus on family-centered communication and strategies of management may achieve optimal synergy of change by targeting different processes. However, this hypothesis remains to be tested. It is not at all clear how best to operationalize a comprehensive theoretical model of intervention. For example, should each theory be given weight in various specific modules based on different theoretical approaches? Alternatively, should one theoretical model be chosen as the primary guiding model for the overall intervention and specific theories identified to guide specific modules of intervention?

Although intervention findings should be used to modify and refine theoretical models, it is equally important that new developments in theoretical models and integration of models be used to guide intervention. Ideally, this process should involve a much closer dialogue among researchers who develop theories, those who conduct psychological intervention research, and those who are interested in the process of developmental change. Clinically relevant perspectives concerning such issues as barriers to change and factors that influence acceptability of psychological interventions to children and families should be included in new theoretical models related to intervention. Moreover, theory refinement should be informed by clinical practice. For example, some theories are well articulated and involve sound psychological principles but may not be readily applicable to practice. Consequently, the clinical significance of the theory-guided interventions is very important. On the basis of my research and clinical experience, theories will need to be focused on highly specific, clinically relevant targets. Chapters 6–10 describe a number of such interventions that focus on specific chronic conditions.

II

PRAGMATIC STRATEGIES

3

RESEARCH DESIGN CONSIDERATIONS FOR PSYCHOLOGICAL INTERVENTIONS

Investigators who design and implement psychological interventions need to make an extraordinary number of decisions and consider any salient methodological issues that relate to the population they wish to treat. The purpose of this chapter is to consider some of these challenges and potential ways of meeting them. To accomplish this aim, I describe a model that takes investigators through the specific decisions that are necessary in designing psychological intervention research and the issues that need to be considered in making them.

INVESTIGATORS' RESOURCES FOR DECISION MAKING

To facilitate the process of designing an intervention study for children with chronic illness, investigators might want to take inventory of their personal and collaborative resources for decision making. One important resource is clinical experience with a particular population, which may be critical in identifying the need for and potential focus of a psychological intervention. For example, my clinical experiences in psychological evaluations of young children who were hospitalized for failure to thrive indicated significant gaps in patterns of clinical care for this population. In particular, hospital-based patterns of clinical care did not address the family members' influences on the child's feeding and nutrition that accounted for the child's condition. These clinical experiences underscored the need for and also informed the development and evaluation of a home-based, family-centered model of intervention designed to promote more adaptive patterns of infant feeding and nutrition (Drotar, Malone, Nowak, Elamin, & Eckerle, 1985).

Other resources that investigators may want to consider in designing psychological intervention studies are colleagues within their own setting or others who have had experience with the population and intervention issues of primary interest. Psychological intervention research takes place in the context of interdisciplinary teams who have a range of expertise and experience with children with chronic illness and their families that will be critical to investigators. In addition, pilot and preliminary studies can be an invaluable resource to inform decision making. It is important for investigators to recognize that decisions that are made concerning the design of psychological intervention research are never ideal, in that they involve difficult trade-offs. For example, a decision to increase sample size may be critical from the standpoint of enhancing statistical power but may necessitate increased resources (e.g., staff time) that may not be realistic based on the available funding. For this reason, investigators need to be knowledgeable about the most critical issues in the design of intervention research yet also be familiar with the pragmatic considerations that are needed to implement the intervention. Investigators may wish to consult relevant published resources for additional information concerning methodological issues in the design and implementation of intervention studies (Drotar, 2000a, 2000b; Kazdin, 1980, 1992, 2000) and reporting and evaluating data from randomized controlled trials (RCTs; Altman, 1996; Altman et al., 2001; Chalmers, Smith, & Blackburn, 1981).

DECISIONS AND CONSIDERATIONS IN SELECTING AN INTERVENTION MODEL

As outlined in Exhibit 3.1, the rest of the chapter describes the specific decisions involved in selecting a psychological intervention model and issues to consider in making these decisions.

Choice of Population and Sample

The choice of which chronic condition to study will depend on the state of the art with respect to the science of psychological interventions

EXHIBIT 3.1
Decisions and Considerations in Selecting a
Psychological Intervention Model

Focus of decisions	Issues to consider
Choice of population and sample	Scientific state of the art Categorical model: specific chronic condition Noncategorical: more than one chronic condition
Scope of intervention	Generalized Selected Targeted
Timing and purpose of intervention: problem duration and severity	Primary prevention Secondary prevention Tertiary prevention
Target participants and model of intervention	Participants Child Parent/child Family system Physicians Teachers Type of intervention Actions involved Target behavior Outcome that is assessed
Intensity and duration	Number of intervention sessions relative to length of intervention Length of intervention
Operational definition of target problem and outcome	Specificity Clinical relevance
Clinical need/significance and target problem	Definition of the target problems/outcomes Incidence and prevalence of target problem Morbidity of target problem Frequency of symptoms Impact on functioning Comorbidity in clinical problems
Clinical experience with the target sample	Description of target problem Feasibility Acceptability What has worked in practice
Evaluating available empirical research	Reviews of empirically supported research Descriptive research concerning processes that affect potential targets of intervention
Role of pilot feasibility/studies	Determining acceptability and feasibility Developing intervention content and structure Determining intensity/duration of intervention Estimation of effect size

(continued)

EXHIBIT 3.1 *(Continued)*

Focus of decisions	Issues to consider
Role of theory	Theory of processes that affect target outcome Theory of change (e.g., how intervention affects outcome) Rationale for expected changes
Choice of research design: Within subject, between group Randomized selection of participants and RCTs	State of the art in intervention research (e.g., what is known vs. interventions with specific populations and unknown about problems) Resources/feasibility Choice of control group
Problems of RCTs	Ethical problems Defining adequate controls Patient and family preferences Regression to the mean Interpreting the source of change Operational issues
Choice of control group	Phase of intervention research Feasibility
Estimation of sample size	Effect size Variability in target outcome
Methods of sampling	Defining inclusion and exclusion criteria
Standardizing eligibility criteria	Methods of quality control across sites of data collection and time
Evaluating impact of selective participation and attrition	Identifying characteristics of participants vs. nonparticipants Identifying characteristics of attrition samples Documenting and describing whether the data are missing at random or not Using statistical methods to limit the impact of missing data
Evaluating intervention fidelity	Documenting how intervention was delivered: participants, content/focus, structure, and process Fidelity checks
Defining and measuring usual or standard care	Documenting content, frequency, and duration of visits
Describing and enhancing adherence to intervention protocol	Define critical tasks needed to accomplish Record whether tasks were accomplished Develop strategies to enhance adherence to the intervention
Selecting measures for intervention studies	Types of outcomes Reliability and validity Sensitivity to target outcome Feasibility and response burden Sensitivity to moderating and mediating effects Generalizability of intervention effects across multiple respondents

(continued)

EXHIBIT 3.1 *(Continued)*

Focus of decisions	Issues to consider
Developing a data-analytic plan	Hypothesis testing Statistical power Analysis of change over time Mediation and moderation of intervention effects
Maximizing scientific opportunities if an intervention shows no effects	Secondary analyses: measurement validation studies Studies of respondents versus nonrespondents to intervention Strategies to integrate data across multiple respondents Prediction of outcomes

Note. RCT = randomized controlled trial.

with that particular condition. Although there is a need to develop and evaluate psychological interventions with each and every chronic pediatric condition, the quantity and quality of the available scientific knowledge base and data vary significantly across different chronic conditions. For example, the number of studies and empirically supported interventions is much greater with chronic conditions such as asthma and diabetes than it is for many other conditions (see chaps. 6–10). Psychological intervention research will generally be conducted with a specific chronic condition because it is necessary to tailor an intervention to the demands and stressors that are specific to a particular chronic condition. However, investigators should also appreciate that a major disadvantage of condition-specific or categorical interventions is the lack of generalizability to other chronic conditions. For this reason, noncategorical interventions that can be generalized across different chronic conditions should be considered (see chaps. 1 and 11).

Scope of the Intervention

Another relevant set of decisions for intervention researchers concerns the model and scope of the psychological intervention relating to pediatric chronic illness (Pless & Stein, 1994). Gordon (1983) described three potential types of interventions with respect to populations that are applicable to such research for children with chronic illness: (a) *generalized* or universal interventions that are provided to all children with a specific chronic illness or children with chronic conditions as a group, (b) *selected* interventions that are offered to a subset of individuals who are at risk (e.g., children and adolescents with chronic illness identified to be at risk for problems), and

(c) *targeted* interventions directed at those at high or demonstrated risk (e.g., children with chronic illness who demonstrate significant psychological adjustment problems such as depression that are clearly interfering with their functioning). The National Institute of Mental Health (1998) described a similar framework with respect to prevention of mental disorders.

Many published psychological intervention studies for children with chronic illness have focused on either selected or targeted interventions. This may reflect the fact that such problems are often the focus of clinical attention. On the other hand, universal interventions such as comprehensive care or psychological support for all children with families with a newly diagnosed chronic condition who are cared for in a setting or community are potentially important from a public health standpoint (Kazak, 2001). However, universal interventions generally require more resources to implement than selected interventions.

Timing and Purpose of the Intervention

The type and severity of problems that are associated with childhood chronic illness are heterogeneous (see chap. 1). Unfortunately, the duration and severity of target problems have not been well defined in many psychological intervention studies. For this reason, decisions concerning the timing and purpose of the intervention are particularly challenging. Such decisions involve two salient questions: (a) When should psychological interventions be timed with respect to the onset of specific psychological adjustment or adherence problems, and (b) what areas should one target (e.g., serious and potentially more entrenched psychological problems, less serious ones, or primary prevention)?

Clinical experiences or pilot data with specific chronic illness populations are important in helping to make decisions concerning the timing of interventions. In addition, when available, scientific data and theory concerning the natural history, duration, and severity of specific psychological and adherence problems in various settings may inform the design of psychological interventions. Other research data that may be useful concern risk factors for the development of adjustment or adherence problems and information concerning factors that are maintaining the problems.

Investigators should consider that newly developed psychological problems may have very different characteristics from those that are long-standing. Moreover, different processes and risk factors (and hence targets of intervention) may be involved in increasing the risk for or triggering the development of clinically relevant problems in psychological adjustment and adherence to medical treatment versus maintaining similar problems once they have developed (Rutter, 2000). For example, some problems related to nonadherence to medical treatment may be influenced by inconsistent parental reinforcement or monitoring of adherence-related behaviors. However, once significant nonadherence problems develop, additional factors such as parent–child conflict may also become a well-reinforced part of the process that helps to maintain the problem (B. J. Anderson & Coyne, 1991). For this reason, the content and structure of psychological interventions that are designed to reduce the probability that adherence-related problems will occur might be expected to differ substantially from those that are designed to limit the health-related and psychological consequences of a well-entrenched problem.

Caplan's (1964) prevention framework is applicable to decisions concerning the timing and purpose of psychological intervention. This model distinguishes among the following types of prevention: (a) *primary prevention*, which aims to reduce the incidence of mental disorders in a community setting; (b) *secondary prevention*, which is defined as reducing the prevalence or duration of disorders that occur; and (c) *tertiary prevention*, which is designed to reduce impairments that may result from mental disorders. On the basis of Caplan's framework, primary preventive interventions are designed to focus on children and adolescents with chronic illness who are at high risk for mental health or treatment adherence problems. Secondary prevention studies focus on reducing the impact of mental health or adherence problems that have already been identified or reducing the functional impact of symptoms (e.g., pain) on children's functioning in different life contexts (e.g., school). Finally, tertiary prevention studies can target reduction of the impact of serious mental health disorders (e.g., major depression or posttraumatic stress disorder in an adolescent with cancer) or health-related morbidity (e.g., serious problems in treatment adherence leading to recurrent ketoacidosis in diabetes) on the functioning of the child or family.

It should be noted that practitioners who provide treatment to children and adolescents with chronic health conditions are generally engaged in secondary or tertiary prevention of mental health and problems with adherence to treatment. On the other hand, programs that provide comprehensive psychological care to all children with a given chronic illness in a given setting provide primary prevention. In this regard, Rapoff (2000) described an interesting model concerning the prevention of problematic adherence to medical treatment. In this model, primary prevention includes comprehensive education, modeling and rehearsing treatment regimen tasks when medications are first prescribed and in an ongoing fashion, and training patients and families to monitor their adherence. These interventions would be provided to all children. In this model, secondary prevention services are given to those patients for whom significant nonadherence to medical treatment has been identified but has not yet significantly compromised health. Such services may involve reeducation, more extensive monitoring, more explicit social reinforcement to promote adherence, and instructing parents in child-rearing strategies. Finally, tertiary prevention services are proposed to be given to patients whose clinically significant nonadherence has deleterious effects on health. Such interventions may include token system programs, contingency contracting focused on specific regimen tasks and consequences, self-management and problem-solving training to anticipate and manage obstacles to adherence, and individual/family therapy to address family or psychological problems that impact adherence (Rapoff, 2000). This innovative model has not been tested for psychological interventions with pediatric chronic illness populations but clearly warrants attention.

Target Participants and Model of Intervention

Another critical set of decisions in psychological intervention research in childhood chronic illness is the selection of the specific model of intervention that will be tested, the participants in the target content or focus of intervention, and the outcomes that are expected to be enhanced (see chap. 1). For example, psychological interventions may involve the child, parent, family, physicians, or teachers. The content or focus of a potential intervention will vary with the specific model of intervention that is being tested.

Pless and Stein (1994) proposed a three-dimensional conceptual model to guide psychological interventions with children with chronic illness and their families that includes (a) target participants (e.g., who is involved, such as child and/or parent), (b) when the intervention is delivered (timing), and (c) the type of intervention. Type of intervention can be subdivided into two main areas: the nature of the actions that are involved in the intervention (e.g., education, support) and the specific target behavior or area of functioning (e.g., adherence to treatment) that is addressed by the intervention. Although target behaviors involved in psychological interventions are often the same as the outcomes that are studied, this is not necessarily the case. For example, in some intervention models, the targets for the intervention (e.g., problem-solving skills) are mediators of intervention effects; that is, behaviors that are expected to influence the primary outcome (e.g., adherence to treatment; Wysocki, Greco, Harris, & White, 2000).

Intensity and Duration of Intervention

The parameters of intensity and duration, which are important in determining the strength of an intervention, are not well understood in psychological interventions, including interventions for children and adolescents with chronic health conditions (Kazdin, 1995, 2000). *Intensity* can be defined as the number of intervention sessions during the specific time period of an intervention. *Duration* is the overall length of the intervention (Kazdin, 1995, 2000). By definition, a chronic illness has a very long, in most cases lifelong, duration, which complicates the decision concerning the intensity and duration of a potential psychological intervention. For example, at what point in the course of a chronic condition is it most effective to provide an intervention to manage a specific intervention (e.g., psychological distress)? What is the optimal intensity of intervention that is needed to enhance outcomes such as adherence to treatment that are both "chronic" and always necessary? Unfortunately, because these variables have not been systematically studied, there are limited data available to guide investigators' decisions about the intensity and duration of psychological interventions in pediatric chronic illness.

From a theoretical standpoint, interventions that are designed to help families respond to specific illness-related crises (e.g., diagnosis of cancer) would be expected to be limited to these crisis periods. On the basis of clinical experience, one might expect that more discrete, less entrenched problems would respond to less intensive interventions than more pervasive and chronic problems. However, more intensive interventions with longer duration are not necessarily more effective. On the contrary, a substantial body of research on psychotherapy with adults suggests that interventions of greater intensity and longer duration do not necessarily result in greater effects (Kopta, Leuger, Saunders, & Howard, 1999).

Given the many choices concerning intervention content, targets, and timing, how do investigators decide which specific model of psychological intervention to test? Moreover, how do they best operationalize a model of intervention interest? As shown in Exhibit 3.1, in making decisions concerning intervention models, investigators need to consider a complex combination of factors, including the operational definition of the target problem and outcome, clinical need and significance, clinical experiences, empirical research, and theory.

Operational Definition of the Target Problem and Outcome

A clear operational definition of the target problem is necessary to develop the intervention model and to enhance potential replicability in the event of a successful intervention. Ideally, target problems should be defined as specifically as possible. For example, frequency of anxiety symptoms above a specific cutoff as measured by a specific scale is a more precise target than "psychological adjustment problem." Unfortunately, there is little consensus concerning the most relevant target problems or outcomes for psychological intervention research in pediatric chronic illness (see chap. 1). For this reason, a critical and comprehensive review of previous research with a specific chronic condition of interest that is informed by clinical experience is necessary to select the operational definition of the target problem, the most clinically relevant outcomes, and measures of the outcome.

Clinical Need and Significance of the Target Problem

Clinical need and significance, which are important in choosing a target problem and in designing an intervention, include the following parameters: (a) the frequency or incidence and prevalence, (b) medical severity or morbidity of the problem, and (c) functional impact of the problem as defined by caregivers and others (Kazdin, 2000). The trade-off between the clinical significance of target problems and statistical power, which can be a very difficult one in designing interventions, needs to be considered. For example, problems that have substantial clinical significance as defined by high levels of severity or functional impact tend to occur less frequently than those that have less clinical significance. Consequently, the sample sizes that are needed to achieve statistical power for high-severity, low-prevalence problems among children with chronic illness may be very difficult to achieve at a single site. On the other hand, there can be important reasons to test interventions for problems that are relatively infrequent but have high severity or functional impairment (e.g., poor diabetes control leading to recurrent episodes of ketoacidosis; see chap. 7). Investigators might wish to consider alternative designs to test interventions for low-prevalence but high-severity problems such as case series or within-subjects designs, especially in the early phases of interventions that are focused on such problems (Linscheid, 2000; Tervo, Estrem, Bryson-Brochmann, & Symons, 2003).

To design psychological intervention studies that are informed by clinical significance, investigators need to understand that the frequency and pattern of psychological or health problems and symptoms can differ greatly from the level of impact of these problems on children's functioning or health-related quality of life. For example, some children with chronic illness with high levels of psychological (e.g., depression) or physical (e.g., pain) symptoms show relatively little dysfunction in various areas of their lives. Others with relatively few symptoms or behavioral problems may demonstrate more serious dysfunction. Moreover, the factors that influence psychological or physical symptoms may differ from those that influence functioning (Palermo, 2000). Consequently, psychological interventions may affect psychological symptoms differently than functional outcomes (Kazdin, 2000; see chap. 11). Therefore, investigators' decisions concerning the target and focus of interventions and relevant outcomes will need to consider relevant differences in the responsiveness of symptoms and functional outcomes to interventions. Interventions that are targeted to reduce symptoms may also enhance functional outcomes (and vice versa). For this reason, where feasible, measures of symptoms as well as functional outcomes should be included in evaluations of intervention outcomes.

Investigators will also need to consider the level and nature of comorbidity in target problems. For example, in conducting a study to reduce the level of anxiety in children with asthma, it is important to consider that some children with high levels of anxiety may also show high levels of depressed mood. Excluding children with high levels of depressive symptoms will help to focus the intervention on the primary target of anxiety. However, excluding children who have depressive symptoms will limit the generalizability of the intervention. Moreover, depending on the level of comorbidity of symptoms of anxiety and depression in a particular sample, the available sample size may also be significantly reduced.

Clinical Experiences With the Target Sample

Clinical experiences and data that describe the target sample in detail are necessary to operationalize target problems and develop a model of psychological intervention. Koocher, McGrath, and Gudas's (1990) clinical experiences with children and adolescents with cystic fibrosis who were referred for problems with adherence to medical treatment underscored the need to develop a typology of adherence problems that reflects clinically relevant individual differences in etiology. For example, Koocher et al. identified one pattern of nonadherence as family dysfunction leading to inconsistent monitoring of the child's treatment. Another was described as a reasoned choice of nonadherence based on understanding of the burdens of treatment versus potential benefits (Koocher et al., 1990). One would anticipate that these different etiological subtypes of nonadherence to treatment would necessitate different intervention strategies. For example, inconsistent parental monitoring of adherence may necessitate behavioral management, whereas reasoned nonadherence may benefit from a cognitive–behavioral approach that involves changing beliefs about nonadherence or side effects of treatment.

Clinical experiences with children and adolescents with chronic health conditions can also suggest ways to engage families effectively in psychological interventions and educate them about the need for these interventions. Parents of children with chronic conditions are more likely to participate in interventions that they believe are applicable to the stresses and problems that they are experiencing and are provided by professionals whom they perceive to be knowledgeable about their and their children's illness-related experiences.

Evaluating Available Empirical Research

Previous psychological intervention research with specific chronic conditions and the field as a whole have established benchmarks against which investigators can test the new or value-added contribution of their intervention model. In addition, reviews of previous research can help investigators identify potential design flaws (e.g., limited statistical power, absence of appropriate control groups, limited description of samples, sample attrition) that have limited previous research and are pitfalls to be avoided (Bauman et al., 1997). Individual studies of psychological intervention with children with specific chronic conditions as well as critical reviews (e.g., the *Journal of Pediatric Psychology* series on empirically supported interventions; Kazak, 1998) or meta-analyses (e.g., Kibby et al., 1999) are important sources of information concerning data on the efficacy of intervention models.

Reviews of Empirically Supported Research

In evaluating the quality of previous intervention research, investigators should consult standards for reviews that have been developed by others. One such option is the standards for empirically supported treatments developed by Division 12 of the American Psychological Association (Chambless et al., 1996, 1998) and adapted by the *Journal of Pediatric Psychology* (Kazak, 1998). Criteria for a well-established intervention include (a) demonstration of statistical significance either in the group designs or between a large series of single-case experimental designs, (b) development of treatment manuals, (c) clear specification of samples, and (d) demonstration of intervention effects by at least two different investigators or investigatory teams. *Probably efficacious* is defined as studies of treatments that have tested as more effective than a control group, or one experiment meeting several of the criteria for well-established interventions (Chambless & Hollon, 1998). The above categorizations of empirically supported interventions are an important step in the field. However, investigators should recognize that standards for such reviews also have weaknesses (e.g., failure to consider effect sizes or the clinical significance of effects) that need to be considered (Drotar, 2002).

Descriptive Research Concerning Processes That Affect Potential Targets of Intervention

Research concerning the processes that affect the development of target problems (e.g., psychological and health behaviors) may also inform the design of intervention research. For example, findings that problematic family reinforcement of pain-related behavior (e.g., paying attention to children's avoidance of activities) contributes to dysfunctional response to chronic pain suggest that interventions designed to reduce the level of dysfunction associated with pain should focus on this reinforcement pattern (Palermo, 2000).

Role of Pilot and Feasibility Data in Developing an Intervention

The considerable methodological advantages of RCTs may tempt investigators to use this design before they have sufficient evidence to conduct such trials. Given the scarcity of intervention research with some pediatric chronic illness samples (see chaps. 6–10), empirical data may be lacking concerning specific models of intervention as well as their feasibility and potential acceptability to participants. For this reason, pilot and preliminary studies of interventions are important potential contributions of such studies and should include the following: (a) determining acceptability and feasibility; (b) developing intervention content and structure, including a preliminary manual; (c) determining the intensity and duration of the intervention; and (d) estimating effect sizes needed to calculate statistical power.

What are some strategies to accomplish pilot and feasibility studies? Case studies and case series, especially those that are conducted with extensive baseline and outcome data, will inform the design of intervention studies (Drotar, La Greca, Lemanek, & Kazak, 1995). Uncontrolled single-group designs in which all participants receive the same intervention can provide critical information concerning the acceptability of interventions to participants and the feasibility of conducting an intervention model in an applied setting. Study designs that include wait-list controls can also provide useful information (Kazdin, 1980).

Role of Theory in Selecting an Intervention Model and Target Outcome

Previous research and clinical experience are clearly relevant to the selection of an intervention model. In addition, theory can be essential in articulating the principles of the intervention and the processes by which an intervention is expected to be effective (see chap. 2). This will help to organize and plan the intervention. Ideally, the choice of intervention model should be guided by a theory that specifies the following: (a) the process by which the target outcome under consideration is expected to be affected by the intervention, (b) the specific way in which the intervention is expected to affect the target outcome, and (c) an explicit rationale for the expected changes (Peyrot, 1996). For example, an investigator who is interested in testing the effect of an intervention to promote adherence to medical treatment in a chronic illness, such as asthma, would ideally want to identify the specific processes that disrupt or facilitate adherence to treatment, how these will be influenced by the intervention model that is being tested, and how the expected changes will affect the target outcomes (see chap. 2).

Choice of Research Design

An investigator's choice of research design will depend on the state of the art of intervention research with a specific chronic condition and the model of intervention that is tested. In some instances, the state of the art of intervention research with a specific chronic condition may be sufficiently advanced that investigators will want to consider an RCT. (See chap. 11 for discussion of the stages of intervention research.) However, in situations in which intervention research is less well developed, an RCT design may be premature, and investigators may wish to consider other options such as within-subject or between-groups designs (see Kazdin, 1980).

Within-Subject Designs

The major characteristic of a within-subject design is that each of the different treatments in the study is presented to each participant (Kazdin, 1980). In most of these designs, separate groups are used so that different treatments can be balanced across separate groups of participants. These designs include (a) crossover designs, in which all participants cross over or are switched to another experimental condition or multiple treatment counterbalanced design that includes more than the treatments, and (b) intrasubject replication designs, which are characterized by presenting and withdrawing treatments over time in the context of continuous observation and a true baseline phase. Options for intrasubject replication designs include the ABAB design, the multiple baseline design, and the simultaneous treatment design, each of which may have applications in chronic illness intervention research (for details concerning specific methods, see Linscheid, 2000; Rapoff, 1999; Tervo et al., 2003).

Between-Groups Designs

In a between-groups design, a group that receives the intervention is compared with a control group (assignment may or may not be randomized). A fundamental decision in between-groups research designs is the assignment of participants to groups for an optimal test of interventions. Ideally, the nature of the assignment should provide assurance that the groups would not have differed without the manipulation (Kazdin, 1980).

Between-groups designs include pretest–posttest control designs, in which the groups are tested before and after the intervention has been concluded; factorial designs; and posttest-only control group designs. Quasi-experimental designs or nonequivalent control group designs can also be useful (Cook & Campbell, 1979). The hallmark of such designs is that owing to various constraints, the investigator cannot meet the requirements of a true experiment with random assignment. In such designs, the methodological advantages of RCTs are well recognized (Cook & Campbell, 1979). The differences in outcomes are attributable not only to the characteristics of psychological interventions but also to the characteristics of participating children and families (e.g., parental education, severity of illness) that may influence target outcomes and limit the validity of the findings. This should be assessed in the analytic plan.

Randomized Selection and Randomized Controlled Trials

Random selection refers to the selection of the sample (in this case, of children with chronic illness) from a broader population. For example, in a study of psychological intervention with children and adolescents with cancer who are depressed, one would want to sample all of the potential available patients with both cancer and depression and identify and recruit the sample so that each individual would have an equal likelihood of being selected.

Random assignment refers to the assignment of participants into groups so that the probability of each participant appearing in any of the experimental groups is equal (Kazdin, 1980). However, it should be noted that although random assignment can result in bias-free group assignment, it does not necessarily ensure equivalent groups. Such bias is more likely to occur in small samples that are characteristic of many studies of psychological interventions in pediatric chronic illness. Consequently, investigators will need to consider that random assignment may not be sufficient to manage threats to validity posed by group differences on variables on relevant outcomes. The threat to validity that is posed by such influences is most problematic for those variables that differ between the intervention and control groups and are also correlated with target outcomes (Greene & Ernhart, 1991). For this reason, investigators may wish to consider a priori stratification of key variables (e.g., severity of the child's illness, age, family socioeconomic status) that are known to be powerful influences on the target outcomes of interest. The choice of stratification variables needs to be selective because available sample sizes generally preclude more than a few variables to be used in this fashion. Alternatively, although it is not as desirable an option, investigators can use various methods to control statistically for relevant variables (Greene & Ernhart, 1991).

Despite their considerable methodological advantages, RCTs involve a number of problems that need to be considered in designing and interpreting findings from studies of psychological interventions of children with chronic illness (C. E. Schwartz, Chesney, Irvine, & Keefe, 1997). Among others, these include the following: (a) ethical problems of including a true no-treatment control group for some clinical problems and (b) problems of defining an adequate control (e.g., the nonspecific effects included in many interventions, such as social support and education, are powerful). For this reason, it may be very difficult if not impossible to construct a nonspecific treatment condition that does not have active therapeutic ingredients.

Another methodological problem with RCTs involves patient and family preferences: Children and families who volunteer to participate in interventions may be different from nonvolunteers (e.g., more competent and more curious) and may also have strong preferences for a specific intervention. Patients and families who are randomized to the treatment they prefer may do better than those who did not receive their preference. Regression to the mean may also be a limitation of RCT designs. For example, if eligibility criteria focus on patients who are below the mean on a given outcome, then the groups may demonstrate higher rates of outcomes over time owing to regression to the mean, irrespective of the intervention effects. Finally, in some RCTs, changes in response to the intervention may be difficult to distinguish from changes due to accommodation to level of function or adaptation to chronic illness. Other scientific challenges of designing RCTs that need to be considered in studies of pediatric chronic illness include operational issues such as randomization procedures, patient accrual, and maintaining quality control (Weinberger et al., 2001; see chap. 4).

Choice of Control Group

One of the most important and difficult issues in psychological intervention research with children with chronic illness concerns the choice of control or comparison groups. To address this issue, investigators need to consider the purpose of the proposed control group (e.g., what do you want to control for?). In the early phases of psychological intervention research, which reflects the state of the art in research with many chronic conditions, investigators will be most interested in documenting whether a specific intervention is effective compared with usual psychological care. Once a specific intervention model has been shown to be effective with a specific target problem within a chronic illness sample, the primary focus of research may shift to the identification of the most effective or active ingredients in the intervention model (see chap. 11).

It is important to recognize that in some situations, investigators' choice of research design for an intervention study may depend as much on available resources and feasibility considerations as it does on scientific issues. Although RCTs with a sufficiently large sample size to achieve statistical power have clear benefits compared with alternative designs, they are not always feasible because of the limitations of available resources. Moreover, they may not be desirable because of the state of the art in a given area of research. For this reason, in some areas of intervention research, smaller scale, non-RCT designs may be an appropriate match to the scientific state of the art. Such studies may demonstrate feasibility and preliminary effects that are necessary to obtain resources for large-scale RCTs (see chap. 11).

Estimating Sample Size

One of the most important and difficult decisions facing investigators is the sample size, which is critical to document the statistical power of an intervention effect. Limited statistical power is arguably the most common reason that psychological interventions show no difference (J. Cohen, 1988, 1992). A critical consideration in calculating statistical power is estimation of the effect size of a potential intervention. The smaller the effect size of an intervention, the larger the sample that is needed to detect it. Ideally, estimates of effect size should be obtained from data concerning interventions on a population and setting that is similar to that which will be tested either from data from previous research or from preliminary studies. Psychotherapeutic interventions, especially cognitive–behavioral interventions with physically healthy children with psychological problems, have for the most part demonstrated moderate to large effect sizes (Weisz & Weiss, 1993). Effect sizes for psychological interventions with children and adolescents with chronic illness are less well established. However, at least one meta-analysis with psychological interventions with children with chronic health conditions has also shown moderate to large effects (Kibby et al., 1998). On the other hand, summary data on effect sizes drawn from studies of many different chronic conditions are not necessarily applicable to specific target outcomes with specific chronic conditions.

In addition to estimating the potential effect size of an intervention, it is also important to understand the variability in the target outcome measures. In general, it will be more difficult to detect intervention differences (and hence a larger sample size will be necessary) for outcomes that show high as opposed to low variability. For this reason, data from preliminary studies or previous intervention studies with a comparable sample are invaluable in estimating variability in target outcomes.

Methods of Sampling

In determining criteria for potential participants in studies of psychological intervention in childhood chronic illness, investigators again face a difficult trade-off in making their decisions about research design. On the one hand, it is important to limit variation in the target population by setting exclusionary criteria and thus enhance the potential internal validity of study findings. On the other hand, such restriction of sample characteristics limits feasibility and generalizability of findings (Drotar & Riekert, 2000). Inclusion criteria focus on the target population and problem and generally include choice of specific chronic condition and category or subgroup of children who demonstrate risk for target problems (e.g., psychological distress).

Exclusion criteria are those that are imposed by investigators to limit variation that might obscure intervention effects or interpretation of findings (e.g., a very broad age range of participants, presence of serious comorbid mental disorders). In the early phases of intervention research, investigators may decide to enhance internal validity of their findings by selecting a more homogeneous population, assuming they can achieve a sufficient sample size in doing so. In the event that an intervention is successful with a target population of special interest (e.g., school-age children with asthma), generalizability of the effects to broader samples (e.g., to adolescents) might become a priority.

Standardizing Eligibility Criteria

Investigators should standardize the implementation of eligibility criteria across the duration of their studies as well as across sites for multisite studies (see chap. 4 for more detail). Methods to accomplish this include the use of detailed checklists that describe each of the criteria and training research assistants to use them.

Evaluating the Impact of Selective Participation and Attrition

Selective participation and attrition can have a critical influence on the internal and external validity of findings. For this reason, investigators need to decide how these issues will be managed and described in published reports (Betan, Roberts, & McCluskey-Fawcett, 1995). Consider a study of an intervention designed to prevent adherence to medical treatment in pediatric asthma: If a disproportionate number of children who had relatively low risk for nonadherence problems participated, a larger sample than initially anticipated would be necessary to demonstrate an intervention effect (R. E. K. Stein, Bauman, & Ireys, 1991). Moreover, the findings would not be generalizable to children with clinically significant problems in adherence to treatment.

Zebracki et al. (2003) described a comprehensive operational definition of nonparticipation dropout and attrition that is useful for psychological intervention research and that includes the following: (a) preinclusion attrition, (b) dropout attrition, and (c) attrition related to intermittent missing data. *Preinclusion attrition* occurs when participants who are otherwise eligible either do not consent to participate or cannot complete the requirement of the protocol prior to randomization. Riekert and Drotar (1999) found that the families of adolescents with a chronic illness such as diabetes who participated in research on treatment adherence demonstrated higher levels of adherence to medical treatment than those who did not participate. *Dropout attrition* results from participants prematurely discontinuing the treatment or study. *Attrition related to intermittent missing data* occurs when participants do not complete various follow-up outcomes. Each of these different types of attrition may be influenced by very different factors and can affect both internal and external validity of study findings (Zebracki et al., 2003). Several methods are now available to investigators to evaluate the impact of missing data on the study findings and to adjust or correct for the influence of missing data. Readers who are interested in this issue can consult Schafer and Graham (2002) for a comprehensive discussion of this topic. Prevention of the various types of attrition is the most proactive strategy for investigators (see chap. 4).

Evaluating Intervention Fidelity

The *fidelity* of an intervention refers to the degree to which the intervention has been delivered in accord with the plan for participants, content or focus, structure, and process of the intervention. Failure to deliver a psychological intervention as intended can be an important reason why the intervention was not found to be effective. For this reason, documenting whether the treatment or independent variable was in fact carried out (e.g., a manipulation or fidelity check) is an important research design consideration in studies of psychological intervention (Bellg et al., 2004). Investigators have several choices to measure fidelity of an intervention: For example, interventionist and family self-report can be used to check on the fidelity of interventions (Bellg et al., 2004). Although tape recording (audio- or videotape) is a superior method because it is less biased, more time and cost are involved in such methods. Audio- or videotapes should be rated by individuals who are unaware of the specific group assignment by using a standardized checklist that describes the key elements of the specific intervention (see chap. 4).

To demonstrate that the intervention was delivered as hypothesized, investigators must document that the intervention group received the key elements of the intervention and the control groups did not. For example, suppose one is testing the effects of a problem-solving intervention to promote adherence to diabetes treatment over and beyond the effects of nonspecific factors such as support and education. Measures of fidelity will need to document that (a) the problem-solving intervention was given as intended, (b) the problem-solving intervention was not given to the control group, and (c) the problem-solving group did not receive a disproportionate frequency of education or support compared with the control group.

Defining and Measuring Usual or Standard Care

Some psychological intervention studies are designed to compare a new experimental model of intervention with usual or standard care. In such circumstances, it is important to develop procedures to define the care that is provided to children with chronic conditions in specific settings. Such data are not routinely available in clinical settings. For this reason, investigators will need to develop a detailed documentation of the content, frequency or intensity, and duration of the visits that are conducted by various staff.

Describing and Enhancing Adherence to the Intervention Protocol

Because many psychological interventions involve children and families' time-consuming and ongoing commitments, their adherence to such procedures should not be assumed. Although there are few data on this issue, my experience in conducting psychological interventions to promote adherence to treatment for cystic fibrosis and asthma indicates that nonadherence to such interventions is common and needs to be documented because it can affect the validity of such studies. Adherence to a psychological intervention protocol may be documented by defining the critical tasks or what behaviors children and families need to accomplish to implement the intervention of interest. A checklist can be developed to record whether these tasks were accomplished (e.g., documentation of completed homework assignments). However, it is often difficult to observe these behaviors directly. Consequently, investigators may need to rely on children's and parents' self-reports. In addition to deciding on procedures to describe adherence to psychological intervention protocols, investigators need to develop strategies to enhance child and parent adherence to intervention (see chap. 4 for more detail).

Selecting Measures for Intervention Studies

Many different issues need to be considered in choosing outcome measures for chronic-illness-related psychological interventions, some of which are considered here (for a more extended discussion of measurement issues, see Drotar, 2000c; Holmbeck, Li, Schurman, Friedman, & Coakley,

2002; Overholser, Spirito, & DiFilippo, 1999; Quittner, 2000; Quittner, Espelage, Ievers-Landis, & Drotar, 2000).

Types of Outcomes

Intervention studies include *primary* outcomes, which are outcomes that are expected to be most sensitive and relevant to the target intervention of interest, and *secondary* outcomes, which are clinically relevant and might also be expected to change in response to change in the primary outcomes. The inclusion of such outcome variables can help to establish the clinical significance of intervention effects. For example, in a study designed to enhance adherence to asthma treatment as the primary outcome, asthma symptoms and the functional impact of asthma on children's quality of life might also be measured because these variables might be expected to change as a function of the intervention and would add to the clinical significance of the findings. The inclusion of secondary outcomes in studies of psychological interventions in pediatric chronic illness needs to be balanced against factors such as the additional response burden that is involved for children and families and the increased likelihood of spurious findings arising from additional tests of intervention effects using multiple measures.

Reliability and Validity

Ideally, outcome measures should be reliable and valid measures of the target outcome of interest and be sensitive to psychological intervention effects in the specific populations of children with chronic illness who are being studied. For this reason, investigators need to consider the validity of potential measures for their sample and target outcomes. Such data can be gathered in pilot and preliminary studies. These pilot and preliminary studies of the reliability and validity of outcome measures are especially important in heterogeneous samples that vary in ethnicity (Walders & Drotar, 2000).

Sensitivity to Target Outcome

Investigators face a difficult decision in identifying measures that are sensitive to specific intervention effects with specific targets in specific chronic conditions. Psychological measures that are well standardized on normative samples may or may not be sensitive to interventions that are directed to the primary target outcome. One example is the Child Behavior Checklist (Achenbach, 1991), which has been used in many intervention studies in pediatric chronic illness. Because the Child Behavior Checklist was designed as a screening measure of psychopathology, it is not necessarily sensitive to psychological intervention effects across a continuum of behavioral symptoms (Drotar, Perrin, & Stein, 1995).

Feasibility and Response Burden

Another set of considerations in the choice of measures concerns the feasibility of measures. Measures create response burden for participants and also involve additional staff time in administration data management and analysis. For this reason, investigators need to weigh the costs versus benefits of alternative measures with respect to feasibility and response burden and document these factors in their pilot and preliminary studies.

Sensitivity to Moderating and Mediating Effects

Additional measures that may be useful include the following: (a) those that are used to describe the sample, including age, parent age and education, family income, illness-related characteristics, and nature of medical treatment; (b) measures of moderators of intervention effects; (c) mediators of intervention; and (d) measures to assess the validity of outcome measures.

Measuring variables such as gender and age that might be expected to moderate individual differences in response to intervention may enhance the value of the study findings. Moderators are especially important to assess when the intervention effects are variable across the sample and less than optimal (Clingempeel & Henggeler, 2002). Mediators are especially important in documenting the process by which an intervention achieved an effect. (For information specifically about relevant issues in choosing and analyzing moderators and mediators of intervention, see Clingempeel & Henggeler, 2002; Kraemer, Wilson, Fairburn, & Agras, 2002; Weersina & Weisz, 2002.)

Generalizability of Intervention Effects Across Multiple Respondents

Because intervention research in pediatric chronic illness involves children and families, data from multiple informants are necessary for optimal tests of intervention. However, inclusion of data from multiple informants raises significant methodological problems and necessitates special data-analytic strategies (see Holmbeck et al., 2002). For this reason, investigators should carefully consider whether they would anticipate effects of psychological interventions to be comparable across parent and child reports. For example, children's self-reports would be expected to be more sensitive than parental reports in psychological interventions that are designed to reduce psychological distress. On the other hand, parents may be more likely to observe nonadherence to medical treatment than are children, especially younger children. In some instances, investigators will decide to include outcome data based on multiple informants such as parents and children. This strategy has the advantage of information concerning multiple perspectives and reducing the potential bias associated with single-informant outcome data. However, the analysis of outcomes from multiple informants raises special challenges that need to be considered (see Holmbeck et al., 2002).

Also significant in measurement of psychological intervention outcomes is generalizability of measures across different cultural groups. Investigators should not assume that measures that were developed and have been applied to culturally homogeneous normative sample or samples of children with chronic health conditions are necessarily valid for culturally heterogeneous samples. This has become an increasingly critical issue given the diversity of pediatric populations in the United States (see Walders & Drotar, 2000). Investigators who are conducting intervention research with ethnically diverse samples of children with chronic illness may need to conduct additional studies of measures, provide translation if necessary, and document acceptability and validity with the sample of interest.

Developing a Data-Analytic Plan

Development of a data-analytic plan should be a consideration in intervention research. Among other issues, plans for hypothesis testing, statistical power, and testing mediation and moderation effects are especially significant.

Hypothesis Testing

The most critical consideration for investigators is to develop an a priori plan to test the primary hypotheses related to the psychological interventions. Hypothesis-driven analyses are necessary to test the following specific effects: Which specific outcomes and variables are expected to be influenced by the interventions? What is the expected size of the intervention effects? What are the hypothesized specific moderators and mediators of the intervention that will be tested?

Statistical Power

The need for sufficient statistical power to test hypotheses concerning the primary study outcomes is a primary consideration (see earlier section, Estimating Sample Size).

Analysis of Change Over Time

By definition, studies that test psychological interventions involve analyses of change over time. Modern advances in data analysis have resulted in methods such as hierarchical linear models that provide more precise estimates of the description of change and can include all available data from participants. These methods reflect considerable advances over more traditional analytic methods such as analysis of variance (Frank, Thayer,

& Hoaglund, 1998; Rogosa, Brandt, & Zimonowski, 1982). In addition, methods such as structural equation modeling provide a more precise estimate of causal models that describe mediating processes of intervention effects than are possible with more traditional models such as multiple regression (Bollen, 1989).

Testing Mediation and Moderation of Intervention Effects

Mediation effects in psychological intervention studies can be tested by using the following steps: (a) Develop the theory that underlies the anticipated intervention effects (e.g., what is the specific process by which the intervention is assumed to be effective?); (b) identify a measure of the hypothesized mediator and incorporate it into the study design; and (c) use formal tests of mediation in data analysis (Holmbeck, 1997). For example, suppose one is interested in evaluating interventions that are based on problem-solving theory that are hypothesized to achieve effects on adherence to treatment by changing the quality of family problem solving. To test this hypothesis, investigators need to include a measure of problem-solving ability at baseline and at subsequent outcome points to determine whether quality of problem-solving ability changed as a function of the intervention and whether these changes were related to hypothesized changes in the primary outcomes (Holmbeck, 1997).

Analyses of moderation effects are designed to determine individual differences in child or family response to psychological outcomes. Such analyses are important because a particular intervention model may have very different effects with subgroups of participants (e.g., more powerful effects with younger vs. older children). To the extent that subgroups have a very different response to an intervention, the results of overall analyses may be misleading. Statistical analyses of mediation or moderation should be planned in advance and ideally guided by the results of previous intervention research, clinical experience, and theory. Separate analyses of statistical power will need to be conducted to determine whether the sample size is sufficient to detect mediator or mediator effects. It is possible that statistical power may be adequate to detect overall intervention effects but not mediation or moderation (J. Cohen, 1988).

Maximizing Scientific Opportunities if an Intervention Shows No Effects

Investigators who conduct research on psychological interventions in childhood chronic illness should also plan for the unpleasant, albeit realistic, possibility that their proposed intervention will not demonstrate effects. The best way to maximize the scientific contribution of a psychological intervention study is to ensure a valid test by having adequate statistical power, applying strong intervention fidelity, limiting contamination across groups, and reducing sample attrition. A finding of no difference in a well-designed, well-powered study can make a significant scientific contribution.

Studies of interventions, especially large-scale studies, present additional opportunities for investigators to contribute to the science of intervention in secondary analyses. Such analyses may include studies of the reliability and validity of measures with chronic illness populations, factors that differentiate and influence the responders versus nonresponders to psychological interventions, and novel strategies to integrate outcome data across different informants (Holmbeck et al., 2002) and prediction of psychological outcomes. Considering as many of these questions as possible in advance of designing the study will maximize the efficiency and effectiveness of these secondary analyses.

Investigators will need to work through a range of decisions concerning their proposed research design. However, even if one is extremely careful in developing a research plan, it may not be possible to anticipate all of the issues that will occur when the research is implemented. This means that investigators may have to revisit their initial decisions in light of the realities of study implementation. The decisions that are made concerning research design (e.g., sample size) depend on the investigators' assumptions about how the study will be implemented (e.g., recruitment; expected sample attrition). However, these assumptions are not necessarily realistic. Issues and strategies in implementation of psychological intervention studies are considered in the next chapter.

4

IMPLEMENTING PSYCHOLOGICAL INTERVENTION RESEARCH IN PEDIATRIC SETTINGS

Suppose you are an investigator who has been involved in clinical work with children and adolescents with asthma for a number of years. You and your colleagues have an idea for an intervention study that will focus on improving asthma education and coping skills to improve the management of asthma. What are the issues that you need to consider to implement this study? The purpose of this chapter is to consider practical and logistical issues in implementing successful psychological intervention research with children and adolescents with chronic illness (Drotar, 2000b; Drotar, Timmons-Mitchell, et al., 2000).

As shown in Exhibit 4.1, there are a number of general categories and specific tasks involved in implementing psychological intervention research with pediatric chronic illness populations. The four general categories are (a) developing a collaborative context and resources for intervention research, (b) managing the logistical challenges of study implementation, (c) implementing multisite studies, and (d) managing unanticipated changes in intervention protocols.

EXHIBIT 4.1
Critical Tasks in Implementing Psychological Intervention Research in Childhood Chronic Illness

1. Developing a collaborative context and resources for intervention research
   - Developing collaborative relationships with medical caregivers and interdisciplinary staff
   - Involving pediatric practitioners
   - Securing resources to support psychological research
   - Conducting pilot and feasibility studies
   - Developing a research team: Key positions
     - Principal investigator
     - Coinvestigators
     - Project coordinator
     - Interventionists
     - Research assistants
     - Practitioners
   - Planning staff-related resources necessary to implement intervention research

2. Managing logistical challenges of study implementation
   - Identifying settings to conduct psychological interventions and data collection
     - Collect data in clinic settings
     - Collect data in home settings
   - Managing sampling issues in psychological intervention studies
     - Estimate numbers of eligible participants and rates of participation
     - Expand sites for recruitment
     - Ensure comparability and accuracy of sampling recruitment in multiple settings
     - Estimate and describe recruitment and retention of participants
   - Managing barriers to family participation and retention
     - Present the study to children and families clearly and carefully
     - Reduce practical barriers to family participation
     - Provide incentives for families to participate
     - Use multiple contacts and reminders for families concerning appointments
   - Managing quality control issues in implementing psychological intervention studies
     - Maintain fidelity and quality control of the intervention protocol
     - Document fidelity of the comparison or control group intervention
     - Document and enhance adherence to the intervention protocol
     - Describe and evaluate planned psychological interventions received by study participants
   - Managing quality control of outcome evaluation
   - Managing data and quality control

3. Implementing multisite psychological intervention studies
   - Evaluating advantages of multisite studies
   - Planning strategies in implementing multisite studies

4. Managing and documenting unanticipated changes in intervention protocols

DEVELOPING A COLLABORATIVE CONTEXT AND RESOURCES FOR INTERVENTION RESEARCH

Developing the collaborative context and resources to develop and implement interventions is critical to the conduct of such research in pediatric settings. For this reason, investigators need to consider the strategies that are described in the next sections.

Developing Collaborative Relationships With Medical Caregivers and Interdisciplinary Staff

Psychological intervention research involving children with chronic illness and their families takes place in medical settings where children and families are cared for by pediatric subspecialists and other professionals. For this reason, to implement their studies, researchers who conduct psychological intervention research with children with chronic illness need to develop and sustain close collaborations with the physicians, nurses, social workers, and other interdisciplinary staff who treat these children. Such collaborations are critical because these professionals' ongoing relationships with children and families can facilitate identification, recruitment, and retention of potential participants in psychological intervention studies (Drotar, 1989, 1995).

Individual teams of professionals who provide care for children with chronic illness in different settings may vary widely in their experience with, attitudes toward, and interest in psychological intervention research. Moreover, they may differ in their experience in working with psychologists and their capacity to facilitate and support psychological intervention research (Drotar, 1995). Psychologists who have worked collaboratively with medical colleagues in research and comprehensive care with children with chronic conditions have a clear advantage as researchers that is based on their close professional relationships and track record. For example, Kazak (2001) described how the close integration between clinical research and practice in her setting facilitated the development of clinically relevant psychological intervention research—for example, studies of the effects of family-centered approaches on reducing procedural pain and psychological distress. However, some psychologist investigators may have good ideas about psychological interventions but have not established close working relationships with the physicians and staff who care for children with chronic conditions and the families in their setting. These investigators will need to build collaborative support with these groups for their research. In some instances, this can be accomplished by providing clinical care for the children and families and consulting with the staff who are providing medical care to this population. Such collaborative experiences are important to establish trust and credibility.

Involving Pediatric Practitioners

Psychologists should appreciate that their goals and assumptions concerning intervention research may not be shared by collaborating medical colleagues. For example, when the idea for a family-centered, problem-solving intervention to promote adherence to treatment among adolescents with cystic fibrosis was presented to one of our medical colleagues, he raised the question that participation in the intervention might actually increase conflict and stress to families because they would have to confront family conflicts that they were not routinely expressing. Because of our enthusiasm for our intervention approach, this was not a point that we had considered. However, in responding to his concern, we acknowledged that it was quite possible that some families would experience increased conflict, at least initially, when difficult adherence-related problems were discussed openly. (This did turn out to be the case.) At the same time, we noted that the intervention was designed to reduce family conflict and enhance communication over the long term.

To facilitate collaboration concerning psychological intervention research, it is important that other professionals' questions and concerns about the research be acknowledged and discussed for one salient reason: The more that pediatricians and other staff can participate in developing and implementing a psychological intervention research project, the more they will support the study as it is implemented. Consequently, involving collaborating colleagues early in the research planning process will often enhance their support for the study. In addition, such close collaboration can facilitate input from the medical staff concerning their opinions about the potential feasibility and acceptability of specific psychological intervention approaches to children with chronic illness and their families.

Securing Resources to Support Intervention Research

Developing the necessary resources to support the time involved in delivering the intervention, recruiting participants, and collecting and analyzing the data is a critical issue. Many clinical care providers operate under extraordinary constraints to see an increasing volume of patients. For this reason, in my experience it is unrealistic to expect medical and other care providers to devote significant amounts of time to such tasks as recruitment of participants unless they are adequately compensated to do so. Consequently, researchers who conduct intervention research with pediatric chronic illness populations need to develop financial and staff resources to facilitate their research. These resources ideally should support the time required of physicians and other staff to help with patient recruitment, administration of the study, and so on.

Developing financial resources to support psychological intervention research is extremely challenging. Most investigators do not have access to large-scale grant support, at least initially, and may need to develop their publications and preliminary studies before they are ready to apply for such funding. How then should such investigators proceed?

Conducting Pilot and Feasibility Studies

One strategy for investigators is to conduct case studies and series that test psychological interventions using single-case or single-group designs (La Greca & Varni, 1993). Conducting such smaller scale preliminary studies also has the advantage of documenting the feasibility of the intervention and its acceptability to children, families, and physicians as well as evaluating the suitability of outcome measures.

Investigators will also need to develop financial resources to support pilot, feasibility, and preliminary studies of psychological interventions with children with chronic illness. One option is to include "start-up" funds for research that are available in some hospitals and academic departments. Other options are available from the National Institutes of Health through the R21, RO1, and K23 career development award mechanisms. Finally, foundations (such as the Lance Armstrong Foundation for pediatric cancer or the American Lung Association for asthma) can provide funding for smaller intervention projects with specific chronic conditions as well as for career development. Psychological intervention research can be an attractive option to funders because it meets a clear need and has the potential for helping children and families directly. Investigators should consider as wide a range of funding options as possible. For this reason, applications to multiple funding sources are desirable. It is ideal to secure funding for psychological intervention research. However, depending on the nature of the study and demands on staff, investigators may be able to implement small-scale intervention research projects without funding if they have access to the time and intellectual resources of undergraduate or graduate students.

Developing a Research Team: Key Positions

Let us suppose you are fortunate enough to have secured funding for your intervention research. What staff will you need? What are the key positions on your project? What should you consider in recruiting staff to fill them? Intervention projects vary widely in focus and in scope, ranging from early pilot and case studies that involve relatively small numbers of children and families to large, multisite intervention trials that involve hundreds of participants. The staffing needs of such different projects will vary with the scope, intensity, and duration of the intervention. Nevertheless, there are generic tasks to consider in each intervention research project that have important implications for staffing. For example, each and every intervention project needs to recruit participants, implement the intervention, measure the effects with outcome measures, organize and conduct data management and analysis, and write the findings up for publication.

Although the specific requirements of an intervention study will determine the staffing needs of individual projects, many psychological intervention studies require interdisciplinary teams. In general, the key positions in psychological intervention research with children with chronic illness and their families include the investigators, project coordinators who organize and manage the study, interventionists who conduct the intervention, research assistants who conduct the outcome evaluations, and practitioners who provide care for the population of children with chronic illness (e.g., pediatricians, nurses, or social workers).

Principal Investigator

The principal investigator (PI) is the catalyst who develops and leads the team conducting the psychological intervention research. The PI is responsible for the overall conduct and management of the study. For this reason, investigators should carefully consider the time and energy that will be required for them to organize the team and implement their study.

Coinvestigators

Depending on the nature of the study, coinvestigators may include physicians who are subspecialists who provide medical care to the patients in the study and provide quality control and oversight for specialized medical procedures needed for outcome assessment (e.g., spirometry to assess pulmonary functioning in pediatric asthma), statisticians, consultants, and psychologist coinvestigators, including offsite investigators in a multisite study.

Project Coordinator

The project coordinator is a singularly important position in psychological intervention research. Coordinators provide the overall organization for the intervention study, facilitate recruitment of children and families, and organize data collection and analysis. In my experience, successful coordinators may come from a range of professional backgrounds as long as they have the critical skills of outstanding organizational ability, interpersonal skills, initiative, and attention to detail.

Interventionists

Ideally, professionals who conduct psychological interventions should have research and/or clinical experience with children with chronic conditions. For this reason, experienced social workers and nurses can be excellent interventionists. However, depending on how structured the intervention is, extensive experience with children with chronic health conditions may not be essential. Moreover, some experienced professionals may have difficulty shifting to a highly structured, research-based intervention protocol. Consequently, for some intervention protocols, graduate students and fellows may be excellent interventionists. Irrespective of their specific professional backgrounds, interventionists need to have the skills to establish and sustain relationships with children with chronic illness and their families.

Research Assistants

Research assistants who help with recruitment and retention and conduct assessments in an intervention study are also central members of a psychological intervention research team. Strong interpersonal skills are a must for such positions. Depending on the nature of the protocol, research assistants often have a great deal of contact with families in helping them complete time-consuming measures that are critical to the study. In addition, a great deal of persistence and patience is often required to manage appointments with children and families for assessment and intervention. For this reason, staff who conduct baseline and outcome assessments should have attributes that are similar to a study coordinator, such as attention to detail and ability to relate to children and families, including children and families from multiple ethnic and social backgrounds, in a sensitive and empathic manner.

Practitioners

Practitioners who provide care for children and adolescents with chronic illness have a number of potential roles in psychological intervention research. These include establishing the diagnosis of a chronic condition and documenting the nature of medical treatment, which is especially critical in studies of intervention to promote adherence to medical treatment. Practitioners also may be critical in referring and informing children and families about intervention research studies. (This task has become especially important given the new guidelines of the Health Insurance Portability and Accountability Act [1996]; see chap. 5.) Finally, practitioners' help is needed in promoting the intervention study to colleagues, residents, and community pediatricians who are in a position to refer children and families to the study. Physician collaborators can also be a fertile source of ideas about relevant target areas for interventions, potential barriers, and ways to implement the treatments in clinical settings. Other practitioners, such as nurses and social workers, can also be extremely helpful to researchers in recruiting potential participants for intervention studies and in contributing ideas concerning the feasibility and acceptability of the intervention model to children and families.

Planning Staff-Related Resources Necessary to Implement Intervention Research

In planning resources for their studies, investigators must develop and budget sufficient funding to support the wide range of multifaceted tasks that are involved in an intervention study so that they will not overload their staff and reduce their effectiveness. Given the demands of research participants, the staff time that is needed to ensure optimal recruitment and retention of participants in psychological intervention studies may be extraordinary. Consequently, resources to support such staff time must be anticipated in planning for the budget and implementation of the study. For example, economically disadvantaged families of children with chronic illness face extraordinary stressors that may limit their capacity to enroll in and follow a protocol for a study of psychological intervention. For this reason, substantial investments of staff time are often required to facilitate participation by families through multiple contacts. Staff who are conducting the intervention should have sufficient time to perform necessary record keeping, participate in supervision, and engage in interventions and outcome assessments that are necessary to implement the protocol.

MANAGING LOGISTICAL CHALLENGES OF STUDY IMPLEMENTATION

Investigators who conduct psychological intervention research need to anticipate a number of difficult challenges in implementation of such research. If these challenges are understood and planned for, investigators will maximize the chances of a successful intervention study and enhance the methodological rigor of their research (see chap. 3). These challenges and potential strategies of management are now considered.

Identifying Space and Settings to Conduct Interventions and Data Collection

Securing the space to conduct interventions and data collection is a basic challenge of psychological intervention studies for obvious reasons. In many pediatric settings, space is at a premium. Moreover, the space that is suitable for medical visits is generally not feasible for psychological interventions. In addition, to enhance the efficiency and validity of data collection, it may be important to ensure that the outcome data are collected in a setting that is different from where the study participants receive their medical care. For this reason, investigators need to secure space for their studies of psychological intervention, ideally by obtaining funding for their research.

In some settings where investigators do not have access to dedicated space in which to conduct their intervention research, and depending on the specific project, it may be possible to use clinic rooms, especially after business hours. However, in my experience, investigators should consider this option carefully, given the considerable logistical and methodological challenges that are involved. For example, data collection in clinic settings imposes additional burdens on clinic staff (e.g., competition for space), potential ethical problems such as assurance of confidential data collection, and challenges for standardizing procedures.

Another potential option for conducting psychological interventions and gathering data is the home setting, which also has the advantage of convenience for families. The home may be the only place to gather data or conduct intervention for some families who cannot reliably keep appointments in hospital settings. Moreover, the home may be the optimal setting in which to gather data that are critical to evaluate the effects of certain interventions. Such data may involve the observation of family interactions during mealtimes that is a critical benchmark of the outcomes of some psychological interventions (e.g., interventions designed to promote adherence to dietary treatment).

However, collection of data in home settings has potential disadvantages. For example, it may be difficult to standardize the structure of data collection or interventions in home settings, which can compromise the integrity of the data and intervention protocol. Home visitation is time consuming, requires additional staff resources, and necessitates reimbursement of staff for travel. Moreover, some families are concerned about their privacy and do not want researchers to visit their homes. For this reason, so that families know what to expect, it is important to inform them in depth of the purpose and content of home visits when this data collection method is used.

One issue that can arise when conducting psychological interventions and collecting data in home settings is that of staff safety. Strategies that can facilitate the safety of home visitors include sending teams rather than one staff member; visiting only during daylight hours; making sure the family who is being visited is expecting the visit, so they can to facilitate the team's entry and exit; and recruiting staff members who match the ethnic makeup of a community as part of the research team.

Managing Sampling and Recruitment Issues in Psychological Intervention Studies

Estimating the available pool of eligible participants in psychological intervention studies is a crucial but difficult task. Investigators will need to work with their practitioner colleagues to identify patients who are followed for the care of chronic illness who meet study criteria and are potential participants in the study. However, the ease of identifying the potential pool of participants depends on the sophistication of record keeping in individual settings and subspecialty groups. In my experience, there is extraordinary variation across settings in the nature of and ease with which patient information can be accessed. For this reason, research assistants' time will often be needed to accomplish the critical task of identifying potential study participants.

Investigators need to consider that rates of participation in psychological intervention studies vary considerably depending on the demands of the protocol, participant characteristics, and the nature of the setting. In my experience, participation rates of 50% or fewer may be realistic for some psychological intervention studies with pediatric chronic illness populations, especially those that involve multiple intervention visits and extended follow-up periods. However, it may be difficult to estimate participation rates, especially for new interventions. For this reason, pilot and feasibility studies can be helpful in providing information concerning participation rates as well as suggesting strategies that can enhance recruitment rates.

Given the limitations in the available numbers of children with specific chronic conditions, it may be necessary for investigators to utilize multiple clinical sites in the same city or region to secure a sufficient number of participants in psychological interventions studies. Depending on the population, setting, and protocol, these options can include other hospitals and community practices in the same community or other clinical settings within the same site (e.g., emergency room or inpatient services). In some studies, it is often critical to cast nets widely in developing potential recruitment sites to secure a reasonable sample size. However, given the additional staff time needed to work with multiple sites, investigators also need to consider the efficiency or yield of recruitment at different sites (e.g., the numbers of participants recruited relative to the time spent). If sites do not yield a sufficient number of participants to justify the staff resources that are provided, investigators may need to reconsider their choice of site.

Because inclusion and exclusion criteria are critical to the interpretation of findings from psychological intervention studies, it is important that these criteria be implemented consistently over the entire duration of the study. Errors in the application of inclusion and exclusion criteria (e.g., participants who were initially thought to meet criteria but do not) are not uncommon, but they are costly because such data cannot be used. Moreover, in the absence of consistent oversight concerning recruitment, there can be significant changes in how criteria for participants are applied across the duration of the study. This can pose a threat to the internal validity of study findings. To ensure standardization of how inclusion and exclusion criteria are implemented, investigators should use detailed forms that describe study criteria and can be applied across settings by different staff. Standardized participant recruitment procedures are also important.

A detailed description of selection criteria (e.g., rationale for inclusions and exclusions, recruitment procedures, and relevant characteristics of the settings from which participants were recruited) is necessary to help other researchers understand the procedures that were used and evaluate findings of psychological intervention studies. Moreover, to facilitate interpretation of study findings, investigators need to describe the demographic and illness-related characteristics of participants versus nonparticipants (e.g., those who were offered participation but did not participate) and the characteristics of participants who began the intervention but did not complete data collection (e.g., dropouts). Participants who did not complete the study should be compared with those who did to identify differences that may suggest sample bias, which is not uncommon in intervention studies (Zebracki et al., 2003).

Managing Barriers to Family Participation and Retention

One of the most challenging issues in psychological intervention research in pediatric chronic illness is how best to enhance family participation and retention in such studies. Parents of children with chronic illness may be highly stressed by job-related responsibilities, the demands of the child's medical care, the care of siblings, and problems with access to transportation that limit their availability to participate and complete research protocols. These parents can be difficult to contact to discuss their potential participation in research. Others may feel threatened by their potential psychological involvement in intervention research, especially if they feel that their parenting or family life will be scrutinized or criticized in some way. Some parents from ethnic minority groups may have special concerns about being harmed or stigmatized by their participation in research (Walders & Drotar, 2000).

To increase sample size and limit bias due to selective participation and attrition (Drotar & Riekert, 2000), which can be a potential methodological problem in psychological intervention research, researchers can implement a number of special procedures to enhance family participation and involvement (Senturia et al., 1998). For example, in the course of implementing several studies of psychological intervention, I have found that it is useful to use standardized scripts in presenting the study to potential participants.

These scripts should include descriptions of (a) the nature of the intervention, (b) what will be required of children and families over the course of the study (e.g., the nature of their time commitment and responsibilities), and (c) what the staff will provide (e.g., the intervention, incentives, reimbursement for transportation). A sufficient amount of time needs to be spent with children and families to discuss the purpose of the interventions, explain the nature of family participation, and answer questions that arise. In addition, a nonhurried, respectful dialogue with families concerning the study requirements will also facilitate their informed consent and comprehension of difficult concepts such as randomization to different groups (Kodish et al., 2004; see chap. 5).

To maximize child and family participation in intervention and reduce attrition, researchers need to anticipate and address a wide range of practical barriers that may limit families' participation. Moreover, it is useful to implement proactive strategies to increase families' access to and participation in intervention research. For example, increasing parents' access to transportation by providing reimbursement for bus fare, coupons for taxis, and payment for parking may increase family participation (Drotar & Robinson, 1999). Flexible scheduling, such as using weekends and evenings, is often critical in intervention studies and is particularly important in involving working family members who are not available during normal business hours, such as fathers. In my experience, family members other than the children and their primary caregivers can be involved in psychological intervention research, but their engagement can only be secured by special efforts involving time and energy to reach out to them and flexibility of appointment times.

For some families, concrete incentives can make a difference in their participation in intervention research. For this reason, where it is feasible to do so, investigators should provide incentives for families to participate in intervention research as well as material incentives—for example, T-shirts or small tote bags with the study's name on it. Incentives that are tailored to the child's age-related preferences may facilitate child and family participation in psychological intervention studies. Irrespective of the types of incentives that are used to enhance child and family participation in psychological intervention studies, it is critical that they be attractive to the participants. At the same time, compensation should not be so excessive as to be coercive (see chap. 5).

To enhance family participation in intervention studies and reduce the level of sample attrition, researchers need a great deal of staff initiative, energy, and persistence to contact families to schedule and remind them of appointments. Moreover, when working with families who have agreed to participate in prospective intervention studies, I have found that it is important to maintain close contact over the course of the research in as many ways as are feasible, depending on study resources. For example, thank-you letters not only provide an expression of appreciation for a family's participation in research but also provide a check on whether the addresses are up to date. Giving families a staff member's phone number for questions sends a clear message about the investigator's interest and commitment. Birthday cards for the child and parents, holiday greetings, or regular phone contacts to inquire about the child's progress are other helpful ways to keep families aware of the study and motivated to participate. To help sustain family members' interest in the study, it is also helpful to send out progress updates or newsletters that summarize findings, results, and implications. Such mailings can also be useful in determining changes in families' addresses. Reminder calls concerning upcoming appointments for intervention and assessments are also important.

To be most effective in maintaining contact with families throughout the course of the intervention studies, I have found it helpful to obtain additional contact information. In my experience, parents are usually willing to give a phone number and address where messages can be left (e.g., their mother's, sister's, or friend's). Such contact information can be critical, given the frequency of moves and phone disconnections in some populations.

Quality Control Issues in Implementing Psychological Intervention Studies

One of the most important considerations in implementing psychological intervention studies with children with chronic illness is the level of quality control of the intervention procedures. A critical quality control procedure, also known as *fidelity*, ensures that the intervention is delivered in accord with the proposed model (Kazdin, 1980). Several strategies are useful in enhancing the fidelity of psychological interventions for children with chronic illness and their families. One strategy is to develop a detailed treatment manual that includes the principles of the intervention and details of procedures for each session. The greater the level of operational detail that is included in an intervention manual, the easier it will be to maintain fidelity of the psychological intervention model that is tested.

In addition to development and use of a treatment manual, investigators need to provide ongoing supervision and feedback concerning the intervention, monitor its implementation, and limit challenges to standardization. For example, no matter how well a psychological intervention is designed, individual children and families may raise special challenges (e.g., problems with adherence to the intervention plan) that may necessitate different approaches to enhance their adherence to the intervention (e.g., different types of incentives). In fact, substantial differences in how individual families accept or respond to interventions are not uncommon. For this reason, studies need to develop strategies of psychological intervention that are responsive to individual differences in child or family perceptions (e.g., level of acceptance of the need for intervention).

Moreover, interventionists who start out by delivering a psychological intervention in accord with the study protocol may also change or "drift" in their delivery. The discrepancy between what is designed and how a psychological intervention is actually delivered may pose a powerful threat to the validity of the study findings. For example, if the key component of a specific intervention is hypothesized to be relaxation training but relaxation training was not given consistently or effectively, this would invalidate the test of the intervention model. For this reason, ongoing procedures for checking the fidelity of psychological intervention should be developed. The most informative procedures include videotapes or audiotapes of the intervention sessions done at intervals across the time of the study (Kazdin, 1980). These should be analyzed by raters who are not aware of the study design or the study group membership of the session they are rating. To facilitate the reliability ratings, these raters should use a detailed structured checklist that includes specific items reflecting the key aspects of the intervention that are operationalized in the manual for the study versus control intervention. Fidelity checks should be conducted with different interventionists across different staff and sessions of the intervention and across different time periods.

The assessment of fidelity of control or comparison group interventions (content, dosage, and timing) is important for a number of reasons. Such documentation is necessary for ethical reasons, that is, to ensure that the medical and psychological care received by the control group will not fall below community standards (see chap. 5). Moreover, in those studies in which a novel psychological intervention is compared with a standard or treatment-as-usual condition, it is critical to obtain an accurate documentation of the new intervention to accurately judge its scientific value-added contribution.

Many participants in psychological intervention studies in pediatric chronic illness may receive interventions that range from supportive, educational sessions from clinic staff to psychotherapy that may affect the interpretation of findings from intervention studies. For this reason, it is important for investigators to document the nature and the frequency of psychological intervention contacts received by participants that are not part of the study protocol. Such information can be used to understand the variation in intervention findings that may be attributable to such contacts. Moreover, frequency of other interventions may be used as a covariate in the data analysis, especially if this variable correlates with the primary study outcome.

Patterns of ongoing clinical contact may also pose serous threats to the internal validity of study findings. For example, it is possible that the intervention and control group families may receive different levels of clinical care in the setting or outside sources (e.g., mental health services). For example, if the comparison group receives a high level of psychological service that may be standard care in some settings, this may influence the target outcomes and reduce the impact of the potential intervention effects. For this reason, unless the comparison group intervention is documented in great detail, it may be difficult if not impossible to evaluate the scientific significance of the proposed intervention.

Other threats to the validity of study findings that need to be detected by fidelity checks include contamination of intervention and control procedures. In some studies, the intervention design may involve testing a novel psychological intervention model compared with a comparison group that receives an alternative but potentially influential intervention with an equivalent number of sessions or "doses." For example, a study may be designed to assess the effects of a new model of behavioral family-centered management to promote adherence to treatment in diabetes compared with a more traditional model of family education and support that has an equivalent number of contacts with children and families. In such studies, the internal validity of the intervention protocol depends on the assurance that the children and families who received the comparison group intervention received the equivalent number of contacts as the experimental group but did not receive the behavioral management intervention. But what if the children in the control group also received behavioral management in visits with the clinic psychologist? This could pose a serious threat to the validity of the study's findings. For this reason, investigators need to provide detailed data documentation of the similarities and differences in the nature and number of intervention sessions and contacts that are received by the intervention group and control groups. Such documentation is also important to reduce or, better yet, eliminate overlap or contamination between the interventions received by the experimental and control groups.

Another important quality control issue in psychological intervention research is the level of child and family adherence to the intervention protocol. It is possible that psychological interventions may be delivered effectively by the research team but not be implemented according to the protocol by children and families. This can be a particular problem for complex psychological interventions that are demanding of participants' time and energies. For this reason, investigators should develop procedures that can monitor children's and family members' response to the intervention and their adherence to psychological interventions.

To document child and parent adherence to psychological intervention protocol, I have used checklists that involve families' behaviors concerning the intervention, including compliance with assignments, assessment of attendance at sessions, and participation and response to the sessions. Such measures are important to allow investigators to ascertain the level of adherence to their intervention procedures throughout the course of their study and take steps to enhance adherence. In addition, such data can be used to analyze whether intervention effects differed as a function of child or family adherence to the psychological intervention protocol.

Investigators should also anticipate problems with adherence to psychological intervention protocols and develop proactive strategies to enhance adherence to treatment. In this regard, child and family participants should be apprised of the importance of their adherence to the protocol at the outset of the intervention and throughout the course of the study. Nevertheless, even if the intervention procedures are well explained, parents and children may not understand all of what is required until they begin to participate. For this reason, it may be very effective to provide families with experience with the protocol by having them participate in assessment procedures prior to final enrollment or assignment to intervention groups (Pablos-Mendez, Barr, & Shea, 1998). Such "run-in" procedures give the child and family an opportunity to experience some of the tasks and burdens associated with the protocol. Families who are able to complete these tasks successfully are randomized to the intervention versus control group, whereas families who are not able to complete these tasks are eliminated from the study. Thus, run-in procedures can serve as a screening procedure that can identify children and families who are unlikely to complete the study protocol.

To make sure there will be sufficient numbers of eventual participants, investigators need a large pool of children and families who are potentially eligible to participate to ensure optimal use of run-in procedures. Depending on how many participants are eliminated by the use of a run-in procedure, the study findings may have limited generalizability.

How can investigators best enhance child and family adherence to psychological intervention studies? In my experience, one of the most important issues in enhancing family adherence to psychological intervention protocols is the quality of the families' relationships with the study staff (coordinators, research assistants). Such staff have the most contact with children and families and provide emotional support to families for their participation in intervention studies. In addition, incentives (money, gift certificates, small prizes) that are given for completion of intervention or outcome assessment visits can also enhance adherence to an intervention protocol but have the downside of reducing generalizability of the psychological intervention model to clinical practice.

Quality Control of Outcome Evaluation Procedures

Investigators who conduct psychological intervention research with children with chronic illness need to develop and implement a plan for quality control of outcome assessment procedures throughout the course of data collection. Some of the procedures, including so-called objective measures that are used to monitor the effects of psychological intervention (e.g., audiotapes, electronic monitors of adherence to treatment; Quittner, Espelage, et al., 2000), are subject to technical errors. For example, questionnaire data, which are commonly used in assessment of outcomes, are subject to error through inconsistencies in administration of procedure, incomplete data, and so on. In my own research, one interesting example of this was the evaluation of pulmonary functioning via spirometry procedures of children with asthma who were engaged in a study of psychological intervention designed to promote adherence to treatment. My colleagues and I found that children's extremely low pulmonary scores at baseline appeared to be inconsistent with their clinical status, which was not only confusing but also a safety concern. When we observed the administration of the test, we found that the research assistant who administered the tests was pressing the computer start key a bit too late, missing the first half second of the child's blow into the spirometer. When the procedure was corrected, this resulted in findings that were more consistent with clinical observation of the severity of the children's asthma. Problems in quality control of procedures and measures that are used to evaluate the outcomes of interventions are inevitable. For this reason, investigators need to develop ongoing quality control procedures that can include observation and review of procedures by investigators and coordinators, videotapes or audiotapes, discussion and review, and forms that standardize data.

Data Management

Data management in psychological intervention studies, especially in large-scale studies, can raise extraordinary challenges. These include managing the accuracy of scoring protocols, data entry, and accurate preparation of reports to describe the progress of the study for funders and the nature of adverse events for data safety and monitoring boards (see chap. 5). Effective data management requires ongoing attention from the entire team. Strategies that are routinely implemented to enhance data management in psychological intervention studies include double data entry, ongoing analyses of the distributions of data including outliers, and the description and summary of adverse events. Readers who are interested in more information on this topic may wish to consult McFadden, LoPresti, Bailey, Clarke, and Wilkins (1995).

IMPLEMENTING MULTISITE INTERVENTION STUDIES

When the financial resources or collaborative relationships for conducting meaningful psychological interventions for children with chronic illness do not exist at a single institution, which is often the case in this area of research, multisite and multicollaborator research represent a potentially viable, albeit challenging, alternative to single-site intervention research (Armstrong & Drotar, 2000). Multisite intervention studies, especially multisite randomized control trials, have advantages such as enhanced external validity; increased statistical power, which is especially important in studies of conditions with low incidence or prevalence; low incidence or prevalence of target outcomes (e.g., morbidity, large variance in the outcome); and more rapid recruitment. Two models of multisite collaboration in intervention studies have emerged: limited institutional collaboration (e.g., studies involving only two or three sites) and large multicenter cooperative group research (Armstrong & Reaman, 2005). Each of these models involves different assets and limitations (for more information concerning the costs vs. benefits of alternative models, see Armstrong & Drotar, 2000).

A detailed discussion of the challenges of multisite psychological intervention research in childhood chronic illness is beyond the scope of this chapter (for more detail, see Armstrong & Drotar, 2000). In brief, the major scientific challenges of multisite interventions studies include the difficulty of maintaining standardized intervention protocols at multiple sites, data management and analysis, and defining usual care. Operational or logistical issues such as site selection, randomization procedures, patient accrual, oversight, and maintaining commitment and enthusiasm from investigators at different sites are also challenges (Weinberger et al., 2001). To address these challenges, the effective conduct of multisite studies requires close collaboration among investigators that includes (a) a regular method of communication among the staff at each site to review procedures, (b) a method of identifying problems that occur and developing a plan to meet them, and (c) reviewing how the plan is operating.

MANAGING AND DOCUMENTING UNANTICIPATED CHANGES IN INTERVENTION PROTOCOLS

The implementation of psychological intervention studies inevitably involves the management of unanticipated events that may affect the scientific integrity of the study. Some of these events may necessitate changes in the protocol to reduce threats to study validity. For example, to reduce dropout or missing data, investigators may need to make changes in procedures for assessments and interventions during the course of their studies to make them more efficient and acceptable to children and families. Whenever such changes in procedures and protocol are made, it is critical to carefully describe precisely what changes were made, when they were made, and why. Such careful documentation will facilitate accurate description of study methods, clear presentation of the study results, and replication of study procedures by other investigators. In addition, substantive changes in the protocol will need to be reported to and approved by the local institutional review board as an addendum to the intervention protocol. In other instances, investigators may encounter unanticipated ethical issues related to informed consent and unexpected adverse events or stressors experienced by research participants. It is important to document these in detail and to develop an ethically sound plan of management. Developing a proactive approach that anticipates and plans for these events is important. A detailed consideration of the ethical issues in the design and implementation of psychological interventions is provided in chapter 5.

5

ETHICAL ISSUES IN CONDUCTING PSYCHOLOGICAL INTERVENTIONS

Suppose you are conducting an intervention research study to determine whether a family-centered intervention would lessen psychological distress in children with cancer. In the first intervention meeting, the parents describe significant marital discord. Despite having agreed to participate in the intervention, the adolescent who has cancer says she feels coerced by her parents into having participated and no longer wants to do so. Moreover, she feels that her cancer has ruined her life and shares her feelings that she might be better off dead. She wants to kill herself but is not sure whether she would act on her feelings. What are your responsibilities as a researcher with respect to the issue of informed consent? What are your responsibilities concerning the adolescent's clinical care?

As shown in this example, psychological intervention research in childhood chronic illness can raise ethical challenges (Drotar, Overholser, et al., 2000; Glantz, 1996; Grodin & Glantz, 1994). The purpose of this chapter is to describe these ethical challenges and approaches to address them.

ANTICIPATING ETHICAL RISKS IN INTERVENTION RESEARCH

Psychological intervention research is by no means inherently benign from an ethical standpoint (Koocher, 2002; Street & Luoma, 2002). For this reason, researchers who conduct intervention studies with children with chronic illness need to anticipate potential ethical problems, take steps to limit or prevent them, and take steps to manage them when they occur. Unfortunately, the challenges that investigators face in anticipating and managing critical ethical issues are heightened by the absence of data concerning the application of ethics to psychological intervention research. For this reason, investigators have important opportunities to discuss the ethical issues in their research, to describe how they were managed, and to formulate suggestions for future psychological intervention research. To facilitate the formidable task of anticipating relevant ethical challenges, Koocher (2002) described a useful model to evaluate the potential risks in clinical psychological research, including psychological intervention research, with children. This model suggests that researchers should consider risks in the following domains: *cognitive* (e.g., threats to intellectual functioning), *affective* (e.g., emotional distress), *biological* (e.g., side effects of treatment), *legal* (e.g., legal consequences to families owing to reporting of abuse and neglect), *economic* (e.g., lost time from work), and *social and cultural* (e.g., stigma from disclosure of HIV).

Participation in psychological intervention research can involve special risks for children and families that need to be considered by investigators. For example, Koocher (2002) noted that there are potential hazards of manualized protocols, such as insensitivity to the needs of individual children and families and the potential of continuing a problematic treatment. In the context of family-centered psychological interventions, children and parents may become distressed when discussing potentially conflict-laden topics. Moreover, participation in psychological intervention research also can be burdensome given the time, energy, and level of emotional engagement that are required for intervention sessions and outcome assessments. Some measures (e.g., videotaping of family interaction) of outcomes of psychological interventions may be threatening and potentially stressful to families. Videotaping and audiotaping also raise special issues related to confidentiality that need to be considered carefully. For example, family members will need specific assurances that such information will remain confidential and will be destroyed after the research has been completed.

ETHICAL ISSUES IN THE DESIGN OF INTERVENTION RESEARCH

The design of psychological intervention research also raises important ethical issues. To understand these, investigators should recognize that control groups in psychological intervention research with children with chronic illness are used in two fundamental ways: (a) to differentiate the effectiveness of a specific intervention model from the natural course of the target problem or from nonspecific or common factors of an intervention approach and (b) to evaluate whether a specific factor or process is responsible for intervention change. To address these issues, investigators may use either a standard-care or treatment-as-usual group or an enhanced-care control group that is designed to achieve a specific purpose (e.g., control for number of contacts).

In clinical trials of treatment, including psychological interventions, one of the most important principles is that of *equipoise*, which is defined as a genuine uncertainty on the part of researchers about the comparative therapeutic merits of the alternative interventions that are being tested (Street & Luoma, 2002). Suppose an investigator wants to test whether a new method of cognitive–behavioral intervention is more effective in reducing psychological distress among the survivors of pediatric cancer than supportive comprehensive care. The scientific merit of the research question and equipoise depends on whether the outcome of the cognitive–behavioral intervention is uncertain.

The principle of equipoise provides a safeguard against the health and well-being of study participants being disadvantaged by their participation in intervention research. For this reason, it is important that the standard-care or treatment-as-usual group that is included in the intervention design be comparable with the current standard of care for the intensity and quality of interventions (medical, psychological, or both) in the setting in which the research takes place.

In addition, participation in a study of psychological intervention should not interfere with access to clinically indicated psychological services that are provided for children and adolescents with chronic illness in a particular setting, even if the availability of such interventions may obscure the interpretation of study findings. For this reason, ethical concerns clearly prohibit the use of no-treatment control groups for clinically significant problems associated with chronic illness (e.g., depression) for which referral and intervention are indicated and reflect the current standard of practice.

On the basis of the above considerations, defining standard care or treatment as usual in psychological interventions for children with chronic illness assumes critical importance, from the standpoints of both ethics and research design. However, in studies of chronic illness, the operational definition of psychosocial "treatment as usual" is complicated by the fact that the intensity and quality of medical and psychological care for children with chronic illness are variable across and within settings. For example, there is generally no standardized protocol for psychosocial services or medical care in clinical settings. Moreover, data that describe the content and intensity of such services may not be readily available in clinical care databases. For this reason, it is important that investigators develop strategies to clearly document current medical and psychological care that are provided to children and adolescents with chronic illness in the setting of their research (Alvirdrez & Arean, 2002). Such documentation is needed to define the services received by a comparison group and hence provide assurance that current community standards of clinical care are being met.

In addition to the treatment-as-usual control group, another design option in psychological intervention research is to compare the efficacy of two alternative treatments that differ in content or structure with treatment as usual (C. E. Schwartz et al., 1997). Such a research design is resource intensive. However, it poses a more rigorous test than a treatment-as-usual design of the value-added effects of a specific model of psychological intervention compared with the support that is inherent in any contact with the child. For this reason, this design may be indicated in areas of psychological intervention research that have progressed to the point at which a primary need concerns identification of the active ingredients of an effective intervention.

ISSUES IN INFORMED CONSENT IN PSYCHOLOGICAL INTERVENTION RESEARCH

One of the most important considerations in psychological intervention research (or any research) is to ensure that adequate informed consent is obtained from participants. The key elements of informed consent include the following: (a) a clear statement that the study involves intervention research; (b) an explanation of the purposes of intervention research (e.g., which hypotheses will be tested and why?); (c) the expected duration of the participants' involvement in psychological intervention sessions and outcome assessments; and (d) clear identification of any procedures that are experimental, such as a new psychological intervention that is being tested (Grodin & Glantz, 1994). To enhance informed consent, information given to potential participants in discussions and consent forms should also describe intervention research procedures, including interventions and outcome assessments, reasonably foreseeable risks, and the potential benefits of the research to participants or others (if they are relevant).

In addition, participants need to understand alternative procedures, such as other interventions that are available to them, the confidentiality of research participation, that their participation is voluntary and can be terminated at any point, and the individuals to contact for questions about procedures and problems that are encountered. For example, consider the intervention study comparing a new cognitive–behavioral intervention to reduce distress among the survivors of childhood cancer with supportive comprehensive care described earlier. Children and families who participate in this study need to understand that (a) a specific new intervention is being tested, (b) their participation is voluntary, and (c) they will still have potential access to the typical comprehensive care and psychological services that are offered in their setting if they choose not to participate. To ensure effective informed consent for children and families with chronic illness who participate in psychological intervention research, investigators need to consider how best to approach parents to obtain their consent for their child's participation and facilitate parent and child understanding of intervention research and study design.

Approaching Parents to Obtain Their Consent for Their Child's Participation

To ensure the family's and child's confidentiality, researchers need to work closely with the child's attending physician and caregivers in accord with institutional review board (IRB) procedures (Phillips, 1996) to develop the most effective and ethically sound strategy to inform them about the intervention study. As of April 14, 2003, all hospitals in the United States are required to be in compliance with the Health Insurance Portability and Accountability Act (HIPAA; 1996) regulations, which has important implications for the way that all research, including intervention research, is conducted in health care settings. The essential new requirement under HIPAA is the restriction on the release of any and all protected health information that relates to the past, present, or future physical and mental health of an individual. For children with chronic illness, this means that only those caregivers who provide ongoing care to the child should have access to their health information, including the child's status as a patient with chronic illness. In settings where psychological intervention researchers are not part of routine care, families would not necessarily have the expectation that the psychologist would know about the child's chronic health condition. For this reason, under such circumstances, in accordance with HIPAA guidelines, psychologists cannot have direct access to patient information to identify participants who may be eligible for research. Moreover, they cannot contact a participant directly unless the family gives consent to the participant's health care provider. In practical terms, what this means is that medical and nursing practitioners who provide clinical care for children with chronic illness and their families will need to contact the family for permission to be contacted about an available psychological intervention research study. On the other hand, in clinical settings where a psychologist meets every family, is part of the routine care for the child, and whose role is understood by the family (e.g., by meeting all children with a new diagnosis of cancer), he or she should be able to contact families directly to discuss their children's research participation. However, it should be noted that the individual IRBs vary in their interpretation of HIPAA regulations.

The new HIPAA regulations have brought about significant changes in procedures concerning recruitment for all research studies, including psychological intervention studies. These new procedures have required investigators to develop different strategies for contacting participants in intervention research. For example, prior to HIPAA, my research team had been identifying potential participants for an adherence promotion study in pediatric asthma by reviewing charts of children who were hospitalized or who had been seen in the emergency room. Subsequent to the implementation of HIPAA, we could not access this information directly and needed to ask practitioners who were providing clinical care to children with asthma to inform families about the study and ask their permission to be contacted by us for their consent. It is clear that such procedures place a greater time burden on practitioners who are already pressed by clinical care demands, and it may be unrealistic to expect practitioners to assume such a burden. In some settings, this may limit investigators' abilities to contact potential participants in intervention studies and hence reduce the numbers of available participants. However, it is possible for investigators to meet the challenge of developing HIPAA-compliant yet user-friendly procedures (e.g., readily available forms that practitioners can give to parents to sign indicating their interest in being contacted by researchers) to facilitate contact with families and to help in recruitment.

Facilitating Parent and Child Understanding of Intervention Research

One of the most important issues for parents and children is to understand the nature of the research-based psychological interventions that will be provided to them and how they will be expected to participate in such interventions. It may be difficult for many parents and children to understand what is involved in psychological interventions because they are less concrete and less familiar than medical treatments such as medications. Psychological interventions are different from medical treatment that involves medication in that the former require a more active level of child and family participation as defined by the time commitment and nature of their involvement (e.g., in family communication, sharing of information about feelings, etc.). Consequently, to make an informed decision about their participation, it is important for parents to understand what is involved in such research. In addition to the ethical importance of informed decision making, an accurate parent and child understanding of what will be required of them if they participate in intervention research may reduce subsequent dropout from research. To facilitate such understanding, investigators may find it helpful to describe psychological interventions in detail with specific concrete examples. Concrete details and illustration of the intervention(s) that the child and family will receive are also important to include in such descriptions because some parents and children may equate psychological interventions with psychotherapy or psychiatric treatment or media-based accounts of psychological treatment.

In addition to helping children and parents understand the nature of the psychological intervention they will receive, it is important to facilitate their understanding of the basic study design, such as the nature of their assignment to alternative interventions in controlled studies or randomized control trials (RCTs; Kodish, Lantos, & Siegler, 1990). For example, if the study involves randomization to different groups, parents need to understand what this means for their family (e.g., that they have an equivalent chance to be included in one group or the other and that this cannot be predicted or controlled by the family). However, concepts such as random assignment to different intervention groups are difficult to understand. Kodish et al. (2004) found that many parents of children with cancer who enroll in RCTs of medical treatment for pediatric cancer do not clearly understand the concept of randomization. Although data are not available concerning parental understanding of randomization to different arms of psychological intervention studies, one might expect that parents who are asked to consent to their children's participation in RCTs of psychological interventions would have a similar difficulty. Potential reasons for the gap in parental understanding of informed consent include ambiguity of investigators' descriptions of the study and barriers to parental understanding, such as differences in culture and ethnicity between parents and investigators (Drotar, Miller, Willard, Anthony, & Kodish, 2004; Kodish et al., 2004; V. A. Miller, Drotar, Burant, & Kodish, 2005).

Another interesting challenge related to informed consent that has implications for psychological intervention research is therapeutic misconception (Lidz, Appelbaum, Grisso, & Renaud, 2004). Research on medical treatment has described the problem that some families may fail to distinguish the consequences of participating in research from receiving ordinary treatment. Families may also erroneously believe that research or treatment intervention is treatment and is inevitably beneficial (Lidz et al., 2004). The possibility that families who participate in psychological intervention also believe in the therapeutic misconception needs to be considered by investigators.

Given the potential for parent and child misunderstanding of intervention research, investigators should not assume that parents or children will easily understand the design of a psychological intervention study and what is required of their research participation. For this reason, it is important for investigators to take proactive steps to enhance parents' understanding of psychological intervention studies. In my experience, researchers may help parents and children to understand their participation in psychological intervention research by using the following methods: (a) using simple, concrete language in the consent and assent forms and conversation about the study; (b) taking time to explain the study in detail; (c) using visual aids such as diagrams to illustrate the study design; (d) providing detailed information about the tasks required in the intervention; and (e) providing the opportunity to ask questions about the study.

Moreover, I have found that it is not correct to assume that parents and children understand the design of intervention research and what is required of their participation just because the procedures have been explained to them. For this reason, it is important that investigators try to determine research participants' levels of understanding. To check parents' and children's understanding of an intervention study, investigators may want to give them an opportunity to describe what will happen in the intervention and what they understand their choices to be (Kodish et al., 2004; Levi, Marsick, Drotar, & Kodish, 2000). Although such additional dialogue adds time to the informed consent process, it provides an excellent opportunity for feedback to correct child and parent misinterpretations about the research. In the long run, such dialogue may enhance the level of trust between researchers and families and reduce dropout.

The Role of Child or Adolescent Assent

Assent, which is defined as the affirmative agreement to participate in research, is distinguished from *consent*, which refers to the autonomous choice to participate in research (V. A. Miller, Drotar, & Kodish, 2004). Assent involves assisting the child or adolescent in developing a clear understanding of the intervention study, including what will be required for participation in the intervention and data collection (e.g., time, energy, and nature of the data), and including them in the decision about research participation. From a strictly legal vantage point, parents can give proxy consent for their child's participation in research on intervention, and the child's own consent is not required (Bartholome, 1989). However, assent is nonetheless important because it provides the vehicle for the child or adolescent's voice to be heard in the decision to participate in psychological intervention research. From a pragmatic vantage point, the quality of child or adolescent assent may also affect the quality of their participation in psychological intervention research. For example, one potential hypothesis is the following: The more the child or adolescent participates in the decision making concerning the study, asks questions about it, and is engaged in the process of communication with investigators, the more he or she will be likely to participate actively and productively in the research.

In some intervention studies, investigators need to appreciate that there may be critical differences between parents' decisions in consenting for the child's or adolescent's participation and the child's or adolescent's assent for his or her own participation. For example, in my experience in studies of psychological interventions to promote adherence to medical treatment, parents often have a much stronger investment in the child's participation in these studies than their child does. In addition, some children and adolescents may have difficulty expressing their lack of interest in participating in psychological intervention studies because they do not want to disappoint or frustrate their parents or investigators.

One example of this issue occurred in the context of the Diabetes Control and Complications Trial (DCCT), which was an RCT that compared intensive treatment involving multiple daily injections of insulin with what was then standard care for Type 1 diabetes (DCCT Research Group, 1993). In the course of working with adolescents and their parents during this 10-year prospective study, my colleagues and I encountered some adolescents who we believe agreed to be enrolled in the trial because their parents wanted them to participate, not because they were fully committed to participating. In this study, parents had a direct investment in their adolescents' participation because they wanted the treatment team to improve their adolescents' adherence to diabetes treatment, which they regarded as more problematic than their children did. The stark contrast between parents' and adolescents' level of interest and investment in the study was not apparent at point of initial consent. However, as the study progressed, some adolescents expressed their opinion, which was obvious in their actions, that they were less-than-enthusiastic participants in this study. We addressed this issue in individual discussions with the adolescents and parents. My experiences in the DCCT suggest that investigators might want to elicit and be aware of potential differences in child or adolescent and parental preferences for psychological intervention in the informed consent process.

Identifying and Managing Constraints on Informed Consent

Given the potential for constraints to be imposed on informed consent in psychological intervention studies, it is helpful for investigators to anticipate such issues and to take steps to prevent them. In this regard, several procedures may be useful. For example, my colleagues and I have found it useful to structure the consent process by having standardized scripts for all the individuals who are conducting informed consent. In addition, we have also found it useful to review the experiences of the staff in informed consent over the course of the study to identify problem areas (e.g., areas of child or parent misunderstanding) and address them.

Unanticipated constraints on informed consent can also be imposed by colleagues who are engaged in clinical care with potential research participants. One example of the above problem occurred in the course of our intervention research with the families of infants with failure to thrive

(Drotar & Robinson, 1999). Early in the course of our study, we learned that some pediatric residents had informed parents whose children were hospitalized for failure to thrive that if they did not participate in the intervention study they could be reported to the Department of Human Services for child neglect. This procedure was a clear ethical problem because it placed undue coercion on families to participate in the study. To address this issue, our staff met with families who were approached in this manner to clarify the implications of their decision to participate versus decline consent concerning their medical care and potential referral to human services (i.e., that they would not be placed in jeopardy of losing medical care or be referred to human services if they did not participate). In addition, we addressed this issue by meeting with residents and faculty physicians to emphasize the need to use appropriate informed consent procedure and give a sample script to physicians that described our informed consent procedure, including our conversation with families about their options. Finally, we instructed our staff to slow the consent process down by asking families to take time to think about their decision before committing to the project and to understand that their participation was truly an option.

OTHER RELEVANT ETHICAL ISSUES IN PSYCHOLOGICAL INTERVENTION RESEARCH

Investigators who conduct psychological intervention research are often working with a team of caregivers. As leaders of research teams, they have the responsibility for ensuring that members of their team carry out the research in an ethical manner. These responsibilities include documenting adverse events, communicating with data safety and monitoring boards, managing participants who demonstrate significant psychological distress, managing child abuse or neglect, managing confidentiality, determining incentives, dealing with ethical issues raised by the use of technology in intervention, and educating and communicating with IRBs concerning intervention research.

Documenting Adverse Events

An important consideration in psychological intervention research in childhood chronic illness is the need to document adverse events (e.g., psychological distress) that can occur in the context of intervention or assessment. In addition, other issues need to be documented, such as the identification of and appropriate referral for clinically significant depression that may not be an adverse effect of the intervention per se. For this reason, it is important for investigators who are conducting psychological intervention research to anticipate such events, keep an ongoing and detailed record of them, and review them with their team. Moreover, it is important to develop a clear plan for management of such events as identification and referral in advance of the study.

Communicating With Data Safety and Monitoring Boards in Intervention Research

To establish ethical standards for the safety and monitoring of data from intervention trials, data safety and monitoring boards (DSMBs) have been established to oversee the ethics of intervention. These DSMBs involve professionals who represent different disciplines, including biostatistics, medicine, psychology, and other fields. The purpose of the DSMBs, which were originally designed for trials of medication treatment but have been extended to include National Institutes of Health–funded trials of psychological intervention, is to provide oversight of the study from the standpoint of patient safety as well as implementation. In this capacity, the DSMB regularly reviews information about the conduct of the study, especially adverse events that may result from the conduct of the intervention, and advises the researchers about the management of these issues and others (e.g., threats to data integrity). The advantages of a DSMB in providing an outside impartial review of study procedures from an ethical vantage point are significant for any psychological intervention study, not only for National Institutes of Health–funded studies. For example, in my experience in conducting a study of psychological intervention with children and adolescents with pediatric asthma, I have found periodic dialogue with the DSMB to be very helpful, not only in anticipating and managing ethical issues but also in dealing with logistical challenges, such as recruitment of participants. For this reason, investigators who are conducting psychological intervention research may wish to consider convening a DSMB that is made up of investigators who are not part of their research team.

Managing Participants With Psychological Problems

It is not uncommon for clinically significant psychological and family problems to be uncovered in the course of conducting psychological intervention research (Hoagwood, 2003). Consequently, investigators should have a plan to provide feedback to participants concerning psychological problems that reach threshold for referral for treatment and provide information to families concerning services that can be accessed. Such a plan is also important because some families may unrealistically expect the research study and staff to provide clinical care for a range of problems (Lidz et al., 2004). For example, in conducting research with mothers of infants who were failing to thrive, my research team notified participants who reported high levels (e.g., above the cutoff scores for clinically significant) of depression or distress on standardized psychological measures concerning this information (Drotar & Robinson, 1999). These research participants were informed about available treatment resources that could help them with their psychological distress if they so chose.

Managing Child Neglect or Abuse

Psychological intervention studies in pediatric chronic illness afford investigators significant additional opportunities to observe problems such as *medical neglect*, defined as the failure to comply with the minimal level of acceptable care that is required for the condition, or child abuse in assessment procedures such as family observation (Bussell, 1994). For this reason, parents of children with chronic illness who participate in psychological intervention research should be informed about the increased risk for observation of neglect that might occur in response to their participation in the research. Psychologists are mandated to report abuse and neglect under the Child Abuse Prevention and Treatment and Adoption Reform Act (1992). Each state has legislation that describes the definition of reportable behaviors. As mandated reporters, psychologist investigators are required to report neglectful and abusive behavior that may be observed by them or members of their team to relevant authorities and to manage the consequences of family reactions and decisions concerning their continued participation in the study. It is both possible and desirable from a methodological vantage point for families who have been reported for neglect or abuse to sustain their participation in psychological intervention. However, in my experience, most parents who are reported for abuse or neglect by investigators become upset and choose not to continue to participate.

Given the importance and complexity of issues related to abuse and neglect, before implementing their study, it can be helpful for investigators to develop a plan for reporting and management of parent neglect or abuse. In most cases, this will involve procedures such as additional evaluation or mandated reporting that reflect the community standards of care for comparable situations.

Managing Confidentiality

Investigators who conduct research on psychological interventions in childhood chronic illness have occasion to observe children and families with intensive methods such as home observations and electronic monitoring of adherence to treatment. One of the more difficult problems involves the issue of reporting problems in adherence to medical treatment that are identified in the course of a study. For example, what if an investigator identifies that a child or adolescent is not doing prescribed medical treatment, on the basis of evidence from self-report or electronic monitoring of adherence? In addressing this difficult question, investigators need to consider the customary procedures (e.g., additional clinical contacts, referral for psychological evaluation and management) that are in place in many clinical settings for the identification and management of adherence-related problems for children and adolescents with pediatric chronic illness. Such procedures may involve identification and referral for psychological services. In cases of serious nonadherence to medical treatment that reflects medical neglect, the family may be reported to child protection services. Similar procedures should be used to manage comparable problems that arise in the context of psychological intervention research.

Another issue that needs to be considered in deciding whether to report nonadherence to treatment relates to the reliability, validity, sensitivity, and specificity of the measures that are used to assess adherence to treatment in intervention research studies. The combination of the inconsistent reliability and validity of measures of adherence to medical treatment in pediatric chronic illness (Riekert & Drotar, 2000) and the inconsistent relationship between adherence to treatment and clinical outcomes (Johnson, 1995) would mitigate against taking clinical action on the basis of research data concerning adherence treatment. Finally, research on adherence to treatment depends on the trust that can be developed between the coinvestigator and research participants, which depends on confidentiality. For this reason, disclosure of problematic adherence behavior in and of itself may not be required of investigators. On the other hand, in some instances, clinically significant nonadherence to pediatric medical treatment may reflect parental neglect. If this is the case, it may well be a reportable act of neglect.

Determining Use of Incentives and Payments for Expenses

Incentives, which can include cash or other materials, are commonly given to participants in psychological intervention research, including children with chronic illness. Such incentives provide fair compensation for one's time, which can be substantial in psychological intervention research, commonly involving multiple visits for intervention sessions and for assessments. In addition, participants' families are often reimbursed for expenses (e.g., travel funds) that are incurred in the course of participation. In determining the level of incentives, investigators need to consider the difficult balance between respect for participants' time and compensation for it and potential coercion (Hoagwood, 2003).

Investigators should consider that individual and community perceptions concerning the difference between fair compensation and coercion can vary as a function of socioeconomic status and culture (Hoagwood, 2003). Moreover, the norms of individual IRBs concerning compensation to research participants can also vary. Investigators may want to consult their IRBs or patient–family advisory boards for guidance concerning the appropriate level of compensation.

Dealing With Ethical Issues in Computer-Based Interventions

The advent of new technologies, such as computer-based psychological interventions, for children with chronic illness (M. A. Davis, Quittner, Stack, & Yang, 2004) that provide options for interventions that are potentially cost-effective may reduce the stigma associated with traditional office-based psychological interventions and increase access to psychological services (Wade, 2004). This exciting new area of psychological intervention provides an opportunity for researchers to describe the ethical issues that are encountered (Wade, 2004). Interventions delivered via new technologies can raise potential ethical issues involving privacy and confidentiality that need to be considered by researchers and practitioners (Fisher & Fried, 2003). For example, the privacy of children and families who participate in psychological interventions via the Internet may be compromised (Wade, 2004). For this reason, strategies to ensure family privacy need to be considered and implemented in such research. In an online intervention group for teens with cancer, for instance, adolescents can be required to have a diagnosis of cancer in order to use the Web site. To implement this requirement, the Web site can provide a downloadable form to be signed by a physician that they send back and a consent form that can be completed online. Such procedures help to ensure both the privacy of the adolescents' information and identity and the accuracy of appropriate inclusion in the group so that participants will be assured they are talking with other teens with cancer.

Another important ethical issue related to the use of computerized technologies in psychological intervention research concerns the potential burden that research participants might experience relating to the ongoing and comprehensive nature of some methods (e.g., computerized daily diaries). To understand the nature of the burden and to implement proactive strategies to reduce the impact, investigators might want to evaluate the extent to which participants experience a burden by conducting pilot studies of these methods and obtaining feedback from participants concerning feasibility and response burden.

Educating and Communicating With Institutional Review Boards About Intervention Research

Investigators should recognize that IRBs in individual settings vary substantially with respect to their experience with psychological intervention research and hence their capacities to evaluate such research. It is possible that IRBs may misinterpret the nature and impact of psychological intervention research and measurement of outcome. For this reason, investigators should appreciate that they are in a position of educating and communicating with IRBs about relevant issues related to psychological intervention research. Such issues may include HIPAA-related issues, informed consent, assent, defining and managing adverse events, and managing the data from outcome assessments.

FUTURE DIRECTIONS IN INTERVENTION RESEARCH ETHICS

Research on psychological interventions in childhood chronic illness will be expanding in response to significant scientific progress. Unfortunately, at present, researchers have very little information about how parents and children understand the nature of psychological interventions and their participation in them. Consequently, investigators who are conducting psychological intervention research have an opportunity to gather important data concerning the ethics of such studies. These data are needed to address a number of important questions, including the following: (a) How do parents and their children with chronic illness understand their participation in psychological intervention research? (b) How do parents and children perceive the risks versus the benefits of their participation in the research? (c) To what extent are parents and children stressed by their participation in the research? (d) What are similarities and differences in parents' and children's appraisals of their participation in the research? and (e) What are the best ways to ensure that children and parents understand the risks and benefits of psychological intervention research? Methodologies that combine interviews of participants and investigators to obtain their perceptions of the research participation and understanding of consent with direct observation of the informed consent process via audiotape have been shown to be useful in conducting research on the ethics of psychological intervention research (Kodish et al., 2004).

Investigators should expect to encounter a range of ethical issues in the course of conducting intervention research. Prompt action to rectify ethical problems is highly desirable, but the specific steps that need to be taken may not be clear. For this reason, investigators should be prepared to seek consultation from other researchers, their IRB, or experts on bioethics when ethical issues arise that may be confusing or difficult. Investigators should consult the guidelines of the American Psychological Association for the ethical principles for psychologists and codes of conduct (American Psychological Association, 2002) and their implications (Fisher, 2004).

Developing systematic approaches to training graduate- and post-doctoral-level researchers to understand, anticipate, and manage ethical issues related to psychological intervention research will be an important future direction. In this regard, I have found the following methods to be useful: (a) regular discussion of ethical issues in individual mentorship of intervention research projects; (b) formal course work on research ethics; (c) seminars in which experienced investigators discuss the ethical issues that they have encountered in their research, including psychological intervention research, and ways that they managed them; (d) courses on research ethics and procedures that are provided by the local IRBs; and (e) opportunities to participate in research that relates to research ethics (e.g., informed consent).

Ongoing continuing education concerning ethical issues that relate to intervention research is also critical. For this reason, investigators should also take advantage of lectures that are offered by IRBs and departments of bioethics. Finally, interested readers might also wish to consult sources that focus on related topics, such as informed consent issues with children and families (Abramovitch, Freedman, Henry, & Van Brunschot, 1995; Koocher & Keith-Spiegel, 1998; Range & Cotton, 1995), rights to privacy and other issues in research with adolescents (Brooks-Gunn & Rotheram-Borus, 1994; Caskey & Rosenthal, 2005), family observational methods (Bussell, 1994), adherence promotion and monitoring (Rand & Sevick, 2000), intervention research with high-risk children and youths (Scarr, 1994), research with children and adolescents with mental health problems (Hoagwood, Jensen, & Fisher, 1996), psychosocial treatment research (Hoagwood, 2003), and research with children with varying cultures and ethnicities (Fisher et al., 2002). The more knowledgeable and prepared investigators are in identifying and managing potential ethical issues, the greater the likelihood that their psychological intervention studies will be conducted in an ethical manner.

III

PSYCHOLOGICAL INTERVENTIONS WITH REPRESENTATIVE PEDIATRIC CHRONIC CONDITIONS: RESEARCH AND CLINICAL APPLICATIONS

6

PSYCHOLOGICAL INTERVENTIONS: ASTHMA

The most common childhood chronic illness, pediatric asthma, is an important chronic health condition from a public health perspective because of its high prevalence, high morbidity, and potential impact on the quality of life of affected children and families (Vinicor, 1998). Nearly 5 million children under the age of 18 years in the United States are affected by asthma (Centers for Disease Control and Prevention [CDC], 1996), and the prevalence, morbidity, and mortality associated with asthma have increased dramatically in recent years (CDC, 1996). The prevalence of asthma is particularly high among ethnic minority youths (Crain, Kercsmar, Weiss, Mitchell, & Lynn, 1998), children and adolescents with obesity, and those with a family history of asthma (Rodriguez, Winkleby, Ahn, Sundquist, & Kraemer, 2002). African American children with asthma have a particularly high disease severity, morbidity, and mortality (National Institutes of Health, 1997; W. R. Taylor & Newacheck, 1992).

Asthma is a chronic respiratory disease that is characterized by intermittent and variable periods of acute reversible airway obstruction (McQuaid & Walders, 2003). Episodic exacerbations involve symptoms that can range from mild to life threatening and can include shortness of breath, cough, wheezing, and chest tightness. During an asthma attack, constriction of the bronchial smooth muscles, swelling of bronchial tissues, and increased mucous secretion narrow the airways and cause breathing difficulty. Asthma attacks are often followed by airway swelling that persists after the initial acute episode has resolved and can result in extended periods of impaired functioning (American Lung Association, 2000) and reduced quality of life even for patients with mild asthma (Hallstrand, Curtis, Aitken, & Sullivan, 2003). Asthma symptoms can be worsened by environmental triggers such as allergens, seasonal factors (e.g., weather changes), and developmental factors. Children with asthma have a high prevalence of functional morbidity related to their symptoms, including school absences, frequent doctor visits, and hospitalizations (W. R. Taylor & Newacheck, 1992). For example, Forrest, Starfield, Riley, and Kang (1997) noted that among adolescents, multiple domains of health status are affected by asthma, particularly by the frequency and severity of recent symptoms.

The economic burden from pediatric asthma related to lost school days has been estimated to total $1 billion each year in the United States (American Lung Association, 2000). The medical costs of problematic asthma management are also extraordinary (McQuaid & Walders, 2003). Data from pediatric patients enrolled in a national health maintenance organization found that enrollees 18 years of age and younger were responsible for nearly half of the overall expenditures for asthma (Stempel, Strum, Hedblom, & Durcanin-Roberts, 1995). A majority of the health care costs for asthma are allocated for a relatively small segment of the patient population who demonstrate recurrent symptoms (D. H. Smith et al., 1997).

MEDICAL TREATMENT

Successful medical management of asthma requires the child and parents to develop knowledge and skills in symptom monitoring and recommended asthma treatment. Medical practice guidelines for asthma, which are based on illness severity and related functional morbidity (National Institutes of Health, 1997), recommend the following: (a) an appropriate and timely response to acute exacerbations of asthma, (b) prevention of disease progression by avoiding asthma triggers, and (c) use of long-term-control medications to reduce underlying airway inflammation. One foundation for implementing current medical practice guidelines involves a written asthma "action plan" that involves medications to prevent symptoms and to reduce acute symptoms as well as instruction regarding appropriate health care utilization on the basis of the severity of symptoms (McQuaid & Walders, 2003). Children and adolescents with persistent forms of asthma characterized by underlying inflammation of the airways generally require both quick-relief medication and long-term-control medication for optimal management (McQuaid & Walders, 2003). Quick-relief medications are used to reduce symptoms associated with bronchoconstriction. In addition, for children with moderate to severe asthma, long-term-control medications (e.g., corticosteroids) should also be taken on a daily basis to control persistent asthma symptoms. However, it should be noted that asthma medications have significant side effects, which may intensify problems with treatment adherence (Creer & Bender, 1995). Side effects of inhaled corticosteroids may include delayed growth acceleration and increased aggressive or oppositional behavior (Creer & Bender, 1995) and effects on memory and mood (Celano & Geller, 1993).

PSYCHOLOGICAL IMPACT OF PEDIATRIC ASTHMA ON CHILDREN AND FAMILIES

Children's experience of living with asthma can include a range of emotional responses and sequelae, including symptoms of fear, panic, and depression (Taitel, Allen, & Creer, 1998). Although many children and adolescents adapt to the stressors associated with pediatric asthma without developing significant psychological problems, a subgroup may experience behavioral adjustment difficulties that may be related at least in part to asthma-related stressors (Klinnert, McQuaid, McCormick, Adinoff, & Bryant, 2000).

Consider the example of Jimmy, a 10-year-old boy with severe asthma who struggles with his anxiety concerning an asthma attack. Several months ago, he had experienced a particularly severe attack that required hospitalization. Since that time, his anxieties have increased, which have interfered with the management of his asthma. For example, he has begun to panic at the first sign of symptoms. In addition, he has limited his activities outside his home because he wanted to make sure his mother is available to help him with his symptoms. Children with asthma who experience anxieties like Jimmy's are not unusual and are in need of intervention. For example, a meta-analysis of 26 published studies of behavioral adjustment of children with asthma found higher rates of behavioral problems, especially internalizing behaviors, among children with asthma compared with healthy children (McQuaid et al., 2001). Psychological adjustment difficulties were most common among children with severe asthma (McQuaid et al., 2001). Such findings underscore the importance of developing psychological interventions that address the behavioral problems associated with pediatric asthma.

Pediatric asthma can also have a significant psychological impact on families (Creer & Bender, 1995; McQuaid & Walders, 2003). In turn, the quality of family resources and relationships may have an impact on the level of control and morbidity in pediatric asthma. Significant relationships among caregivers, mental health, and children's asthma morbidity have been identified. For example, the National Cooperative Inner-City Asthma

Study (NCICAS) found a relationship between hospitalization rates for children with asthma and caregiver mental health problems (Weil et al., 1999). Psychological and family dysfunction, problematic asthma management, and asthma-related morbidity can be clustered together and result in problematic outcomes. For example, family dysfunction, especially disorganization in family leadership and routine, may limit adherence to medical treatment and aggravate the frequency and severity of asthma symptoms, necessitating additional visits to the emergency room and even hospitalization in some instances. In turn, the burdens imposed by these asthma symptoms and the necessary treatment may cause additional stresses and burdens for families. For this reason, family-centered psychological interventions are important in the promotion of psychological adaptation and illness management in pediatric asthma (Creer & Bender, 1995).

ILLNESS MANAGEMENT AND TREATMENT ADHERENCE

Successful asthma management requires children and family members to engage in a wide range of behaviors, such as avoiding asthma triggers, taking medication(s) to prevent asthma attacks, responding to asthma exacerbations with appropriate pharmacologic or medical attention, and keeping regular follow-up appointments (Creer, 1998). However, successful adherence to the demands of ongoing asthma treatment is difficult for many children, adolescents, and their parents for several reasons. One primary reason is that asthma symptoms are unpredictable (Creer, 2000): Children and adolescents may have relatively long periods of time without experiencing any symptoms. Such symptom-free periods may cause the child and parent to believe that the child either no longer has asthma or has a very mild form. Consequently, many children and families may be unprepared to manage unpredictable exacerbations of asthma symptoms when they occur. Depending on the child's condition, when asthma symptoms do occur, they can be severe and potentially life threatening, requiring prompt and effective action to limit their impact and preclude treatment in emergency room or inpatient settings.

A related clinical feature of pediatric asthma is the extraordinary individual variation in the severity and course of the condition. Such variation necessitates the development of an individualized treatment plan designed to prevent acute symptoms and manage flare-ups as well as chronic airway inflammation (National Institutes of Health, 1991, 1997). Such treatment plans also need to be updated in response to changes in the child's symptoms and response to treatment. Although written treatment plans for asthma can reduce asthma morbidity, including the frequency and recidivism of emergency room visits, they may not be consistently provided to children because of barriers to care. This may result in both inadequate prevention of symptoms and problematic management of acute symptoms (McQuaid & Walders, 2003).

Child and family nonadherence to asthma treatment plans and problematic management can have significant clinical consequences, such as increased illness complications, excessive functional morbidity, elevated health care costs, and even fatal asthma attacks (Birkhead, Olfaway, Strunk, Townsend, & Teutsch, 1989). Children and adolescents with asthma who typically demonstrate a combination of severe disease, treatment nonadherence, and poor health management skills are very costly to the health care system (McQuaid & Walders, 2003). Milgrom et al. (1996) found that the overall rate of adherence to treatment in pediatric asthma was only 58%, and that nonadherence to asthma treatment was associated with disease exacerbations. Halterman, Aligne, Auinger, McBride, and Szilagyi's (2000) study of a nationally representative sample of children with moderate to severe asthma found that many children, including those who had been hospitalized multiple times, did not receive adequate therapy, which related partly to treatment nonadherence. Only about one fourth of the sample had taken a maintenance asthma medication during the past month (Halterman et al., 2000).

Taken together, the morbidity and costs of problematic asthma management and nonadherence underscore the need to develop and evaluate psychological interventions to enhance adherence to asthma treatment and limit or prevent asthma symptoms. In particular, psychological interventions are needed to help families and health care providers surmount barriers to adherence to pediatric asthma treatment, especially for economically disadvantaged, minority children and adolescents with asthma, who face special barriers to effective adherence to treatment and illness management (Celano, Geller, Phillips, & Zimen, 1998; Milgrom & Bender, 1997; Walders, Drotar, & Kercsmar, 2000a, 2000b).

A large number of barriers to asthma adherence treatment have been identified, including inadequate access to medical care (Crain et al., 1998), environmental triggers (McQuaid & Walders, 2003), limited knowledge of asthma (Zimmerman, Bonner, Evans, & Mellins, 1999), delays in receiving emergency treatment for acute asthma attacks (D. H. Smith et al., 1997), erroneous parental health beliefs about asthma symptoms and their management (Farber et al., 2003; Peterson-Sweeney, McMullen, Yoos, & Kitzman, 2003), health provider and system barriers (Mansour, Lanphear, & DeWitt, 2000), family dysfunction (K. B. Weiss & Wagener, 1990), poverty (R. Evans, 1992), and family allocation of asthma management tasks (Walders et al., 2000a). Yoos, Kitzman, and McMullen (2003) noted that parents' diminished treatment expectations and fears about anti-inflammatory medications were barriers to the use of medically appropriate anti-inflammatory medication use. Minority parents were more likely than nonminority parents to view asthma as unpredictable and uncontrollable and to have negative attitudes toward anti-inflammatory medications. Pradel, Hartzema, and Bush (2001) found that many children lacked understanding of the categories of asthma medications and also reported problems with the medication, such as bad taste, lack of effectiveness, and side effects. Psychological interventions designed to enhance treatment adherence and family management of asthma may focus in one way or another on identifying some of the above barriers and reducing their impact on management.

REVIEWS OF PSYCHOLOGICAL INTERVENTIONS FOR PEDIATRIC ASTHMA

Over the past 20 years, a range of psychological interventions designed to enhance the management of pediatric asthma, including adherence to treatment, have been published. Wigal, Creer, Kotses, and Lewis (1990) reviewed 19 educational and self-management programs. These included programs such as Open Airways (D. Evans et al., 1987) that have been developed for application with a broad spectrum of patients across a number of settings. In addition to providing education, many of these programs involved a wide range of psychological interventions, such as goal setting, goal monitoring, relaxation training, self-efficacy and control, behavioral management, and parent guidance. Wigal et al. (1990) concluded that when asthma management skills were performed as part of these interventions, children and parents could accept greater responsibility for the management of asthma, prevent and manage asthma attacks more effectively, and hence have a functional impact on asthma. However, this review did not critically evaluate the methods of individual studies, include data based on observation of children's and parents' asthma management skills, consider the implications of contradictory findings of interventions, or describe effect sizes of the studies that were reviewed.

Bernard-Bonnin, Stachenko, Bonin, Charette, and Rousseau (1995) conducted a meta-analysis of randomized controlled trials (RCTs) that were designed to teach self-management to reduce the impact of asthma-related morbidity. The programs that were reviewed focused on teaching self-management in an interactive manner (rather than by mailings or audio-visual aids) and included outcome variables related to one or more of the following morbidity variables: emergency room visits, hospitalizations, hospital days, asthma attacks, and school absenteeism. On average, the 11 RCTs that fit the criteria were rated as fair in overall quality on the basis of Chalmers et al.'s (1981) criteria. Analyses of effect sizes indicated that for the most part, teaching of self-management skills did not reduce school absenteeism, asthma attacks, hospitalizations, or emergency room visits. Bernard-Bonnin et al. (1995) cautioned that several methodological limitations may have affected the findings and their interpretation in the studies reviewed. For example, most studies included children with mild to moderate asthma in which the potential range for reduction of morbidity was low and did not stratify on severity. One example was Clark et al.'s (1986) intervention, which found no difference in the effects of health education for the sample as a whole but had significant effects among children with previous hospitalizations.

In addition, the conclusions based on the studies considered in this review were limited by (a) the imprecision in the outcome measures, which could be influenced by many variables other than control of asthma symptoms, and (b) the variation in the structure of the teaching programs across different studies (Bernard-Bonnin et al., 1995). Nevertheless, the major conclusion of this review—that even comprehensive teaching programs did not necessarily result in behavioral changes in the management of asthma—has informed the design of psychological interventions (Bernard Bonnin et al., 1995).

McQuaid and Nassau's (1999) review of 14 studies of psychological intervention designed to reduce psychological symptoms in pediatric asthma concluded that frontallis electromyograph biofeedback was a well-established treatment, relaxation training was probably efficacious, and family therapy intervention was promising. In a more recent review, Haby, Waters, Robertson, Gibson, and Ducharme (2005) reviewed RCTs or controlled clinical trials of children (involving 1,407 patients) who presented to the emergency room for symptoms of asthma. Compared with the control conditions, which involved usual care or lower intensity education, formal education did not reduce subsequent emergency room visits, hospital visits, or unscheduled visits. Haby et al.'s (2005) conclusions were similar to those of Bernard-Bonnin et al. (1995): that education alone was not sufficient to improve asthma management and that effective psychological intervention needs to focus on behavioral change. Finally, Haby et al. identified two major methodological problems in the studies reviewed: (a) wide variability in the nature of intervention and control group interventions and (b) inconsistent or problematic reporting of measures and analysis of outcomes.

Finally, Lemanek et al.'s (2001) review indicated improvements in both adherence and health outcome (e.g., peak flow rates, asthma symptoms) as well as good treatment acceptability in eight studies of interventions designed to enhance adherence to medical treatment in pediatric asthma (Baum & Creer, 1986; da Costa, Rapoff, Lemanek, & Goldstein, 1997; Eney & Goldstein, 1976; Holzheimer, Mohay, & Masters, 1998; LeBaron, Zeltzer, Ratner, & Kniker, 1985; N. A. Smith, Seale, Ley, Mellis, & Shaw, 1994; N. A. Smith, Seale, Ley, Shaw, & Bracs, 1986; Weinstein & Cuskey, 1985).

Lemanek et al.'s primary conclusions were that behavioral strategies and educational strategies were promising interventions, organizational strategies (e.g., simplifying regimens or increasing health care decisions) were probably efficacious, and multicomponent treatment packages needed more research to determine their efficacy. However, Lemanek et al. noted that the findings of the studies they reviewed were limited by methodological problems such as lack of controls and follow-up and problems in measurement of adherence. Moreover, none of the empirically supported interventions reviewed focused on minority children.

Despite the recognition of the impact of psychological and behavioral factors on the health and well-being of children and adolescents with asthma (McQuaid et al., 2001; McQuaid & Walders, 2003), relatively few studies have focused on improving the psychological adaptation of children with asthma as the primary target outcome. One example of such an intervention is Perrin, MacLean, Gortmaker, and Asher's (1992) RCT that assessed the efficacy of a combined education, stress management, and contingency coping intervention. Stress management included relaxation training, which emphasized deep breathing through guided imagery and muscle relaxation. Contingency coping training targeted specific difficulties that children encountered in coping with their asthma and emphasized alternative choices of action, including coping strategies. Children who were randomized to the intervention group had fewer behavioral problems and less frequent internalizing symptoms compared with controls.

EXAMPLES OF STUDIES OF PSYCHOLOGICAL INTERVENTIONS FOR PEDIATRIC ASTHMA

In the following sections, some specific examples of studies of psychological interventions in pediatric asthma are described, including computerized self-management approaches, home-based approaches, tailored approaches, and large-scale RCTs. These examples illustrate the broad range of intervention approaches that have been used to enhance the quality of asthma management and improve adherence to treatment.

Computerized Self-Management Approaches

Guendelman, Meade, Benson, Chen, and Samuels (2002) conducted a randomized trial of an interactive, computerized self-management and education program, the Health Buddy, which was designed to enable children to assess and monitor their asthma symptoms and quality of life and to transmit this information to health care providers through a secure Web site. Control group participants used an asthma diary. Activity limitations were lower for children who were randomized to the Health Buddy intervention. Moreover, the intervention group was likely to report problematic peak flow readings and to make urgent calls to the hospital and had greater improvements in adherence and self-care. Although the absence of data concerning costs and long-term outcomes of the intervention is a limitation to eventual application of this model of intervention, the results are promising enough to warrant replication with more extensive samples.

Home-Based Approaches

Some recent approaches to asthma intervention have focused on conducting interventions in home settings to provide access for difficult-to-reach children with asthma and their families. For example, J. V. Brown et al. (2002) found that a home-based education program for low-income caregivers of young children with asthma was associated with less bother from asthma symptoms, more symptom-free days, and better caregiver quality of life on follow-up for very young (ages 1–3 years) children but not for older (ages 4–6 years) preschoolers.

Tailored Approaches

S. Bonner et al. (2002) described an RCT in an urban Latino and African American intervention that provided patient education to children with asthma based on a readiness-to-learn model and facilitated interactions between patient and doctor. Readiness to learn was operationalized on the basis of four dimensions ranging from symptom avoidance (e.g., failure to recognize asthma as a chronic disease and habituation to persistent symptoms) to self-regulation, which was defined as family application of a stepped action plan when symptoms changed and discussion of the efficacy of asthma treatment during regular consultation with physicians. Family education addressed basic learning needs of children with asthma by improving their perception of asthma symptoms, persistence using asthma diaries, and peak flow measures. The physician intervention focused clinicians' attention on patients' diary records and peak flow measures and encouraged physicians to use stepped treatment action plans. The intervention group showed improvements on knowledge, health beliefs, self-efficacy, adherence, and decreased symptoms and activity restriction.

Large-Scale Randomized Controlled Trials of Asthma Management

Vulnerable subgroups such as low-income minority children encounter special barriers to asthma management that need to be addressed in psychological interventions (Mansour et al., 2000; Warman, Silver, McCourt, &

Stein, 1999). The NCICAS conducted a randomized multisite RCT with a large sample ($N = 1,034$) that was designed to minimize days in which asthma symptoms (e.g., wheezing) were evident as measured by 2-week recall at 2-month intervals over a 2-year follow-up period among children ages 5 to 11 years with asthma (R. Evans et al., 1999). An asthma risk assessment tool was used to structure a tailored comprehensive educational intervention. Families were assigned to either this individualized intervention conducted by master's-level social workers that was tailored to each family's asthma risk profile (e.g., exposure to allergens, allergen sensitivity, smoking, access to care) or a control group involving usual care. Participants in the intervention had fewer symptom days, especially among children with severe asthma, and fewer hospitalizations than in the comparison group. These changes were sustained in the 2nd year of the program. R. Evans et al. (1999) concluded that individualized problem-solving approaches may be particularly useful in working with inner-city children and their parents who may encounter multiple barriers to asthma management, such as economic uncertainty, environments with high allergen levels, multiple caretakers, and stressors, each of which may divert their energies away from attention to asthma management.

As a follow-up to the NCICAS study, the CDC sponsored implementation of the NCICAS asthma counselor model in 22 sites across the United States in clinical settings (P. R. Wood, Sadof, Kercsmar, & Kattan, 2004). Thus far, these data have demonstrated the feasibility of implementing the NCICAS model on a large scale, for example, among high-need, inner-city children with asthma who are enrolled in interventions conducted by an asthma counselor outside the research setting (P. R. Wood et al., 2004). On the other hand, retention of participants and completion of all intervention components was difficult to achieve, and there was high turnover of asthma counselors. These findings suggest that the NCICAS intervention model (R. Evans et al., 1999) will be difficult to implement on a wide scale unless the barriers to delivering the intervention model in nonresearch settings are identified and addressed (P. R. Wood et al., 2004).

RECOMMENDATIONS FOR CLINICAL CARE

Pediatric psychologists in a number of settings provide services to children and adolescents with asthma, including children and families who are nonadherent to treatment and have recurrent problems with symptomatic management. In other settings, social workers may provide supportive services to families as well as counseling and mental health services to selected families. At some large, nationally recognized treatment programs for children with asthma, such as the National Jewish Hospital, psychological services, including assessment and intervention, are provided routinely to children and families. In addition, pediatric psychologists meet regularly with the medical treatment team as part of the team and consult routinely with physicians who are managing the services (B. Bender, personal communication, July 21, 2004).

McQuaid and Walders (2003) described a number of salient roles for pediatric psychologists in facilitating psychological interventions in the context of comprehensive pediatric asthma management. These include the following: (a) asthma education for patient and family (e.g., recognition of knowledge deficits and referral to asthma education problems, development of new educational resources or refinement of existing programs that incorporate behavioral management), (b) identification and treatment of psychosocial barriers to effective asthma management by enhancing problem-solving skills (Wade, Holden, Lynn, Mitchell, & Ewart, 2000), and (c) application of psychosocial intervention techniques such as problem-solving methods, family-centered interventions, or relaxation training and biofeedback. It will be important to describe the clinical effectiveness of these strategies in future case reports, case series, and program evaluations using quantitative methods.

Creer (2000) developed a model of self-management skills for pediatric asthma based on extensive clinical care and research experience that has application for psychological interventions including preventive management in clinical care settings. This model divides self-management skills into three domains: *prevention*, including adherence to medication advice as prescribed, prevention of acute episodes of illness, and preventive health; *management of an acute episode*, including treating the episode systematically in accord with a prescribed plan and taking medications correctly and in a timely manner; and *prevention and management of acute episodes*, including self-directed behaviors such as self-statements, self-management skills such as self-monitoring and decision making, and coping skills. Creer also identified the key behaviors that are necessary for self-management that are utilized by children with asthma (and other chronic conditions) and their families. These include (a) goal selection for a treatment plan; (b) information collection, such as recording data concerning asthma symptoms; (c) information processing, such as identifying asthma symptoms and evaluating their significance for treatment; (d) decision making concerning whether to take a rescue medication; (e) actions, such as taking asthma medication; and (f) self-reactions, including evaluating one's performance during asthma tasks.

Support for various elements of Creer's (2000) self-management model, including decision making, has been found in clinical observations of the development of a self-management program in asthma (Creer et al., 1988). In 5-year posttreatment interviews, children and families reported that they had become increasingly skilled at taking appropriate actions to manage their asthma on a day-to-day basis as well as asthma attacks. Families also described greater efficiency of decision making and asthma management in that they had become increasingly able to reduce the number of their treatment-related actions, taking only those steps that were absolutely necessary to limit an asthma episode. Moreover, families had become increasingly able to tailor their treatment approach to the severity of an episode and the situation in which it occurred. Empirical support for self-efficacy as an aspect of adaptive self-management in asthma was shown by increased confidence in performance of self-management skills over the course of a 5-year follow-up as well as an increase in positive expectancies of asthma outcomes (Creer et al., 1988). For example, children and families were more likely to believe that if they managed their condition as they had been taught, they could make a difference in its outcome.

Empirical research on Creer's (2000) model needs to be extended in a number of ways. For example, it will be important to incorporate key elements of the model (e.g., decision making, acquisition and performance of self-management skills) in models of comprehensive care for asthma as well as for other chronic conditions. In addition, it will be important to use objective measures to assess the key illness-related outcomes, such as treatment adherence and morbidity, and to monitor the child's progress in chronic illness self-management in response to comprehensive care. Key advantages of Creer's model are that the concepts are applicable to a range of chronic conditions, and the model can be used as a template to operationalize self-management interventions and test their efficacy on illness-related morbidity.

RECOMMENDATIONS FOR RESEARCH DIRECTIONS

Future research concerning psychological interventions in pediatric asthma should build on the considerable progress that has been made. Bernard-Bonnin et al. (1995) recommended greater emphasis on controlled evaluation of behavioral interventions and inclusion of behavioral outcomes in studies of psychological intervention in pediatric asthma. McQuaid and Nassau (1999) recommended greater specification and measurement of the effect of psychological interventions for pediatric asthma and potential moderators of treatment such as physiologic reactivity to stress or asthma symptoms triggered by emotional stress. On the basis of their review of RCTs of interventions in pediatric asthma, Haby et al. (2001) recommended the following: (a) developing stronger, more comprehensive interventions that involve a written action plan and regular medical review; (b) testing behavioral methods such as self-monitoring and reporting outcomes in units that are suitable for meta-analysis; and (c) evaluating the characteristics of individual studies of interventions (e.g., scope, timing, duration, and setting of the intervention) that might be expected to affect individual differences in outcomes.

The results of these reviews are consistent in their recommendations for a greater emphasis on behavioral interventions as opposed to strictly educational interventions and for a greater emphasis on measurement of behavioral outcomes. Investigators may tailor specific behavioral interventions to the specific problems experienced by individual children and families (McQuaid & Walders, 2003). For example, relaxation training may be especially important for those children and parents who become so anxious at the first sign of an asthma attack that they have difficulty accomplishing the next appropriate step in their treatment plan (McQuaid & Nassau, 1999). Cognitive–behavioral approaches that involve identification and reframing of problematic beliefs about the lack of effectiveness and side effects of medications may be effective for children and parents whose health beliefs pose a barrier to asthma management. Family-based problem-solving interventions may be useful for those families who need help in developing more effective problem-solving strategies to surmount specific barriers to asthma management, including more effective distribution of management tasks among family members (e.g., a balance between child self-management and parental involvement; McQuaid & Walders, 2003).

One priority area for future research concerns studies of clinical effectiveness of psychological interventions that have been shown to be empirically supported in clinical settings (e.g., what interventions are feasible and effective to use in clinical settings?). Such research would be an important companion piece to studies of medical treatment (e.g., specialist medical care, asthma action plans, and comprehensive education outreach support), some of which have shown efficacy and effectiveness with economically disadvantaged children and their families (R. Evans et al., 1999; Kelly et al., 2000).

Future research should also develop and evaluate psychological interventions that focus on enhancing the psychological adaptation of children with asthma, including the reduction of psychological distress that affects the control of asthma symptoms and children's management of acute exacerbation of symptoms. For example, relaxation training that involves the use of breathing techniques and progressive muscle relaxation to reduce autonomic arousal and emotional distress may be an effective model for distressed children (McQuaid & Nassau, 1999), especially if combined with training in problem solving and coping. In this regard, Perrin et al.'s (1992) comprehensive intervention approach, including stress management (e.g., relaxation training and training in coping with specific asthma-related problems), bears replication in larger samples in different settings.

Another set of future research directions includes refinement of methods of evaluation (e.g., increased specificity in the description of interventions) and measurement of outcomes (e.g., adherence to treatment; Lemanek et al., 2001). The use of electronic monitoring devices to assess adherence is an important development, although the technical and measurement problems associated with these technologies need to be addressed (Quittner, Espelage, Ievers-Landers, & Drotar, 2000). Other areas include specification and testing of the mechanism of processes that account for successful interventions (see McQuaid & Nassau, 1999; Lemanek et al., 2001). Because most studies did not specify a model by which psychological interventions were expected to work, it was not always clear why interventions that were found to be effective worked (McQuaid & Nassau, 1999).

Future psychological interventions should also focus on improving children's psychological adaptation and functioning in various settings (e.g., school) in addition to improving physical symptoms and morbidity associated with asthma, because this impact is a neglected area. As noted by Lehrer, Feldman, Giardino, Song, and Schmaling (2002), models of psychological interventions that have shown positive effects on various outcomes with adults that might warrant evaluation with children and adolescents include symptom perception training (Stout, Kotses, & Creer, 1997) and written emotional expression (Smyth, Stone, Hurewitz, & Kaell, 1999).

One of the most important future directions concerns the implementation and evaluation of psychological interventions in the clinical care of children with asthma. This is a complicated issue for several reasons. Large numbers of children are affected with asthma of different levels of severity, which raises challenges for deployment of services. In many settings, children and families with the most serious problems in management and nonadherence to treatment may be the ones who are referred for psychological services. These patients certainly may benefit from psychological interventions. However, assuming scarce mental health resources, providing services to these high-risk problem patients can divert clinical attention away from providing ongoing services to a wider population in a preventive model as part of a comprehensive care approach (Drotar, 2001).

What might such preventive models look like? Cognitive–behavioral strategies are ideally suited for pediatric asthma interventions, given their emphasis on reducing stress, anxiety, and deficits in behaviors such as problem solving that may affect asthma morbidity (Wade et al., 2000). Cognitive–behavioral techniques can be used to adapt problematic behaviors (e.g., treatment nonadherence) that are often characteristic of patients who experience difficulty coping with asthma (McQuaid & Walders, 2003).

As an example of a psychological intervention that is potentially feasible in clinical care, Walders et al. (in press) conducted an RCT of an interdisciplinary intervention for pediatric asthma at an urban tertiary-referral pediatric hospital. In this study, 185 patients who lacked a written treatment plan for asthma and presented with asthma-related emergency department visits (two or more) and/or hospitalization (one or more) in the past year were randomized to a comparison group receiving standard care or an interdisciplinary intervention group. All of the participants received written asthma management plans and peak flow meters. The intervention group also received additional asthma education, an asthma risk profile assessment, brief problem-solving therapy, and access to a 24-hour asthma hotline. Over the year follow-up, the intervention group demonstrated less frequent health care utilization than the comparison group. Both groups demonstrated significant reduction in asthma symptoms and improvements in quality of life.

Another area for future care is development and evaluation of clinical psychological interventions designed to manage the problem of high levels of asthma morbidity. A relatively small number of children with asthma account for the largest number of hospital admissions, emergency room visits, and health care costs. Many of these children have the most problematic constellation of risk factors that may require the most intensive programs. Bratton et al. (2001) found that multidisciplinary care in a short-term outpatient treatment program, which was designed to reduce costs and emphasize family management, was associated with a significant improvement in functional severity of asthma, perceived competence in asthma management, and quality of life for both caregiver and child compared with a previous program that involved long-term hospitalization. Medical data demonstrated a significant improvement in the use of corticosteroid medication, emergency room visits, hospital days, and use of medical care encounters (Bratton et al., 2001). Although this was an uncontrolled study, it demonstrates the potential of psychological interventions with children and adolescents who present with high levels of morbidity.

FUTURE CHALLENGES IN CLINICAL CARE AND RESEARCH IN PEDIATRIC ASTHMA

Creer and Bender (1995) noted several paradoxes in the understanding and management of asthma that will require the concerted attention of researchers and practitioners. First, increasing numbers of children and adolescents experience asthma and its impact, thus increasing burdens on society for asthma management and prevention of morbidity. Second, the newer and more effective treatments for asthma that have been developed are beneficial but have side effects that need to be understood by providers and families. Third, although new and more effective medical treatments for asthma are available, they are not being used consistently by physicians and families of children with asthma because of barriers related to education and practice. Finally, responsibility for asthma management has shifted dramatically from physicians to parents and children who are asked to monitor asthma triggers, to evaluate information about their symptoms and treatment, and to make sophisticated decisions concerning asthma management.

The implications of the above paradoxes are considerable. For example, psychologists and other professionals need to develop strategies for teaching much more sophisticated self-management skills to children and families. This will create a significant demand for psychological services to be integrated with programs for pediatric asthma in various pediatric centers. However, the prevalence and unpredictable nature of asthma pose considerable challenges for such proactive programs. Moreover, the targets of behavioral research and preventive intervention will need to be expanded to include adherence to medication regimens and the promotion and maintenance of environmental control of asthma triggers. Again, this will pose considerable challenges to the development of comprehensive intervention models that involve universal primary prevention, targeted secondary prevention, or indicated tertiary prevention services (Creer & Bender, 1995).

Creer (2001) also described several important future challenges with respect to asthma management that involve consumers and practitioners. These challenges include (a) understanding the needs of consumers of care (e.g., children and adolescents with asthma and their family members), (b) identifying the processes of management and benchmarks of outcomes that will meet these needs, (c) identifying best practice standards of asthma treatment and indicators to measure performance, (d) establishing performance expectations that are monitored and compared with performance, and (e) providing feedback to providers and consumers.

To achieve these objectives, the clinical care programs of the future for children and adolescents with asthma and their families will need to include outcome data that will evaluate how well a program provides necessary care and eliminates unnecessary care; benchmarks of programs that provide new and innovative (e.g., enhanced self-management) versus traditional interventions; and routine, repeated measures of critical outcomes (e.g., how well a program reduces the need for medical services and hospitalizations). Finally, such programs will need to apply this knowledge in routine clinical care to achieve better health and psychological outcomes for children and adolescents with asthma and their families. These needs for program evaluation create extraordinary opportunities for psychologists and other professionals who are interested in pediatric asthma.

7

PSYCHOLOGICAL INTERVENTIONS: DIABETES

Type 1 diabetes mellitus (DM1), also known as insulin-dependent diabetes mellitus, is among the most common of chronic pediatric illnesses, occurs in 1 in 600 children (Wysocki, Greco, & Buckloh, 2003), and is recognized as an important public health problem (Vinicor, 1998). This condition results from autoimmune destruction of pancreatic islet cells that produce insulin, which results in permanent insulin deficiency. Treatment involves either multiple daily insulin injections or the use of an insulin pump, which infuses a constant rate of insulin through a catheter, with additional doses before meals (Boland, Grey, Oesterle, Fredrickson, & Tamborlane, 1999).

Type 2 diabetes mellitus (DM2), also known as noninsulin-dependent diabetes mellitus, now accounts for 10% to 20% of new cases of diabetes, especially in African American, Native American, and Hispanic youths (American Diabetes Association, 2000; Bradshaw, 2002). In contrast to insulin deficiency, which occurs in DM1, DM2 is characterized by insulin resistance, which impairs cellular uptake of insulin and often progresses to islet cell failure and insulin deficiency, with symptoms similar to those of DM1. In some instances, DM2 can be managed with diet and exercise alone or with oral medications, although many youths require insulin injection treatment. Both DM1 and DM2 carry the long-term risks of complication to the heart, kidneys, eyes, and nerves (Wysocki et al., 2003).

Large-scale randomized control trials (RCTs), such as that conducted by the Diabetes Control and Complications Trial (DCCT) Research Group (1993), have shown that risks for complications of DM1, including damage to the eyes, heart, kidneys, and nerves, increase as a function of levels of hemoglobin HbA_{1C}, which is a measure of the average blood glucose levels in the prior 2 to 3 months. Maintaining near-normal HbA_{1C} can reduce the risks of complications to levels that equal those of the general population (DCCT Research Group, 1993). These findings clearly heighten the need to develop efficacious psychological interventions to promote adherence to treatment and increase control of HbA_{1C}.

Given increased prevalence based on increasing rates of pediatric obesity, DM2 is recognized as a critical public health problem (Pinkas-Hamiel et al., 1996; Young-Hyman, 2002). In future years, there will be increased emphasis on developing effective psychological interventions to manage as well as prevent this condition. There is, however, a much more extensive scientific knowledge base concerning psychological interventions of DM1. For this reason, this chapter focuses on DM1. Nevertheless, many of the methods and principles of psychological interventions that are successful with children and adolescents with DM1 will also be applicable to those with DM2.

MEDICAL TREATMENT REGIMEN

The medical management of DM1 requires a complex and multifaceted series of tasks, such as self-monitoring of blood glucose before meals and at bedtime, and adjustment of medical regimens accordingly. Maintenance of near-normal HbA_{1C} is important to long-term health (DCCT Research Group, 1993). Consequently, recommended treatment for DM1 includes insulin regimens involving three or more daily injections or use of insulin pumps as well as making insulin adjustments in response to diet or exercise or both. Insulin management also involves detection and correction of abnormally high (hyperglycemia) or low (hypoglycemia) blood glucose levels, each of which can cause symptoms that can reduce quality of life (QOL) for affected children and adolescents and increase the level of family burden. Prolonged hyperglycemia, which results from underdosing or omitting insulin injections or oral medications, overeating, or infections, can lead to hospitalization for diabetic ketoacidosis (Gray, Marrero, Godfrey, Orr, & Golden, 1988). Hypoglycemia, which results from injecting too much insulin, undereating, or extraordinary physical exertion, results in symptoms such as trembling, nausea, sweating, dizziness, and confusion. Mild to moderate hypoglycemia is treated by ingesting carbohydrates, whereas severe hypoglycemia is treated by injection of glucagons, a hormone that blocks insulin and raises blood glucose (Wysocki et al., 2003).

Modern dietary treatment regimens for DM1 and DM2 require eating a specified number of grams of carbohydrates at each meal and a scheduled snack. In addition, persons with DM1 and DM2 may eat limited quantities of refined sweets as long as they are included in the daily carbohydrate allowance and blood glucose targets are reached. Regular exercise is also important in the management of DM1 and DM2 because it may reduce insulin requirements, promote cardiovascular health, facilitate weight control, and enhance psychological well-being (Wysocki et al., 2003).

PSYCHOLOGICAL IMPACT OF TYPE 1 DIABETES ON CHILDREN, ADOLESCENTS, AND THEIR FAMILIES

From the standpoint of psychological impact, one of the important features of DM1 is the multifaceted and demanding treatment regimen that involves insulin treatment, diet, and exercise (Johnson, 1995). Rubin and Peyrot (2001) identified several clinically relevant sources of stress among children and adolescents with diabetes. These included (a) being deprived of food because of dietary restrictions; (b) problems in monitoring blood glucose, such as pain and frustrations concerning unpredictable blood glucose levels; (c) concerns about taking insulin, including fears of hypoglycemia; and (d) conflict with parents and professional caregivers about diabetes management. Such stressors may be the focus of clinical attention among children and adolescents with diabetes who are referred for psychological intervention.

Mellin, Neumark-Sztainer, and Patterson (2004) identified five themes of challenging concerns among the parents of adolescent girls with DM1: (a) parental worries about DM1, including long-term complications; (b) parent–adolescent conflicts regarding DM1 management; (c) psychological impact of DM1 on parents and other family members; (d) parent–adolescent conflicts that are unrelated to DM1 management; and (e) difficulties regulating blood sugar in specific situations, such as in sports and social activities. Because such stressors can affect the quality of parent–child relationships, they are logical targets for psychological intervention. Other potential targets of intervention for children and adolescents with DM1 focus on emotional concerns. For example, B. J. Anderson (2002) described the wide range of emotional reactions that are experienced by parents and family members of children and adolescents with DM1 and DM2, such as guilt, blame, financial concerns, loss of a normal lifestyle for family members, and fears (e.g., of diabetes-related long-term complications or low blood glucose).

Family and child reactions to DM1 may need to be addressed in psychological interventions, as shown in the following case example. Sam is a 9-year-old with DM1 who presents with behavioral problems. At home, he has resisted taking responsibility for his diabetes management and continually argues with his mother about it. Sam's mother has been highly stressed by Sam's behavior and does not have an effective strategy to manage his behavior. Sam's parents disagree about how to manage his behavior and his illness. His father believes that Sam's mother is overprotective. However, his mother believes that his father just does not understand him. This family would benefit from family-centered intervention that focuses on enhancing communication and problem solving.

Although diabetes-related stressors such as those identified in Sam and his family are common, it is important to recognize that such stressors do not necessarily result in clinically significant psychological or psychiatric disorders, either in children with DM1 or family members. Johnson's (1995) review found that children and adolescents with DM1 demonstrated patterns of general psychological adjustment that were comparable with that of healthy peers. Nevertheless, some children and adolescents with DM1 are at increased risk for psychiatric problems such as depression, anxiety, and eating disorders. These problems are frequent reasons for clinical referrals for psychological evaluation and intervention for this population. In a prospective study, Kovacs, Goldston, Obrosky, and Bonar (1997) found that about 25% of youths had an episode of major depression, and 13% had anxiety disorders 10 years after onset of diabetes. Some adolescents with DM1 may also be at higher risk for the development of eating disorders because of the weight gain associated with insulin treatment (Colton, Rodin, Olmsted, & Daneman, 1999) and the focus on diet required in diabetes management (Antisdel & Chrisler, 2000). Finally, the symptoms associated with DM1, such as low blood sugar, may also affect children's cognitive development. Children with early DM1 onset (before 5 to 7 years of age) may be at risk for developing learning disabilities (Ryan, 1997).

Interrelationship of Psychological Stressors and Physical Health in Type 1 Diabetes

Psychological factors can affect the physical health of children and adolescents with diabetes in ways that have potential implications for targeting psychological interventions. For example, mental disorders, such as depression and eating disorders, may interfere with diabetes management, affect the level of overall blood sugar control, and eventually cause severe hypoglycemic and hyperglycemic episodes or recurrent diabetic ketoacidosis (Rubin & Peyrot, 1992).

Another potential pathway of psychological influence on the physical health of children and adolescents with DM1 involves the impact of stress on glycemic control. Such pathways of influence can be direct (e.g., triggering a physiological state of arousal including increased output of counterregulatory hormones), indirect (e.g., disrupting self-care routines and lowering gylcemic control; Peyrot & McMurry, 1985), or a combination of direct and indirect influences. It should be noted that none of these hypothesized pathways have been studied extensively. However, Hanson, Henggeler, and Burghen (1987b) found that among adolescents with DM1, stress had a direct effect on glycemic control and was not mediated by regimen adherence. In addition, interventions such as relaxation training may reduce stress and hence improve blood sugar control. For example, behavioral interventions, such as problem-solving or coping skills training, may improve glycemic control by enhancing the quality of self-management behaviors (Rubin & Peyrot, 1992).

Adherence to Treatment for Type 1 Diabetes

Given the complex treatment regimen for DM1, it is not surprising that adherence to treatment is a significant clinical problem as well as a potential source of psychological stress for children, adolescents, and families. Although effective regulation of blood glucose levels can prevent a wide range of diabetes-related complications (DCCT Research Group, 1994), it is by no means the norm, especially for adolescents and young adults with DM1 (Wysocki et al., 2003). Clinically significant problems with adherence to diabetes treatment (Schmidt, Klover, Arfken, Delamater, & Hobson, 1992) as well as declines in treatment adherence have been described among adolescents and young adults (Wysocki et al., 2003). For this reason, the promotion of adherence to medical treatment to DM1 is an important target for psychological intervention.

SUMMARY OF REVIEWS OF PSYCHOLOGICAL INTERVENTIONS FOR TYPE 1 DIABETES

Compared with psychological intervention research on other pediatric chronic conditions, psychological intervention research on DM1 has a much longer history. A wide range of psychological interventions for psychological adjustment and adherence-related problems for children with DM1 have been evaluated and summarized in reviews, including meta-analyses. The results of these reviews are now summarized.

Padgett, Mumford, Hynes, and Carter (1988) conducted a meta-analysis of 93 studies of 7,451 adult, child, and adolescent patients that tested the effects of nine intervention types: (a) didactic education, (b) enhanced education (e.g., behavioral emphasis), (c) dietary instruction, (d) exercise instruction, (e) self-monitoring instruction, (f) social learning and behavioral modification, (g) relaxation training, (h) individual counseling by mental health professionals or clinicians, and (i) peer support. Patient education, diet instruction, and self-monitoring instruction were the most commonly reported interventions in this review. An overall mean effect size (ES) of 0.51 was found for the interventions as a whole. Diet instruction (ES = 0.68) and social learning interventions (ES = 0.57) demonstrated the strongest effects. In addition, for the most part, psychological interventions demonstrated the greatest effects on knowledge and physiological outcomes (e.g., metabolic control). In contrast, psychological outcomes did not show significant ESs in response to intervention. Variables such as number of intervention visits, sex, and age did not correlate with mean ES, whereas overall ratings of the study quality were inversely related to ESs. Methodologically weaker studies (e.g., that were uncontrolled) had higher ESs (Padgett et al., 1988). Recommendations for future research based on this review included greater use of control groups; more reliable measures of outcomes, especially for treatment adherence; and studies of long-term effects of intervention (Padgett et al., 1988). However, it should be recognized that children and adolescents were less well represented than adults in the intervention studies included in the review.

Rubin and Peyrot's (1992) review of psychosocial problems and interventions for children, adolescents, and adults with DM1 found empirical support for the efficacy of behavioral interventions such as coping skills, training, peer modeling with children and adolescents, support and stress management interventions, and family group interventions. However, these authors also identified salient methodological problems such as flawed study designs (e.g., no control groups, small sample size, and limited statistical power), samples that were unrepresentative of the diabetes population as a whole, limited outcome measures, and lack of clarity concerning factors that account for intervention change.

Two reviews of psychological intervention research in children and adolescents with DM1 were published as part of the *Journal of Pediatric Psychology* series on empirically supported treatments. McQuaid and Nassau's (1999) review of 7 studies of psychological interventions designed to reduce the frequency and impact of physical symptoms in DM1 concluded that future research was needed to determine the efficacy of interventions such as psychoanalysis, social skills training, and stress management. Lemanek et al.'s (2001) review of 11 studies of psychological interventions designed to enhance adherence to treatment in DM1 concluded that operant learning procedures and multicomponent, self-management interventions were categorized as probably efficacious. In contrast, cognitive–behavioral self-regulation was characterized as promising.

The Psychosocial Therapies Research Group (Delamater et al., 2001) reviewed key research findings concerning psychological interventions for DM1 separately for children and adults. This expert group concluded that family-based behavioral intervention procedures such as goal setting, self-monitoring, positive reinforcement, behavioral contracts, supportive parental communications, and appropriate sharing of responsibility for diabetes management resulted in improvements in the parent–adolescent relationship (B. J. Anderson, Brackett, Ho, & Laffel, 1999; Wysocki, Harris, et al., 2000), regimen adherence, and glycemic control (B. J. Anderson et al., 1999; Satin et al., 1989). Moreover, psychoeducational interventions with children and their families designed to promote problem-solving skills and increase parental support early in the disease course demonstrated improved longer term glycemic control (Delamater et al., 1990). Peer group support and problem-solving interventions were associated with short-term improvements in glycemic control (B. J. Anderson et al., 1989; Kaplan et al., 1985).

Other noteworthy effects of psychological interventions for children and adolescents with DM1 described by Delamater et al. (2001) were as follows. Adolescents with intensive diabetes treatment who received coping skills training demonstrated improved glycemic control and QOL (Boland et al., 1999; Grey et al., 1998). Other studies have demonstrated that stress management and coping skills training models have resulted in reduction in diabetes-related stress (Boardway, Delamater, Tomakowsky, & Gutai, 1993) and improved social interaction (Mendez & Belendez, 1997). However, ESs for these interventions were not reported, which limits the degree to which the power and clinical significance of these intervention effects can be evaluated.

It is important to note that the methodological problems and barriers that were identified by Delamater et al. (2001) were similar to those identified by Rubin and Peyrot (1992) nearly a decade earlier (i.e., small samples conducted at specific sites and measurement issues). Delamater et al. also described salient methodological problems such as use of glycemic control as the sole measure of intervention effectiveness, failure to target subgroups (e.g., by age, socioeconomic status, or ethnicity) in the intervention approach, the need to generalize study findings to clinical care, and the need to document the cost-effectiveness of psychological interventions in clinical settings.

Hampson et al.'s (2000, 2001) systematic reviews of research concerning behavioral interventions for adolescents with DM1 identified 64 reports of empirical studies, including 24 RCTs and 35 controlled studies (non-RCTs), and calculated ESs for 18 studies. The mean ES of 0.33 across all outcomes indicated that interventions had a small- to medium-size effect on diabetes management. The most commonly used interventions identified in this review included skills training (46%), family-centered interventions (26%), dietary interventions (20%), and problem-solving interventions (20%). Interventions were most commonly targeted to groups (46%) as opposed to individuals (23%) or families (14%). Where specified in the study methods, the interventions were most likely to be conducted by psychologists (30%), nurses (27%), or physicians (15%; Hampson et al., 2000, 2001).

Consistent with Delamater's (2002) review, the most common (71%) intervention outcome in Hampson et al.'s (2001) review was blood sugar control, followed by measures of individual or family functioning (57%; e.g., self-efficacy for diabetes management, family conflict, diabetes-specific stress, and QOL). Knowledge was assessed in 26% of the studies reviewed, whereas diabetes self-management behaviors, such as adherence to prescribed dietary regimens, were less commonly assessed (11%). The majority of the studies that were reviewed (63%) did not include any follow-up assessment after assessments conducted immediately after the intervention (Hampson et al., 2000).

With respect to the strength of intervention effects for different categories of interventions, the largest mean ESs (0.37) were obtained for psychosocial outcomes (e.g., psychological distress) compared with ESs for blood sugar control (0.33), self-management (–0.15), or knowledge (0.16). It is important to note that the mean ES for theoretically based interventions (0.47) was significantly larger than the mean ES for atheoretical interventions (0.06; Hampson et al., 2000).

Methodological limitations of studies that were reviewed by Hampson et al. (2000) included small sample sizes and relative absence of theoretically informed studies, longer term follow-up and cost-effectiveness studies, and description of the maintenance of intervention effects in clinical care settings. Hampson et al. (2000) also noted that in general, the interventions that were reviewed had modest effects. On the other hand, even relatively modest effects of interventions on blood sugar control were found to improve the health of children and adolescents with DM1 if they were sustained over a period of time (Hampson et al., 2000). Finally, it should also be noted that some psychological interventions were delivered in conjunction with diabetes education and skills-enhancement interventions received by children and families at the time of the diagnosis of DM1. This limited the degree to which intervention effects could be attributed to specific psychological intervention models (Hampson et al., 2000).

EXAMPLES OF STUDIES OF PSYCHOLOGICAL INTERVENTIONS IN PEDIATRIC TYPE 1 DIABETES

The results of previous reviews underscore the efficacy of several models of psychological interventions for patients with DM1. In this section, specific examples of representative psychological interventions that were designed to enhance illness management and psychological adaptation in children and adolescents with DM1 are described.

Individual Behavioral Management Approaches

Mendez and Belendez (1997) evaluated the effects of a behavioral program to increase treatment adherence and to improve stress management in adolescents with DM1 by using a quasi-experimental pretest–posttest design with a nonequivalent control group. A total of 12 intervention sessions encompassed a wide range of procedures, including instruction, blood glucose discrimination training, role-playing, relaxation exercises, self-instructions, problem-solving strategies, and homework, among others. The results showed such significant positive changes in the experimental group as diabetes knowledge adherence, management of daily hassles, ease of social interactions, glucose testing, blood glucose estimate errors, and so on, and these improvements were maintained at a follow-up 13 months after the end of the program. On the other hand, the program had no effect on either diet and physical exercise or glycemic control.

Grey et al. (1998) conducted an RCT to determine whether a behavioral intervention (coping skills training [CST]) combined with intensive diabetes management improved metabolic control and QOL in adolescents who received intensive therapy for DM1. Adolescents received either intensive diabetes management with CST or intensive management without CST. CST included a series of small group measures designed to teach adolescents coping skills by social problem solving, social skills training, cognitive–behavioral modification, and conflict resolution. Adolescents who received CST had lower HbA_{1c}, had better diabetes self-efficacy, and were less upset about coping with diabetes than adolescents who received intensive management alone. In addition, adolescents who received CST found it easier to cope with diabetes and experienced less negative impact of diabetes on QOL than those who did not receive CST. The coping skills intervention had durable effects on metabolic control and QOL (Grey, Boland, Davidson, Li, & Tamborlane, 2000).

In an RCT, Howells et al. (2002) studied changes in self-efficacy for self-management in adolescents with DM1 participating in a negotiated telephone support (NTS) intervention developed using the principles of problem solving and social learning theory. Adolescents were randomized into three groups: continued routine management, continued routine management with NTS, or annual clinic with NTS. The second and third groups received an average of 16 telephone calls per year. After 1 year, the participants in the two intervention groups showed significant improvements in self-efficacy, but there was no difference in glycemic control in the three groups.

Family-Centered Approaches

Laffel et al. (2003) evaluated an ambulatory, family-focused intervention designed to enhance glycemic control, minimize diabetes-related family conflict, and maintain QOL in youths with Type 1 diabetes. Children and adolescents were assigned to a family-focused teamwork intervention or to standard multidisciplinary diabetes care. Patients in both study groups were seen at 3- to 4-month intervals and were followed prospectively for 1 year. Families exposed to the family-focused teamwork intervention maintained or increased family involvement significantly more than families who received standard care. In multivariate analysis, the family teamwork intervention and the daily frequency of blood glucose significantly predicted HbA_{1c}. The teamwork group reported no increase in diabetes-related family conflict or decrease in QOL.

Wysocki et al. (2001) found that behavioral family systems therapy, which was designed to enhance blood sugar control and adherence to treatment, improved family communication skills and reduced family conflict but did not result in improvements in adherence to treatment. Additional studies of behavioral family systems therapy have been conducted by Harris, Harris, and Mertlich (2005) and Harris and Mertlich (2003) with adolescents with poorly controlled diabetes. Although the initial posttreatment evaluation indicated decreases in general family conflict, diabetes-related family conflict, and behavior problems, evaluation at 6-month follow-up demonstrated that initial posttreatment improvements were no longer present for any of the variables assessed. Metabolic control remained unchanged from baseline to initial posttreatment as well as at 6-month follow-up (Harris et al., 2005).

Ellis, Frey, et al. (2005) and Ellis, Naar-King, et al. (2005) studied whether multisystemic therapy (MST), an intensive, home-based psychotherapy, could decrease rates of hospital utilization and related costs of care among adolescents with poorly controlled DM1. Adolescents were randomly assigned to receive either MST (duration of 6 months) or standard care. The MST treatment lasted approximately 6 months, and all participants were followed for 9 months. Intervention was associated with significant improvements in frequency of blood glucose testing (Ellis, Frey, et al., 2005; Ellis, Naar-King, et al., 2005). In addition, intervention participants had a decreasing number of hospitalizations from the baseline period to the end of the study, whereas the number of inpatient DM1 sessions increased for controls. Medical care costs were also lower for adolescents receiving MST. However, use of the emergency room did not differ in the groups. Correlational analyses indicated that decreases in inpatient DM1 sessions were associated with improved metabolic control for participants who received MST and not standard care (Ellis, Frey, et al., 2005; Ellis, Naar-King, et al., 2005). These findings suggest that MST has the potential to decrease inpatient DM1 sessions among adolescents who are nonadherent to medical treatment for DM1, which is an important clinical problem that is referred to pediatric psychologists.

RECOMMENDATIONS FOR FUTURE INTERVENTION RESEARCH

Reviews of psychological intervention research in DM1 have provided important research-related recommendations that are summarized here. A priority in future research will be to improve the power and sustainability of the effects of psychological interventions on the medical and functional outcomes of children and adolescents with DM1 and DM2. One way to accomplish this would be to test the efficacy of strategies that combine components of psychological interventions that have been shown to be effective in previous studies (e.g., family problem solving and behavioral management). Other priorities involve improving the methodology of intervention studies by including larger samples and analyses of factors that mediate positive intervention change (Rubin & Peyrot, 1992).

Delamater et al. (2001) described the following research priorities that focus on tailoring psychological interventions to individual differences in children and adolescents with DM1 or DM2. These priorities included the following: (a) testing psychological interventions for children and adolescents with DM1 who are undergoing critical developmental transitions (e.g., transition to adolescence, transition to adulthood), (b) evaluating interventions for high-risk patients who demonstrate poor regimen adherence and response to risk factors such as psychopathology and family dysfunction, and (c) conducting interventions that are tailored to culturally diverse populations of children and adolescents with DM1 and DM2.

Studies of Clinical Effectiveness of Interventions

A critical mass of psychological intervention research has been conducted for children and adolescents with DM1 and have shown the efficacy of cognitive–behavioral and family-centered interventions. Norris et al.'s (2002) review of the clinical effectiveness of diabetes self-management education conducted in community settings underscored the need for additional research on the clinical effectiveness of interventions in home, camp, and school settings. Specific recommendations from this review included the following: (a) identifying effective components of the intervention that is delivered in the home settings, (b) evaluating the optimal intensity and duration of interventions and person to deliver the interventions, (c) identifying those who would benefit most from interventions (e.g., racial and socioeconomic moderators of intervention effects), and (d) conducting comprehensive assessment of intervention outcomes that are tailored to the setting. In addition, Delamater et al. (2001) recommended an increased focus on documenting clinical significance of psychological intervention studies for DM1 and DM2 (e.g., studies of cost-effectiveness, social acceptability, long-term follow-up) and inclusion of measures of individual and family functioning and health-related QOL to complement the typical outcomes of blood sugar control.

Hampson et al. (2000) carried out a study based on the work of Glasgow, Vogt, and Boles (1999) in which they evaluated the extent to which the psychological interventions with the largest ESs reported in their review could be applied to health care settings (see chap. 11, this volume, for more extensive discussion of applications of interventions). The intervention studies that produced the largest ES in each of the categories, and any study that produced an ES of at least 0.30 in more than one category, were identified as candidates for potential application in health care settings (Hampson et al., 2000). In the category of psychosocial interventions, B. J. Anderson et al.'s (1999) intervention model, which encouraged parent–teen responsibility for sharing diabetes tasks, produced the largest ES (0.72) on parental ratings of unsupportive behavior and family conflict. The potential of this intervention to be adapted in clinical settings was judged as being high for the following reasons: The majority (76%) of eligible families who attended a specialist clinic participated, the nurse-led intervention can be conducted as part of routine medical care, and a written intervention protocol is available.

The largest ESs for blood sugar control (1.18 and 2.03) were obtained in a study by Satin et al. (1989) that involved six weekly multifamily group therapy sessions with a professional group leader to address issues of living with diabetes and improving adherence. Nevertheless, Hampson et al. (2000) concluded that widespread adoption of this intervention would be unlikely for the following reasons: Participation rates were not reported, the intervention requires a professional group leader trained in group therapy, and intervention depends on the degree of parents' willingness to attend numerous sessions and to conduct a demanding simulation (including injecting saline solution and blood testing).

The largest ES on diabetes-related knowledge (0.47) was demonstrated by Pichert, Snyder, Kinzer, and Boswell's (1994) study in which adolescents at summer camp attended four nurse-led group sessions, were taught theoretical principles of anchored (problem-focused) instruction, and discussed a video depicting a person with diabetes taking a daylong boat trip that included numerous problems for diabetes management. However, owing to its highly specific content, this intervention approach was expected to have limited applicability to clinic settings (Hampson et al., 2000).

The intervention evaluated by Grey, Boland, Davidson, Yu, and Tamborlane (1999) was the only one to report an ES of at least 0.30 for psychological outcomes (e.g., measures of coping and self-efficacy) and blood sugar control. Grey et al.'s intervention model included training in coping skills in groups attended by adolescents and led by nurse practitioners, which was provided as an adjunct to intensive insulin therapy. The potential for clinical application of this intervention model was rated as good, based on the fact that the majority (71%) of eligible adolescents from a specialized diabetes clinic agreed to participate and the detailed manual that was used to implement the study (Hampson et al., 2000).

Hampson et al.'s (2000) review suggests that the choice of psychological interventions to be tested in studies of clinical effectiveness should be guided by the clinical applicability of the intervention (Clement, 1995; Glasgow et al., 1999). In addition, as suggested by Rubin and Peyrot (1992), studies of clinical effectiveness would be enhanced by data concerning the types of behavioral and psychological problems encountered among children and adolescents with DM1 or DM2, the prevalence and intensity of different types of interventions that are delivered in clinical care, and the characteristics of practitioners (Rubin & Peyrot, 1992).

Economic Costs Versus Benefits of Comprehensive Diabetes Education and Support

Another relevant area for future research includes studies of the economic costs of various methods of diabetes education, including those that focus on children and adolescents who are newly diagnosed with DM1. For example, Dougherty, Soderstrom, and Schiffrin (1998) conducted a study of the cost of intensive home care including insulin and diabetes self-management for a group of children and adolescents ages 2 to 17 years who were newly diagnosed with DM1. Following diagnosis and hospitalization to stabilize their metabolic control, home-care patients were discharged whereas traditional care patients remained hospitalized for insulin adjustment and self-management education. Home-care intervention included visits by a specially trained nurse who was also available by phone. Blood glucose control was lower for the home-care patients at 24 and 36 months, and costs of the program were lower as well. Because this study was conducted in Canada, it is not directly applicable to the U.S. health care system.

To address this need for studies in the United States, Cuttler et al. (2004) conducted a study that compared intensive outpatient management, which included nursing education and support, medical care, nutritional education, crisis support, and anticipatory guidance by a psychologist, with traditional inpatient management of children and adolescents who were newly diagnosed with DM1. The outpatient management program was much less costly, but the programs had comparable effects on health and psychological well-being. No group differences were found on initial follow-up at 3 months or at 6- and 12-month outcome on blood sugar control, knowledge, child and family adaptation, or QOL.

Studies of costs and benefits of comprehensive care interventions for children and adolescents with DM1 and DM2 might be expanded to studies of psychological interventions. In this regard, important but as-yet-unanswered questions are raised by whether the inclusion of psychological interventions in medical care results in a reduction in costs of medical care. For example, the inclusion of psychological interventions in comprehensive medical care programs for children and adolescents with DM1 and DM2 may result in cost savings from lower health care utilization, reduction of the time required by physicians and nurses, and reduction of complications due to DM1. To my knowledge, this hypothesis has yet to be tested in formal studies of cost-effectiveness. On the other hand, Ellis, Frey, et al. (2005) and Ellis, Naar-King, et al. (2005) demonstrated that as an intensive psychological intervention, MST resulted in decreased numbers of hospitalizations and lower costs of care for children and adolescents with DM1 with histories of recurrent ketoacidosis and frequent health care utilizations.

IMPLICATIONS FOR CLINICAL CARE

The clinical relevance of addressing psychological factors in the management of DM1 is well recognized (B. J. Anderson & Rubin, 2002). Clement (1995) defined diabetes self-management as the process of providing the person with diabetes with the knowledge and skills needed to perform self-care, manage crises, and make lifestyle changes that are needed to successfully manage their diabetes on a day-to-day basis. For children and adolescents, this requires a family-centered approach in which parents and children are involved collaboratively. Moreover, the approach involves a number of different professional disciplines with expertise in a range of clinically relevant areas.

In many clinical settings, diabetes self-management education has evolved to include comprehensive programs, some of which include psychologists. Specific standards for such education include the following: (a) assessment of educational needs; (b) comprehensive instruction tailored to needs and deficiencies; (c) communication with physicians; (d) use of behavioral management strategies, including reinforcement of adaptive self-management behaviors; and (e) instruction in the use of self-monitoring of blood glucose data (Clement, 1995).

To address the above needs, a number of centers have integrated the services of pediatric psychologists and other professionals (e.g., social workers) into the ongoing comprehensive care of children and adolescents with diabetes (B. Anderson, Loughlin, Goldberg, & Laffel, 2001). In this regard, Rubin and Peyrot (1992) noted, on the basis of their experience, that the typical interventions used by psychologists at individual centers ranged from short-term coping-focused interventions for distress to intensive individual and family therapy. On the other hand, standards for the allocation of psychological intervention services for DM1 and DM2 in clinical settings have not been established and are challenging: Rubin and Peyrot highlighted the tension between the mandate to deliver short-term interventions for problems of high prevalence and low acuity versus those that are needed to manage infrequent but serious, potentially life-threatening problems such as recurrent ketoacidosis.

Comprehensive psychological interventions that are designed to enhance management and improve dietary regimens and exercise behavior for DM2 will assume increasing priority given the prevalence of this condition (American Diabetes Association, 2000). For this reason, increasing attention should be given to developing and testing psychological interventions with children and adolescents with DM2 in clinical care settings and in RCTs (Pinkas-Hamiel et al., 1996). One example of this is the multisite Treatment Options for Type 2 Diabetes in Adolescents and Youth (TODAY) study, which has been designed to test the efficacy of new interventions compared with treatment as usual. The two new interventions are medication (metformin) treatment and a combination of medications (e.g., metformin and rosiglitasome) along with intensive lifestyle intervention involving behavioral change in nutrition and exercise and the effect of these treatments on the glycemic control and rate of weight gain of adolescents with DM2 (National Institute of Diabetes and Digestive and Kidney Diseases, 2003).

Targeting Interventions in Clinical Care for Type 1 and Type 2 Diabetes

Taken together, the data from these studies and reviews indicate that various psychological intervention strategies can be effectively tailored to the specific burdens and illness management issues that are encountered in DM1 and DM2 and delivered in the context of clinical care. For example, cognitive and behavioral interventions involving coping skills and problem solving may be useful in managing the stressors associated with DM1 and in enhancing adherence to treatment. In addition, family-centered cognitive–behavioral interventions are also effective in enhancing adherence to treatment in DM1 and may need to be incorporated into clinical care (Laffel et al., 2003).

Experienced psychological practitioners and researchers have summarized useful recommendations for incorporating clinical psychological interventions in the routine medical care of children and adolescents with DM1 and their families. For example, Wysocki (in press) has recommended the following: (a) ensure that behavior change specialists work closely with the other members of the diabetes team and have thorough knowledge about diabetes and its treatment, (b) make routine use of behavior modification to enhance diabetes management, (c) provide consultation with patients and families concerning effective behavior management soon after the diagnosis of diabetes, and (d) conduct routine psychological screening of youths and families and give diabetes health care professionals specific criteria for referring families for psychological services.

Delamater's (2002) recommendations for clinical care focused on strategies to help the parents of children with DM1 accomplish the following tasks: (a) develop realistic expectations concerning their children's responsibility for self-management, (b) facilitate competent self-care attitudes in their children, and (c) understand and manage their children's social adjustment and self-esteem. In addition, Delamater suggested a number of proactive psychological interventions that can be implemented in a preventive approach. These included helping parents and children to manage critical issues such as acceptance of the diagnosis of DM1 and its implications, manage their psychological reactions to the diagnosis, learn skills related to diabetes management such as avoiding and treating hypoglycemia, and develop realistic attitudes toward glycemic control. As with other chronic conditions, effective clinical management of DM1 is best tailored to the developmental needs of children and adolescents. For example, adolescents have special needs to be involved in their diabetes care in collaboration with parents (B. J. Anderson & Rubin, 2002; Rubin, 2002).

Improving the Delivery of Medical Care for Type 1 and Type 2 Diabetes

A final set of recommendations for clinical care of DM1 and DM2 also involve the clinical application and delivery of medical care and psychological interventions to vulnerable subgroups of the population. For example, the consensus of experts who evaluated the status of behavioral research with adults (Glasgow, Hiss, et al., 2001) concluded that health care delivery and psychological interventions have not been as effective in reaching vulnerable segments of the DM1 and DM2 populations, such as patients who are elderly, minority, or of low socioeconomic status. Similar conclusions can be drawn for the medical and psychosocial care of children and adolescents with DM1 or DM2.

To address the above need, Glasgow, McKay, Piette, and Reynolds (2001) recommended a population-based systems approach to care delivery for DM1 and DM2. This approach includes the following key elements: (a) continuity of care and health surveillance, (b) patient-centered collaborative goal setting, and (c) consistent follow-up visits that are focused on key medical outcomes. Some of these recommendations are applicable to children and adolescents, many of whom are cared for by diabetes subspecialists. For example, research concerning health care utilization during early adulthood suggests that young adults with DM1 visit health care providers infrequently for routine or preventive services and are far more prone to utilize health care services episodically or in response to specific crises (Bartsch, Barnes, Jarrett, & Lindsey, 1989). One reason is that once adolescents with DM1 establish independence from their families, they may withdraw from regular health care supervision (Olsen & Sutton, 1998).

There are at least three important but as yet unanswered questions that relate to the delivery of psychological interventions in the clinical care of children and adolescents with DM1 or DM2 that should be considered in the future research and clinical care agendas. First, what is the most effective way to integrate behavioral principles into routine medical care for children and adolescents with DM1 or DM2? Second, what is the optimal role of the psychologist in comprehensive care for children and adolescents with DM1 or DM2? Third, what is the best way to finance comprehensive medical care involving psychological services for children and adolescents with DM1 or DM2? These are complex questions that have no easy answers. Nevertheless, addressing these salient questions will improve the clinical care and outcomes of children and adolescents with DM1 or DM2.

8

PSYCHOLOGICAL INTERVENTIONS: PEDIATRIC CANCER

Pediatric malignancies include a range of conditions such as acute lymphoblastic leukemia (ALL); central nervous system (CNS) tumors; lymphomas; and soft tissue, bone, and eye tumors (Stehbens, 1985). Although cancer is a relatively rare disease, occurring sometime between birth and age 20 in 1 out of every 330 children and adolescents in the United States (Ross, Severson, Pollock, & Robinson, 1996), it is the leading cause of death by disease for children in the United States under age 15 (Ross et al., 1996). However, advances in cancer treatment over the past 30 years have improved the overall 5-year survival rate for children and adolescents to nearly 75% (Vannatta & Gerhardt, 2003). Compared with many other pediatric chronic conditions, pediatric cancer has several special clinical features: It is life threatening and includes highly intensive medical treatment that encompasses distinct stages. These features have salient implications for psychological interventions.

MEDICAL TREATMENT

The medical treatment of pediatric cancer is complex and arduous and, depending on the specific type of cancer, can involve chemotherapy,

Catherine Cant Peterson made significant contributions to the writing of this chapter and in the creation of the table.

radiation, and/or surgery. For example, most children with ALL, the most common form of cancer, are first treated with a month-long course of chemotherapy to induce remission, followed by 8 to 12 months of intensive continuous therapy, which can be administered by injection, lumbar puncture, oral medication, or a combination of these. After these chemotherapy cycles are completed, patients begin maintenance therapy, which is characterized by a shift to multiple orally administered medications for 2 to 3 years. Children with cancer in the United States are often treated in the context of controlled clinical trials, which include standardized protocols that are administered across multiple clinical sites. Finally, another relevant clinical feature of cancer is that in contrast to other chronic conditions (e.g., diabetes, cystic fibrosis), the majority of children and adolescents are considered "cured" of cancer once they have remained in remission for 5 years, though adverse late effects of cancer can occur after completion of treatment (Vanatta & Gerhardt, 2003).

Many children and adolescents with cancer experience multiple intrusive and painful diagnostic procedures. For example, children and adolescents may undergo bone marrow aspirations involving inserting a needle into the bone and lumbar punctures involving inserting a needle into the spinal fluid. They also undergo venipunctures that are administered over multiple periods of time and may engender significant psychological distress as well as nonadherence (DuHamel, Redd, & Vickberg-Johnson, 1999). In addition to experiencing the pain and anxiety associated with medical procedures, children and adolescents also must manage aversive side effects associated with radiation and chemotherapy treatments, including fatigue, diarrhea, hair loss, and posttreatment nausea. After multiple chemotherapy treatments, some children and adolescents may develop anticipatory nausea (DuHamel et al., 1999). The impact of these stressful experiences (e.g., psychological and physical symptoms) comprises relevant targets of psychological intervention (Kuppenheimer & Brown, 2002).

Other functional consequences of cancer and its treatment can include missed school days and social activities, physical limitations, and problems in cognitive functioning (Butler, 1998; Carey, Barakat, Foley, Gyato, & Phillips, 2001; Mulhern, Hancock, Fairclough, & Run, 1992). Children may also have problems in cognitive functioning that are associated with the CNS effects of cancer-related treatment, effects of tumors of the CNS, and treatment for these tumors (Armstrong & Briery, 2004). In addition, children who experience tumors of the CNS may demonstrate slowed processing speed and perceptual motor and memory difficulties (Armstrong & Briery, 2004; Butler & Mulhern, 2005; Moore, 2005). These deficits may affect learning and performance in school that can be stressful for children and families and require psychological intervention (C. C. Peterson & Drotar, in press).

Children and adolescents with cancer must manage the psychological challenges of transitions in phases of medical treatment. For example, school reentry and social reintegration with peers after hospitalization and intensive treatment can be challenging (Varni et al., 1993). Further, the transition from cancer treatment to survivorship can elicit psychological distress, such as perceived vulnerability and worry about relapse (Koocher & O'Malley, 1981). The impact of cancer on children's functioning in life contexts such as school is also a relevant focus of psychological intervention (R. T. Brown, 2004; Clay, 2004).

PSYCHOLOGICAL IMPACT ON CHILDREN AND ADOLESCENTS

The psychological stress, treatment-related side effects, and functional deficits associated with pediatric cancer threaten children's social adjustment (Katz, Rubinstein, Hubert, & Blew, 1988) and emotional well-being (Kazak, 2001). However, considerable variation in the degree and nature of psychological adjustment problems associated with pediatric cancer has been observed. In general, studies that have used control groups, multiple information sources, and standardized measures have identified fewer psychological problems among children and adolescents with cancer than less well-designed studies (Noll et al., 1996; Vanatta & Gerhardt, 2003).

As noted by Vanatta and Gerhardt (2003), longitudinal studies suggest that children who have been recently diagnosed with cancer initially experience increased levels of distress associated with their psychological response to the hospitalization and initiation of treatment, invasive procedures, and intensive chemotherapy compared with healthy comparison children (Sawyer, Antoniou, Toogood, & Rice, 1997; Sawyer, Antoniou, Toogood, Rice, & Baghurst, 2000). On the other hand, the majority of children and adolescents with cancer do not experience psychological problems that are serious enough to disrupt their functioning following completion of cancer treatment (Sawyer et al., 1997, 2000). Similar to other children with chronic illness (Lavigne & Faier-Routman, 1992), children and adolescents with cancer with the highest risk for peer-related difficulties are those whose illness treatment has affected the CNS or who have obvious changes in physical appearance (Reiter-Purtill & Noll, 2003). Taken together, the results of research on psychological adjustment of children and adolescents underscore the need to target psychological interventions at stages of cancer treatment that engender the most significant levels of distress for children with cancer and their families. Moreover, the needs of particularly vulnerable subgroups of children and adolescents with cancer (e.g., the most distressed children) ought to be addressed in interventions (Vanatta & Gerhardt, 2003).

Survivors of pediatric malignancies remain at risk for a recurrence, and a minority develop a secondary cancer within 20 years of their initial diagnosis. Children who have completed treatment for cancer and are considered cured remain at increased risk for adverse late effects, including endocrine and thyroid complications (e.g., growth problems, obesity, and reproductive difficulties); cardiac, pulmonary, renal and urological, gastrointestinal, ocular, and dental problems; and impairments and functional limitations (e.g., diminished stamina). These effects may not be apparent immediately after completion of cancer treatment but can emerge years later (Vanatta & Gerhardt, 2003). A wide range of psychological adjustment patterns have been identified among the survivors of pediatric cancer. Rates of posttraumatic stress disorder (PTSD) have been reported in approximately 5% to 12% of childhood cancer survivors and 20% of young adults (Kazak, Alderfer, Streisand, Simms, & Rourke, in press; Kazak et al., 2001). Rates of subclinical levels of distress are even more frequent (Kazak, Alderfer, Streisand, et al., in press). These data indicate that psychological distress can be an important focus of psychological intervention for survivors of pediatric cancer. The psychological impact of pediatric cancer and associated treatment in children is illustrated by the problems experienced by Cassandra, a 16-year-old with a history of ALL who has successfully completed cancer treatment and is about to begin the maintenance phase of treatment. Cassandra has recently developed symptoms of anxiety and avoidance of peer relationships, which have caused her and her family a great deal of distress. She reports feeling anxious without knowing why. However, in more in-depth interviews, she reports nightmares and flashbacks that relate to experiences with treatment for her cancer. She and her parents are also very fearful of recurrence of cancer as treatment ends. Cassandra's problems will require psychological intervention.

IMPACT OF PEDIATRIC CANCER ON PARENTS AND FAMILY MEMBERS

Given the arduous nature of treatment for this life-threatening condition, providing care and support for their children and adolescents with cancer places extraordinary demands on parents and family members (Sahler et al., 2002). Not surprisingly, prospective studies have indicated that parental distress, particularly anxiety and depression, are higher immediately following diagnosis of cancer for both mothers and fathers compared with controls or norms. However, symptoms typically decline to normal levels after the first year (Kupst et al., 1995; Sawyer et al., 1997). For example, Steele, Long, Reddy, Luhr, and Phipps (2003) found that the perceived stress and psychological distress reported by mothers of children with cancer decreased over the initial 6 months of diagnosis, but caregiver burden remained stable. Rates of PTSD among parents of pediatric cancer survivors range from 5% to 25% (Kazak et al., 1997; Manne, DuHamel, Gallelli, Sorgen, & Redd, 1998). In addition, mothers and fathers have been found to have significantly higher levels of posttraumatic stress symptoms (PTSS) than parents of never-ill children (Kazak et al., 1997, 1998). Similar posttraumatic stress symptoms have been described in siblings of survivors (Alderfer, Labay, & Kazak, 2003). Parents have also reported feelings of uncertainty and loneliness after the cessation of their children's cancer treatment (Dongen-Melman et al., 1995) as well as concerns about their child's future development and opportunities (Greenberg & Meadows, 1992). The stressors and burdens experienced by family members in response to pediatric cancer present important opportunities for psychological intervention, including preventive interventions (Kazak, 2005).

ADHERENCE TO MEDICAL TREATMENT

Curing cancer and preventing cancer relapse can reduce morbidity and save lives. However, modern pediatric cancer requires a complex, burdensome regimen that necessitates patient adherence to a lengthy course of therapy that may be very difficult for many children, adolescents, and their parents to manage effectively (Nachman, Sather, & Buckley, 1993). Much of the most arduous medical treatment provided during the intensive phase of chemotherapy for pediatric cancer is administered by medical staff. For this reason, there is less opportunity for nonadherence. On the other hand, the transition to maintenance therapy includes a shift to orally administered medication, which involves much less direct supervision and control by medical caregivers and hence much more independent responsibility on the part of parents and adolescents than the intensive medical treatment phase. For example, standard maintenance therapy for ALL, the most common form of cancer, includes four medications: daily oral mercaptopurine, weekly oral methotrexate, a 5-day oral steroid course every 28 days, and a single dose of intravenous vincristine each month taken over 1 to 2 years. The overall burden of treatment adherence as defined by numbers and doses of prescribed medication, coupled with the increased level of responsibility that is assumed by children, adolescents, and parents for managing treatment, underscores the risk of nonadherence during the maintenance phase of treatment.

In fact, available evidence suggests that many children and adolescents with ALL do not take their oral medication in accord with their prescribed treatment regimens. Moreover, as is the case for other chronic pediatric conditions, nonadherence to treatment for cancer, including ALL, is much higher among adolescents than among younger children (Festa, Tamaroff, Chasalow, & Lanzkowsky, 1992; Lau, Matsui, Greenberg, & Koren, 1998; Tebbi et al., 1986). In a recent study, Kennard et al. (2004) used a blood assay to detect nonadherence to prophylactic oral trimethoprim/sulfa methotazole (Bactrim) among adolescents with cancer, including ALL, and found that 27% of patients had no detectable medication. Survival rates were lower in the group of patients categorized as nonadherent. Finally, at least two reviews (Davies & Lilleyman, 1995; Partridge, Avorn, Wang, & Winer, 2002) and a report by the International Society of Pediatric Oncology Working Committee on Psychosocial Issues have also underscored the scope and clinical significance of nonadherence to treatment among adolescents with cancer (Spinetta et al., 2002). Given the necessity of treatment adherence for achieving a cure (Relling, Hancock, Boyett, Pui, & Evans, 1999), these data underscore the importance of providing psychological interventions to prevent or limit the frequency of nonadherence to pediatric cancer treatment.

REVIEWS OF PSYCHOLOGICAL INTERVENTIONS FOR PEDIATRIC CANCER

Given the frequency of painful procedures (injection, lumbar puncture) that are experienced by children and adolescents with cancer, psychological interventions that are designed to lessen the pain and distress associated with treatment-related procedures are particularly important with this population. There has been a sufficient body of empirical research on procedure-related interventions to warrant several published reviews. For example, Powers's (1999) review of intervention studies for procedure-related pain, the majority of which focused on pediatric cancer, concluded that cognitive–behavioral therapy, including a range of methods (e.g., breathing exercises, relaxation imagery, filmed modeling, behavioral rehearsal reinforcement, and active coaching), was a well-established treatment. McQuaid and Nassau (1999) reviewed 10 studies of psychological interventions designed to reduce the physical symptoms associated with cancer side effects and concluded that interventions such as imagery with suggestion could be classified as well established, distraction with relaxation as probably efficacious, and video-games as promising.

Kuppenheimer and Brown (2002) conducted an in-depth review of the findings of cognitive–behavioral, pharmacological, and combination interventions that have been designed to facilitate relief of distress during cancer-related procedures. Cognitive–behavioral interventions were demonstrated to be efficacious in managing procedural distress by enhancing children's and adolescents' sense of self-efficacy when exposed to painful procedures. Moreover, these interventions were noted to have the advantages of safety and shorter recovery time than either anesthesia or pharmacotherapy (Kuppenheimer & Brown, 2002). On the other hand, the findings of cognitive–behavioral interventions were noted to be limited by small sample sizes, failure to control for the length of time since cancer diagnosis, previous experience with procedures, overreliance on a single outcome measure, and use of comprehensive approaches, which made it impossible to identify the specific intervention components that were most effective.

It should be noted that pharmacological interventions were found to be relatively safe and effective when administered by medical personnel but may cause side effects and involve significant recovery time (Kuppenheimer & Brown, 2002). However, systematic controlled empirical studies of their efficacy or effectiveness have generally not been conducted. For example, only one or two clinical trials have been conducted with medications (Kuppenheimer & Brown, 2002).

The studies that have compared cognitive–behavioral interventions with pharmacological interventions have generally indicated that pharmacotherapy is no more effective than cognitive–behavioral interventions in the management of distress (Kuppenheimer & Brown, 2002). However, Kazak, Penati, et al. (1996) found that children who received cognitive–behavioral interventions had less distress than children who received pharmacological interventions only. Kuppenheimer and Brown (2002) suggested that pharmacological and cognitive–behavioral interventions offer distinct benefits and disadvantages. Finally, it has been suggested that tailoring cognitive–behavioral interventions on the basis of characteristics such as children's age (Jay et al., 1987; Kazak et al., 1996), developmental level, length of time since diagnosis, and experience with procedures may be valuable (Kuppenheimer & Brown, 2002).

EXAMPLES OF PSYCHOLOGICAL INTERVENTIONS FOR PEDIATRIC CANCER

The empirical support for psychological interventions designed to enhance the mental health and treatment adherence of children with cancer is not as extensive as it is for interventions designed to alleviate distress during painful procedures. Nevertheless, psychological intervention approaches have been developed and tested to promote social skills, school reintegration, and psychological adaptation of survivors and parents. To my knowledge, detailed systematic reviews of such research have not been published. However, the results of published psychological interventions that are designed to reduce the psychological impact of pediatric cancer are shown in Table 8.1. Specific

TABLE 8.1
Description of Psychological Interventions in Pediatric Cancer

Authors	Intervention and design	Sample	Frequency	Follow-up	Measures	Intervention effects	
						+ Significant	− Nonsignificant
				Social skills training			
Barakat et al. (2003)	Communication skills, empathy, conflict resolution, cooperation	13 (8–14 years), mixed brain tumors (single group study)	6 weekly small group sessions	6 weeks (1 year total study)	Social skills and competence (child, parent, teacher reports; CBCL) internalizing, externalizing, and adaptive behavior (child, parent, teacher reports)	Child-reported social competence, parent-reported total competence, and child-reported internalizing, and symptoms	Self-reports of externalizing behavior
Varni et al. (1993)	Problem solving, assertiveness training, handling teasing versus standard school reintegration (education, support, conferences, classroom presentations)	64 (5–13 years), mixed cancer	3 individual 60-minute sessions plus 2 booster sessions	9 months	Child depression, anxiety, self-esteem, perceived social support, parent-reported behavioral and emotional problems, social competence.	Behavior problems improved more in social skills group, reported reduced state anxiety, increased social support, and reduced behavior problems (6 months) and reduced behavior problems	Social competence (9 months)
				School reintegration			
McCarthy et al. (1998)	School reentry program (including meeting with school personnel and parents, meeting with classmates, and teaching doll and videotape for younger children)	10 (5–13 years), diagnoses not reported	Meeting with school personnel: 30–60 minutes; meeting with classmates: 15–45 minutes	Up to 1 year post-intervention	Parent and teacher concerns postintervention; evaluation of program	Evaluations of the program were all positive	Parent and teacher concerns about child's health, safety, and academic progress; children's concerns about keeping up with school activities

Study	Intervention	Sample	Duration	Timing	Outcome measures	Results	Focus
Katz et al. (1988)	Preventive education with medical and school staff, hospital-based liaison, counseling, preparation of child and parents, presentations to school personnel and classmates, follow-up	49 (5–17 years) in intervention group, 36 in comparison group; mixed cancer (excluding brain tumor)	Not reported	1–15 months between pre- and posttesting for intervention group	Child behavior problems, social competence, depressive symptoms, self-perceived social–physical–cognitive competence, age-appropriate school behavior	Intervention group increased in competence between pre- and posttesting, and competence ratings were higher than for the control group. Intervention group had better teacher-reported adjustment and higher competence than control group.	Depression
Katz et al. (1992)	Preventive education with medical and school staff, hospital-based liaison, counseling and preparation of child and parent, presentations to school personnel and classmates, follow-up	49 (5–17 years), mixed cancer	Not reported	Not reported	Parent, child, and teacher evaluation of helpfulness of school reintegration intervention	Children rated favorably, and parents rated as important and useful in attaining goals of school reentry. Teachers rated favorably across several areas, including knowledge gained, social acceptance of child, effectiveness of intervention.	
Cognitive–behavioral interventions: Cancer survivors							
Hoekstra-Weebers et al. (1998)	Cognitive–behavioral identification and challenge of automatic thoughts, problem-focused coping, communication, and assertiveness skills versus standard care	81 (intervention, n = 39; control, n = 42; children 0–16 years), mixed cancer	Eight 90-minute sessions	6 months post-diagnosis	Psychological functioning, state and trait anxiety, social support, intensity of emotions		Psychological functioning and social support

(continued)

TABLE 8.1 (Continued)

Authors	Intervention and design	Sample	Frequency	Follow-up	Measures	Intervention effects + Significant	Intervention effects – Nonsignificant
					Cognitive–behavioral interventions: Cancer survivors		
Hudson et al. (2002)	Educational–behavioral intervention (including health behavior training) versus standard care	266 (intervention, *n* = 131; standard care, *n* = 135; 12–18 years), mixed cancer	Single session (duration not reported)	1 year	Health protective behaviors (e.g., health practices): health knowledge; perceived susceptibility, benefits and barriers		Health protective behavior or beliefs
Kazak et al. (1999)	Group family cognitive–behavioral intervention (mothers, fathers, survivors and siblings)	19 families (children 10–17 years), mixed cancer (single group study)	Four 1–1.5-hour sessions in one day (5 hours therapeutic contact)	1 day	PTSS, parent state and trait anxiety, child anxiety, family functioning (structure and organization, worldview)	Decreased PTSS symptoms and anxiety for all family members; improved family functioning in structure and organization and worldview reported by family members	
C. E. Schwartz et al. (1999)	Psychosocial intervention (including support, education, recreation)	22 (18–29 years), mixed cancer (vs. 54 healthy controls)	3-day weekend	3-day intervention; 3 months total study	Health-related QOL, psychological well-being	Increased QOL (postintervention), perceived QOL (3 months)	Physical health, mental health
Tyc et al. (2003)	Risk counseling intervention (tobacco use, including educational video; goal setting; more intense counseling; and follow-up) versus standard care	103 (10–18 years), mixed cancer (RCT)	One 50–60-minute session with telephone reinforcement	12 months total study	Knowledge, perceived vulnerability, intentions to use, perceived positive effects of tobacco	Knowledge, perceived vulnerability, and intentions improved in intervention group	

Cognitive–behavioral interventions: Parents

Study	Intervention	Sample	Format	Duration	Measures	Results	
Sahler et al. (2002)	Problem-solving skills training (mothers) versus usual psychosocial care	92 mothers (tx, $n = 50$; control, $n = 50$; children 3–14 years), any cancer (RCT)	Eight 1-hour individual sessions	8 weeks	Social problem-solving skills (cancer specific); positive–negative mood	Improved mood, increased rational and constructive problem solving, and decreased negative problem orientation (treatment group)	
Sahler et al. (2005)	Problem-solving skills training versus usual psychosocial care	436 mothers (tx, $n = 217$; control, $n = 230$; children 3–14 years), any cancer	8-hour individual sessions	3 months	Social problem-solving skills (cancer specific); positive–negative mood	Improved constructive problem solving, lower dysfunctional problem solving and depressed mood	Psychological distress, total problem-solving score
Streisand et al. (2000)	Stress management for mothers (including education, relaxation, communication) versus standard care	22 mothers (children 2–16), bone marrow transplant	One 90-minute session	3 weeks post-transplant	Daily stress and parenting stress, adherence to intervention techniques	Intervention techniques used more frequently	Stress outcomes

Note. Empty cells indicate that the data are not available. CBCL = Child Behavior Checklist; PTSS = posttraumatic stress symptoms; tx = treatment condition; RCT = randomized controlled trial; QOL = quality of life.

examples of published studies of psychological intervention for children and adolescents with cancer are now described.

Social Skills Training Approaches

Investigators have found promising results for comprehensive social skills training interventions. Barakat et al. (2003) found that social skills training, including communication skills, conflict resolution, and cooperation, delivered in a group resulted in improved child- and parent-reported social competencies in children who were treated for brain tumors and thus who were at particular risk for social problems (Mulhern et al., 1992).

Varni et al. (1993) compared a social skills training model that included problem solving, handling teasing, and assertiveness training with standard school reintegration, including education, support, conferences, and classroom presentations. Groups from both models demonstrated reduced anxiety and behavioral problems following intervention and increased social support, as well as reduced behavior problems and increased school competence at 6- and 9-month follow-up. The social skills group demonstrated greater improvement on behavioral problems and social support than the standard-care group.

School Reintegration Approaches

Several studies have found empirical support for interventions designed to facilitate children's reentry or reintegration into school settings following the phase of intensive treatment for cancer. Katz et al. (1988) found that children and teachers gave favorable ratings (knowledge, social acceptance) to a school reintegration intervention, including preventive education with medical and school staff, hospital-based liaison, counseling and preparation of child and parents, and presentations to school personnel and classmates. Katz et al. (1992) tested a school reintegration program that involved preparation of the child for return to school, conferences with school personnel, classroom presentations, and communication skills, and they found improvements in behavioral symptoms and school adjustment in children with cancer compared with a control group. Finally, McCarthy, Williams, and Plumer (1998) found that parents and teachers rated a school reentry program that involved meeting with school personnel and parents and meeting with classmates as positive.

Other relevant school-based interventions for children and adolescents with cancer involve advocacy for special education services under the Individuals With Disabilities Education Act (1997) for identified developmental or learning disorder for children with chronic health conditions (Armstrong & Briery, 2004). Moreover, both parents and teachers need to understand the late effects of cancer treatment on children's learning and school performance. Richardson, Nelson, and Meeske (1999) described a program that has provided advocacy training to teach parents to understand their children's legal rights to school programs, to communicate with their children's teachers concerning their children's progress, and to monitor the educational support received by their child on an ongoing basis.

Cognitive–Behavioral Approaches: Cancer Survivors

An emerging body of psychological intervention research has focused on the survivors of cancer. Two of these have focused on health risk. For example, Hudson et al. (2002) tested a behavioral education intervention on 266 cancer survivors ages 12 to 14 years that focused on promotion of health protective behaviors. No differences were found between the intervention and control groups. In addition, Tyc et al.'s (2003) randomized controlled trial (RCT) of a brief (less than 1 hour) educational intervention delivered by telephone demonstrated that at 1 year (but not at 6 months) postintervention, adolescent survivors who received the intervention showed increased knowledge of smoking risks, reported more perceived vulnerability, and indicated less intent to smoke cigarettes than did control participants.

C. E. Schwartz, Feinberg, Jilinskaia, and Applegate (1999) found that psychosocial intervention including support, education, and recreation was associated with increased quality of life (QOL) immediately postintervention among young adult and adult survivors of cancer but decreased QOL at 3-month follow-up. No changes were noted in physical or mental health.

In a single group pilot study, Kazak et al.'s (1999) test of cognitive–behavioral intervention on 19 families found decreases in PTSS and anxiety for all family members (mothers, fathers, survivors, and siblings). They also found improved family functioning (e.g., cohesion, clarity of leadership) and worldview (e.g., life engagement, optimism).

Cognitive–Behavioral Approaches: Parents

In recent years, several different interventions that involved cognitive–behavioral methods designed to reduce the level of distress experienced by parents of children with cancer have been tested. In an RCT, Sahler et al. (2002) found that problem-solving therapy as a means of reducing stress and its psychological impact on the parents of children with cancer were found to be more effective than treatment as usual. Specifically, they found reduced negative affectivity and increased problem-solving skills, including rational and constructive problem solving and decreased negative problem orientation for mothers of children currently in treatment. Strongest support was shown for treatment effects immediately after the intervention was completed (Sahler et al., 2002). Most recently, Sahler et al. (2005) found that differences in some measures of problem-solving skills and distress levels persisted to 3-month follow-up. Young, single mothers demonstrated the greatest benefits of intervention.

Hoekstra-Weebers, Heuvel, Jaspers, Kamps, and Klip (1998) tested a comprehensive cognitive–behavioral intervention that involved identification of automatic thoughts and training on problem-focused coping, communication, and assertiveness skills. They found no effect of the intervention on psychological functioning or social support.

Finally, in a pilot study, Streisand, Rodrigue, Houck, Graham-Pole, and Berlant (2000) found that a single-session stress management intervention (including relaxation education and communication) did not reduce general or parenting stress in mothers whose children were undergoing bone marrow transplantation. On the other hand, they found more frequent use of, and improved adherence to, intervention techniques in the intervention group.

Taken together, the results of studies suggest promising results of social skills training, school reintegration interventions, and cognitive–behavioral interventions. Moreover, such interventions have been shown to be feasible and acceptable to families as well as to demonstrate positive effects on a range of outcomes with both children and parents. The feasibility and acceptability of such interventions are particularly important because cancer is such a burdensome illness that it may be difficult for families to manage the time and energy demands of psychological intervention. Although the results are not consistent across studies, and more controlled studies are needed, there is clearly sufficient evidence to warrant replication and extension of these findings in larger samples of RCTs.

Preventive Intervention Approaches: Survivors and Families

Descriptive studies that have indicated significant levels of psychological distress among children with pediatric cancer and their parents and have also indicated psychological dysfunction such as PTSD among a subset of this population (Vanatta & Gerhardt, 2003) have underscored the need to implement and evaluate psychological interventions designed to reduce psychological distress and symptoms. Recently, Kazak and her colleagues have conducted promising preventive family-centered cognitive–behavioral interventions with children with cancer and family members, as well as interventions designed to reduce the impact of PTSS (Kazak, Alderfer, & Rodriguez, in press; Kazak, Simms, et al., in press). In an initial report of feasibility and outcome from a pilot study of a three-session intervention for caregivers of children newly diagnosed with cancer, Kazak, Simms, et al.

(in press) described the outcomes for families who were randomly assigned to the intervention or treatment as usual subsequent to learning of their child's illness. The study design included pre- and 2-month postintervention assessments of state anxiety and PTSS. The intervention was found to be acceptable to families, and preliminary outcome data demonstrated trends in the predicted direction (e.g., reduced anxiety and PTSS) for family outcomes.

The Surviving Cancer Competently Intervention Program (SCCIP) integrates cognitive–behavioral and family therapy approaches, drawing heavily on adaptations of the Adversities–Beliefs–Consequences (A-B-C) Model (Seligman, 1990), and multiple family discussion groups approaches (Gonzalez, Steinglass, & Reiss, 1985). The SCCIP consists of four sessions within 1 (weekend) day for a group of families. During the two morning sessions, separate groups (of survivors, mothers, fathers, siblings) identify beliefs about cancer and its treatment and learn and practice the A-B-C Model and reframing. In the afternoon, two sessions link individuals' beliefs to how these beliefs affect the family and promote or hinder ongoing developmental growth for the children and families.

Kazak, Alderfer, et al. (in press) conducted a randomized waitlist control trial of the SCCIP intervention with 150 adolescent survivors and their mothers, fathers, and adolescent siblings. Significant reductions in intrusive thoughts for fathers and in arousal for survivors were associated with treatment. These data provided support for the importance of engaging multiple members of the family in psychological interventions.

Interventions to Promote Adherence to Pediatric Cancer Treatment

One of the most salient gaps in intervention research on pediatric cancer concerns research on interventions to promote adherence to treatment. To our knowledge, no adherence-related intervention studies with children or adolescents with cancer have been reported in the peer-reviewed literature. This area represents a significant need in future intervention research.

FUTURE DIRECTIONS FOR PSYCHOLOGICAL INTERVENTION RESEARCH

Kuppenheimer and Brown (2002) recommended the following strategies to enhance the research in pain management concerning cancer-related medical procedures: (a) compare combinations of pharmacotherapy and cognitive–behavioral therapy; (b) examine components of cognitive and behavioral therapy to determine which are most effective in managing pain; (c) study how individual differences in developmental level, cognitive skills, and gender mediate and moderate response to cognitive–behavioral and pharmacological interventions; (d) evaluate consumer satisfaction; (e) document availability and access to services; and (f) describe the costs, benefits, and economic impact of services.

In her review of evidence-based interventions for children with cancer, Kazak (2005) identified several needs for future intervention research, including (a) greater emphasis on interventions that stress enhancement of competencies in children with cancer and their families as opposed to targeting psychopathology; (b) emphasis on integration of research practice and testing psychological interventions that are linked to the levels of psychological risk that are encountered by families; (c) developing interventions concerning the end of life or bereavement (Kazak & Noll, 2004); (d) developing interventions for siblings; (e) extending research, including intervention research to ethnic minority families; and (f) interventions that can be delivered using technology.

In addition to Kazak's (2005) recommendations, I suggest the following: to develop and evaluate programs (e.g., anticipatory guidance) that educate caregivers about neurodevelopmental late effects at the conclusion of treatment, which may reduce burdens when they arise, and interventions that help parents to understand and advocate for their child's needs in improving school reintegration (Peterson & Drotar, in press). Moreover, similar to Kazak et al. (1999), a family burden prevention program that includes cognitive–behavioral family intervention to address anxiety or posttraumatic stress may prevent declines in QOL and enhance the social and emotional competence of pediatric cancer survivors who experience late effects (Peterson & Drotar, in press). To accomplish the recommendations that have been set forth in this agenda, researchers will need to address salient methodological challenges of intervention research in pediatric cancer (Patenaude & Kupst, 2005). Among others, these include sample size, self-selection of participants, difficulty of achieving longer term follow-up, and the need for comprehensive measurement of outcome (Patenaude & Kupst, 2005).

CLINICAL CARE RECOMMENDATIONS

The progress that has been made in medical and psychological research in pediatric cancer in recent years, coupled with the numbers of psychologists who are now working with children and adolescents with cancer and their families, presents important opportunities to develop and evaluate ongoing approaches to clinical care. These include comprehensive and preventive comprehensive care, facilitation of school reentry and functioning, interventions to remediate cognitive deficits, and comprehensive care for cancer survivors.

Comprehensive and Preventive Psychological Care

Practitioners have recommended that psychological services for children and adolescents with cancer be integrated at all phases of treatment (Powers, Vannatta, Noll, Cool, & Stehbens, 1995). Key ingredients of these services include continuity of care and a family-centered approach. Special emphasis should be clinical application of pain management and management of side effects, including behavioral and cognitive approaches, which have been shown to be effective (Kuppenheimer & Brown, 2002; McGrath, Finley, & Turner, 1992).

In their recommendations for psychosocial care for children with cancer and their families, Noll and Kazak (2004) described how crucial it is to establish the importance of psychosocial care by introducing the members of the comprehensive care team, including psychologists, at the outset of treatment and hence communicating to families that psychosocial care is necessary for everyone, not only families with serious psychological problems. This introduction also sets the stage to involve a psychologist or psychosocial team member in medical conferences with families to provide support and clarification. Moreover, ongoing communication and contact with families are necessary to provide continual support and to assess the psychological adjustment of parents, siblings, and children to determine the need for intervention at various points of stress or dysfunction.

Other recommendations for psychosocial care include (a) preventive family-centered psychosocial interventions (e.g., developing routines, parental monitoring, and reinforcement) to promote adherence, school reentry, and psychoeducational planning and (b) assistance with the extraordinary stressors of relapse or, in some instances, the death of a child from cancer (Noll & Kazak, 2004). Families who have experienced the death of a child from cancer may be at psychological risk. Kazak and Noll (2004) have developed specific recommendations for families whose children have died from a childhood illness such as cancer.

Practitioners who are interested in more detailed practical advice for psychosocial interventions for children with cancer and their families should consult Noll and Kazak (2004). In addition, Woznick and Goodheart (2002) published a comprehensive guide to facilitate parents' coping with their children's cancer that contains practical advice and a wealth of useful information on a range of topics (e.g., coping; reducing stress; working with the medical team, teachers, and insurers; and facilitating pain management, self-esteem, and child development).

Facilitation of School Reentry and Functioning

School reintegration services (e.g., encouragement for children and adolescents to return to school as soon as possible, contact with school staff to let them know about the child's illness, and proactive management of school-related problems that may occur) are an important component of ongoing psychological care for children and adolescents with cancer (Drotar, Palermo, & Barry, 2003). For children whose cancer treatment puts them at risk for cognitive deficits, assessment of cognitive and academic deficits (e.g., baseline and follow-up serial neurodevelopmental evaluations assessing global and specific cognitive functions) can be important to document deficits that may require interventions. For example, children with significant neurodevelopmental late effects of their treatment may benefit from team meetings and revised individual education plans each new school year to prevent school failure and psychosocial sequelae of learning problems (Peterson & Drotar, in press). The effectiveness of school liaison teams within pediatric oncology centers may be enhanced by the consistency of communications with parents and school staff about school accommodations and school-related advocacy (Armstrong & Briery, 2004; Peterson & Drotar, in press).

Finally, compensatory psychological and educational interventions that involve accommodation including special education in the school setting and technological supports may be very helpful to pediatric survivors of cancer who demonstrate cognitive late effects. Examples of such compensatory intervention include providing children with access to books on tape for reading requirements, use of computers to modify the amount and complexity of text presented to the child, and oral rather than written testing (Armstrong & Briery, 2004).

Interventions to Remediate Cognitive Deficits

The evaluation of pharmacological interventions designed to reduce the side effects of pediatric cancer is a new research direction (Armstrong & Briery, 2004). For example, clinical trials of medical treatment designed to evaluate the effectiveness and safety of stimulant medications such as methylphenidate to reduce the attentional and organizational problems among children treated for central nervous tumors have shown preliminary efficacy (S. J. Thompson et al., 2001). Another approach is cognitive rehabilitation, which involves repetitive exposure, using computer-based tasks, to behavioral and learning tasks that are hypothesized to strengthen neural pathways, thus promoting recovery of functioning. Preliminary data with children with cancer have indicated that cognitive rehabilitation improved attention as measured by a continuous performance test but not cognitive abilities or school performance (Butler & Copeland, 2002).

Comprehensive Care for Survivors of Pediatric Cancer

Long-term survivor clinics can provide a focused, comprehensive, multidisciplinary team approach to late effects of cancer (see section on psychological adjustment) and other long-term follow-up issues, such as fear of relapse and QOL (Oeffinger & Hudson, 2004). Brief screening or consultation for neurodevelopmental and medical late effects and psychological distress for survivors and their families may be helpful in planning ongoing school-based interventions (Peterson & Drotar, in press). In addition, the comprehensive clinical care of survivors may also need to address the impact of medical and neuropsychological late effects of pediatric cancer on psychological adjustment in the family system, including survivors, siblings, and parents, as well as interactions between dyads (Peterson & Drotar, in press). Early assessment of family-level risk factors (e.g., misunderstanding of late effects, high conflict) could facilitate the development of targeted prevention efforts (Kazak et al., 1999). Finally, family members could benefit from psychological interventions that are designed to enhance coping with survivorship, particularly for those survivors with ongoing late effects, such as managing conflict, distress, and anxiety about relapse and enhancing family cohesion, adaptability, and QOL (Patenaude & Kupst, 2005).

INTEGRATING RESEARCH INTO CLINICAL CARE

Kazak (2005) noted that despite promising evidence of efficacy of psychological intervention approaches with children with cancer and their families, there is little consistency in the degree to which such interventions have been integrated into the ongoing care of children with cancer in various settings. There are many reasons for this, one of which is the lack of a proactive, logical method to allocate psychosocial services to this population. To address this need, Kazak et al. (2003) proposed a three-tiered model of psychosocial need and care based on public health models (Gordon, 1983; National Institute of Mental Health, 1998), using the concepts of universal, selected, and targeted psychological interventions (see chap. 2). On the basis of this model, *universal* interventions would focus on helping well-functioning children and families cope with typical cancer-related stress. *Selected* interventions would focus on families who have indicated, on the basis of excessive burden and stress as well as inadequate coping skills, that they are at risk for psychosocial problems. *Targeted* interventions would be provided to families who demonstrate significant and persistent psychological distress or social difficulties and other indicators of high risk (e.g., family stressors). It should be noted that targeted interventions are the most common within current patterns of psychosocial intervention at most centers. The assumption behind the tiered model of psychosocial care, which to my knowledge has not been tested, is the following: If those families at highest risk for psychosocial distress during treatment can be identified reliably at diagnosis and interventions developed and implemented to match these levels of risk, psychosocial care for the population of children and adolescents with cancer would be more effective and cost-efficient (Kazak et al., 2003).

To facilitate implementation of the tiered model of psychosocial care, Kazak and colleagues have developed a measure, the Psychosocial Assessment Tool (PAT), to evaluate the degree of psychosocial risk and predict the health care utilization costs associated with treating patients and families at different levels of risk (Kazak et al., 2001, 2003). The PAT measure covers a number of relevant areas: family structure (e.g., marital status), family resources (financial impact on employment), social support, child knowledge, school functioning (e.g., attendance, school placement), child emotional and behavioral concerns (e.g., diagnoses based on the American Psychiatric Association's [1994] *Diagnostic and Statistical Manual of Mental Disorders* [4th ed.]), child maturity for age, marital and family problems, family beliefs (e.g., about health care), and other stressors.

Kazak et al. (2003) studied the use of the PAT with the families of 125 children who were newly diagnosed with cancer and completed the measure at diagnosis and 3 and 6 months later. Oncologists and nurses completed an analogous measure of perceived family psychosocial risk at diagnosis and at 3 and 6 months postdiagnosis. Oncology social workers reported types and intensity of psychosocial interventions provided 3 and 6 months postdiagnosis. The PAT identified three subsets of families who presented with varying levels of psychosocial risk at diagnosis, in accordance with the tiered model of psychosocial risk (i.e., universal, selected, and targeted). In general, there was moderate concordance among families', oncologists', and nurses' reports of psychosocial risk. The PAT scores at diagnosis predicted 3-month PAT scores and psychosocial resource use at 6 months postdiagnosis, controlling for demographic and disease factors. Research is proceeding on the development and testing of psychosocial interventions that match family risk level as an effective and cost-efficient approach to working with families of children with cancer to address their concerns and promote short- and long-term adjustment (Kazak et al., 2003).

Kazak (2005) also recommended integrating empirically supported psychological interventions that combine treatment modalities (e.g., pharmacological and psychological, cognitive–behavioral, and family systems) into the routine clinical care of children and adolescents with cancer (Kazak, 2001; Kazak & Meadows, 2000). As is the case concerning comprehensive care for other chronic pediatric conditions, there is considerable site-to-site variation in how well and how frequently psychological services are integrated with medical care for children and adolescents with cancer. In many settings, children with cancer are seen on referral only, and it is extremely rare for settings to provide integrated multidisciplinary psychological care on a routine basis. For this reason, it will be important to describe and evaluate the effectiveness of the delivery of psychological services in the context of multidisciplinary care to children and adolescents with pediatric cancer and their families in a range of clinical settings. Moreover, the clinical effectiveness of new specialized approaches to psychosocial care such as school-based programs, including reentry and compensatory intervention (Armstrong & Briery, 2004), and comprehensive care programs for survivors of children with cancer (Oeffinger & Hudson, 2004) need to be evaluated. Studies of clinical effectiveness of these services represent an important opportunity for researchers and practitioners.

9

PSYCHOLOGICAL INTERVENTIONS: SICKLE CELL DISEASE AND JUVENILE RHEUMATOID ARTHRITIS

One of the hallmark features of sickle cell disease and juvenile rheumatoid arthritis is recurrent pain, which, along with other clinical manifestations of these conditions, needs to be addressed in relevant psychological interventions. This chapter considers psychological interventions that have been described and studied for these two chronic conditions.

SICKLE CELL DISEASE

Sickle cell disease (SCD) is a spectrum of inherited disorders, each of which involves a mutation in the hemoglobin that causes normal red blood cells to take on a sickle shape, thus obstructing blood flow oxygen to tissues and organs. This condition affects primarily African Americans (M. J. Bonner, Gustafson, Schumacher, & Thompson, 1999; National Heart, Lung, and Blood Institute, 1996). A wide range of medical sequelae and complications are associated with SCD. These can include anemia; extreme pain;

Dawn Witherspoon and Kathy Zebracki made significant contributions to the writing of this chapter and in the creation of the tables.

acute and chronic tissue injury; frequent urination, enuresis, and increased fluid intake needs; malnutrition, particularly iron and protein deficiencies; and opthalmological complications (Bonner et al., 1999). Cerebrovascular accidents, including both overt and "silent" strokes (e.g., those that are identified by brain imaging rather than overt neurologic signs), which occur in some children and adolescents, can significantly disrupt learning and school performance (R. T. Brown, Armstrong, & Eckman, 1993).

Acute pulmonary events are a major cause of both mortality and hospitalization (Kirkpatrick & Bass, 1989). In addition, poor or absent spleen function can prevent clearance of bacterial organisms, resulting in potentially life-threatening infections (Lemanek, Ranalli, Green, Biega, & Lupis, 2003). Skeletal complications, which are also common in individuals with SCD, include weakened bones that easily fracture and degenerative joint disease that involves chronic pain and disability. Bilirubin stones, resulting from the increased blood cell turnover in SCD, form in the gallbladder and cause pain; jaundice; and, if untreated, infection. Children and adolescents with SCD who receive recurrent transfusions are at risk for hepatitis virus infection, chronic liver injury, and life-threatening liver failure. Males may experience prolonged painful erections due to sickling within the penile tissues. Delayed growth and sexual maturation due to the demands of profound anemia are associated with SCD. Amenorrhea and infertility are not uncommon in women with SCD (Lemanek et al., 2003).

Recurrent pain is a hallmark clinical characteristic of SCD. Children and adolescents with SCD may experience multiple pain episodes or vaso-occlusive crises per year, which can last 1 to 3 or more days or be chronic (Lemanek et al., 2003). SCD-related pain occurs most commonly in an extremity, in the back, the chest, or the abdomen. Recurrent pain can interfere with a range of important activities, including academic (i.e., completing school assignments, school attendance), sleep, and social activities (Gil, Porter, et al., 2000). The frequency of acute and recurrent pain in SCD and the impact on children's functioning in a range of relevant life contexts are important potential targets of psychological intervention (Palermo, 2000; Powers, 1999).

Medical Treatment

As noted by Lemanek et al. (2003), advances in the understanding of the pathophysiology of SCD in supportive medical and comprehensive care and early identification via newborn screening have improved the quality of life and life expectancies of children and adolescents. Over the past 2 decades, the use of daily penicillin prophylaxis and more aggressive treatment for patients with fever have reduced the number of early deaths and have improved life expectancy in children with SCD.

Hydration and analgesia are used to manage acute SCD complications, and nonsteroidal anti-inflammatory medications and patient-controlled analgesia units are also used in SCD treatment (Lemanek et al., 2003). Transfusions are indicated for the management of strokes, pulmonary complications, and chronic pain. The repeated use of hydroxyurea, which increases protective fetal hemoglobin levels, has helped to reduce the length of hospital stays, the frequency of vaso-occlusive crises, and transfusions (Charache et al., 1995).

The typical pain management protocol for SCD includes hydration, nonsteroidal anti-inflammatory drugs (e.g., ibuprofen), and opioids if the pain is not relieved (e.g., Tylenol with codeine). In a number of centers, a wide range of pain management strategies, such as massage, distraction, and relaxation techniques, have been incorporated into pain protocols for children and adolescents with SCD (Lemanek et al., 2003). In addition, more routine implementation of empirically supported pain management interventions in clinical care (e.g., coaching children and adolescents to control their pain; Gil et al., 1997; Gil, Porter, et al., 2000) has been an important development.

Psychological Impact of Sickle Cell Disease on Children and Adolescents

Recent studies have shown that children and adolescents with SCD are at risk to develop psychological distress (Gartstein, Short, Vannatta, & Noll, 1999; R. J. Thompson, Gustafson, Gil, Godfrey, & Murphy, 1998), which is a clinically relevant focus of psychological intervention. Studies of individual differences in the psychological functioning of children and adolescents with SCD have documented a relationship among coping strategies, psychosocial adjustment, and health care use (Lemanek et al., 2003). In general, children whose coping is characterized by negative thinking and passive strategies are less active in school and social situations, use more health care services, and demonstrate more psychological problems than those who consistently demonstrate more active coping function (Gil, Williams, Thompson, & Kinney, 1991).

Such maladaptive coping patterns may be an important focus of psychological interventions that are designed to reduce their functional impact. For example, consider Raymond, an 11-year-old with SCD who presents with recurrent pain crises. Although Raymond and his family have been quite distressed about his episodes of pain, they have never learned effective ways of managing his pain. They react with anxiety and take him to the emergency room at the first sign of pain. It has been very difficult for Raymond or his family to manage his pain once it starts. Moreover, Raymond's parents have begun to limit his activity as much as possible because they believe it will intensify his pain. As a consequence, he has missed a great deal of school and interaction with peers. Psychological intervention is needed to help Raymond and his family develop more adaptive coping and pain management skills.

The neuropsychological functioning of children and adolescents with SCD is vulnerable to the effects of the illness and hence is a potential target of psychological intervention (R. T. Brown et al., 2000). As noted by Lemanek et al. (2003), global and specific deficits in attention but no differences in academic achievement have been found in comparisons of youths with SCD who have not shown evidence of stroke (Noll et al., 2001). M. J. Cohen, Branch, McKie, and Adams (1997) found that children with left-hemisphere stroke demonstrated impairments in verbal intellectual functioning as well as deficits in language in immediate auditory memory compared with children who suffered right-hemisphere stroke. Among children with SCD who had been referred for learning disabilities, those with a history of clinical or silent stroke demonstrated less adequate sustained attention compared with those who had suffered a stroke (M. J. Cohen et al., 1997). Deficits in neurocognitive functioning, which can be associated with neurologic complications of SCD, may also affect school performance and academic achievement. For example, Schatz, Brown, Pascual, Hsu, and DeBaun (2001) found that a greater percentage of children with SCD who had experienced silent stroke were retained or received special education compared with children with SCD without silent stroke and their siblings. Finally, in a meta-analysis, Schatz, Finke, Kellett, and Kramer (2002) found deficits on measures of general intelligence in children and adolescents with SCD, even in the absence of cerebral infarction. Measures of specific abilities (e.g., language, memory) were more impaired than IQ scores. Taken together, these findings underscore the need for routine assessment of cognitive functioning and ongoing psychoeducational planning and intervention for children and adolescents with SCD (M. J. Bonner, Hardy, Ezell, & Ware, 2004; Drotar, Palermo, & Barry, 2003).

Psychological Impact on Families

The nature and frequency of medical symptoms and complications as well as the medical treatment associated with SCD place considerable burdens on parents. Not surprisingly, increased psychological distress has been documented in parents of children and adolescents with SCD compared with parents of healthy children (R. J. Thompson, Gil, Burbach, Keith, & Kinney, 1993; R. J. Thompson, Gustafson, & Gil, 1995). Several studies have described specific sources of parental distress and concern. For example, parents of children with SCD have reported greater concerns about their children's health and about being perceived as different from peers compared with parents of healthy children (Noll, McKellop, Vannatta, & Kalinyak, 1998). Ievers-Landis et al. (2001) conducted a situational analysis for caregivers of children with SCD who described a wide range of problems and burdens. Almost all caregivers reported experiencing challenging and upsetting problems with helping their children manage their nutrition, minimize the frequency of pain episodes, and express feelings about having SCD. Nutritional problems were more frequently reported for younger children (Ievers-Landis et al., 2001). On the basis of data from focus groups, Mitchell, Kawchak, et al. (2004) found that children's poor appetite and its potential impact on nutrition and children's health were particular concerns for parents of children with SCD, who generally addressed these problems without consulting health professionals. For this reason, psychological interventions designed to help manage the salient parenting and family burdens associated with SCD may be very helpful to families (Mitchell, Kawchak, et al., 2004).

Adherence to Medical Treatment

Given the demanding nature of medical treatment for SCD, it is not surprising that high rates (49%–79%) of nonadherence to treatment have been identified in this population (Pegelow, Armstrong, Light, Toledano, & Davis, 1991) for the overall treatment regimen as well as penicillin prophylaxis (Teach, Lillis, & Grossi, 1998). Barakat, Smith-Whitley, and Ohene-Frempong (2002) found varying rates of nonadherence depending on the specific treatment-related task. For example, adherence to medication for SCD was higher than adherence to recommended pain management approaches. On average, across the different domains of treatment adherence, there was only 50% agreement between treatment recommendations and parent-reported adherence-related activities (Barakat et al., 2002). These findings suggest that problematic adherence to medical treatment is an important potential target for psychological interventions in pediatric SCD.

Reviews of Interventions With Children and Adolescents With Sickle Cell Disease

Two reviews of psychological interventions with children and adolescents with SCD have been conducted and are summarized here. Collins, Kaslow, Doepke, Elkman, and Johnson's (1998) narrative review documented preliminary support for cognitive–behavioral approaches, behavioral contracting, coping skills training, and educational and family support programs as well as additional study of moderators of intervention effects such as the child's age, developmental stage, gender, and socioeconomic status and the therapist's race.

Recently, E. Chen, Cole, and Kato (2004) conducted a critical review of 22 studies of psychological intervention targeted at pain and adherence-related behaviors of children, adolescents, and adults with SCD. These authors used Chambless and Hollon's (1998) criteria to evaluate the level of empirical support that was obtained for the following categories of interventions: teaching, cognitive–behavioral methods, behavioral change, and social support. Gil and colleagues' studies on cognitive coping strategies (e.g., calming self-statements, relaxation, and distraction) in children (Gil et al., 1997) and adults (Gil, Carson, et al., 2000) with SCD met criteria for probably efficacious interventions to reduce pain. These studies included controls and random assignment of families, and in some instances the studies controlled for time spent with the therapist.

Behavioral change interventions, such as behavioral contracting, education, and rewards for behaviors that were incompatible with pain, have been shown to enhance coping skills (Hazzard, Celano, Collins, & Markov, 2002) and adherence to antibiotic regimens for SCD (Berkovitch et al., 1998) in single group studies. On the other hand, cognitive–behavioral interventions demonstrated a relatively weak impact on adherence behaviors, and social support interventions did not meet criteria for empirically supported interventions. Finally, Kaslow et al.'s (2000) family psychoeducational intervention demonstrated improvements in knowledge but not in psychological adjustment or family functioning.

Examples of Psychological Interventions in Sickle Cell Disease

In this next section, examples of studies of psychological interventions that have found positive effects in designs ranging from single group studies to randomized controlled trials (RCTs) are described and are summarized in Table 9.1.

Cognitive–Behavioral Approaches

Gil et al.'s (1997, 2001) RCTs of a behavioral intervention (vs. standard care) that included relaxation, imagery, and calming self-statements found a decrease in negative thinking at 1-week follow-up and increased coping strategies and decreased pain on further follow-up. No differences were found, however, on illness-focused coping strategies or on anxiety and depression. Broome, Maikler, Kelber, Bailey, and Lea's (2001) RCT of children with SCD found that relaxation training was associated with decreased health care utilization for children and adolescents and increased adaptive coping among adolescents.

TABLE 9.1

Psychological Interventions for Children and Adolescents With Sickle Cell Disease

Authors	Target population	Sample	Design and content	Sessions No.	Sessions Length	Sessions Duration	Outcomes	Findings + Significant	Findings − Nonsignificant
			Educational interventions						
Hazzard et al. (2002)	Child	N = 110; 47 children with SCD and 63 with asthma; 58% male; 98% African American; age range 8–18 years (M = 11.7)	STARBRIGHT world computer network; interactive health education, opportunities to interact with other hospitalized children online (uncontrolled design)	1–3	3.5–4 hours	3 days	Disease-related knowledge, perceived social support from peers, coping skills	Increased perceived social support, decreases in negative coping skills	Change in disease knowledge
Kaslow et al. (2000)	Family	N = 39, age 7–16 years (M = 10.25), 24 female	Psychoeducational intervention, manualized, educational activities; RCT intervention compared with treatment as usual	6+	1 hour/ session	6 weeks, 6-month follow-up	Disease knowledge, psychological adjustment, social functioning, support, family functioning	Increased disease knowledge (parent and child), maintained at 6-month follow-up (child)	Psychological adjustment, social functioning and support, family functioning
Applegate et al. (2003)	Family	92 parent–child dyads, child age 7 years, 54% male	Parents' questions were written down and given to them as reminders; random assignment to oral instruction or written instruction condition	1	Approximately 5 minutes	One-time intervention	No. of questions asked by parents or children of their physician		Total no. of questions

(continued)

TABLE 9.1 (Continued)

Authors	Target population	Sample	Design and content	Sessions No.	Length	Duration	Outcomes	Findings + Significant	– Nonsignificant
			Cognitive–behavioral interventions						
Gil et al. (1997)	Child	N = 49; age range 8–17 years; 24 girls, 22 boys	Deep breathing, relaxation, pleasant imagery, calming self-statements, randomly assigned to coping skills group or control	1 session, 1 brief follow-up	45 minutes	1 week	Daily coping, resource utilization	Decreased negative thinking (pre- to posttest)	Reports of active coping
Gil et al. (2001)	Child	N = 46, age range 8–17 years (M = 11.96)	Extension of Gil et al. (1997)	2	45 minutes	2 to 3 weeks after baseline 1-month follow-up	Laboratory pain task; structured interview; depression, anxiety, and coping strategies	Decreased negative thinking and reporting of low-level pain (posttest); increased coping attempts (1-month follow-up)	Negative thinking; illness-focused strategies; reporting of pain, anxiety, depression (1-month follow-up)
Broome et al. (2001)	Children and adolescents	N = 65 children, (mean age = 9.2 years), and N = 32 adolescents (mean age = 15.3 years)	Randomized children into three groups: relaxation, art therapy, attention–control; randomized adolescents into two groups: relaxation, art therapy	9	Not specified	Baseline, post-intervention, and 12-month follow-up	Coping strategies, pain management, emergency room health care visits	Decreased emergency room and sickle cell clinic visits for adolescents in the relaxation and art therapy groups, increase in total no. of coping scores; child reported	No. of coping strategies or effectiveness

			Combined behavioral–pharmacological intervention						
Powers et al. (2002)	Family	M = 3, 9-year-old boy, 12-year-old girl, 10-year-old boy	Family-based cognitive–behavioral management, education, relaxation, pharmacological strategies	6	90 minutes	18 weeks (including 3-month follow-up)	Pain, coping, daily functioning, coping strategies, questionnaire, Daily Pain and Activity Diary	Decreased negative thinking (n = 3); increase in coping attempts (n = 1)	No increases in coping attempts (n = 2)
			Social support interventions						
Chernoff et al. (2002); Ireys, Chernoff, DeVet, & Kim (2001)	Family	N = 136, children (age range 7–11 years); four illness groups: diabetes mellitus, SCD, cystic fibrosis, moderate to severe asthma; SCD, intervention, control	Community-based, family support intervention; "experienced mothers" and child life specialist; telephone contact and face-to-face face visits; special family events; Family-to-Family Network (links mothers with other mothers of older children with same illness)	7 visits	60–90 minutes	15 months	Child outcomes: personal adjustment, depression, anxiety, self-perception, roles and skills; maternal outcomes: depression, anxiety, psychiatric symptom index	Child: modest positive effects of the intervention on promoting adjustment; mother: posttest anxiety scores were lower in the experimental group	Child: no effect of the intervention on measures of anxiety, depression, or self-esteem; mother: no change in depression scores for experimental group mothers
			School-based intervention						
Koontz et al. (2004)	Child, school	N = 24, age range = 8–12 years	Discussion of SCD and complications with school faculty; presentation of age-appropriate information about SCD to the child's classmates; SIP compared with RS control group	1 in-service teacher session, 1 in-service peer session	1 hour	1-month follow-up calls until end of school year	Disease knowledge, consumer satisfaction, self-concept, school absences	Children, peers, and teachers showed significantly more disease knowledge; teachers showed greater satisfaction with interview; children had fewer school absences than the RS group	Self-concept satisfaction with intervention (children and caregivers)

Note. Empty cells indicate that data were not available. SCD = sickle cell disease; RCT = randomized controlled trial; SIP = school intervention program; RS = routine services.

Educational Approaches

In a single group study, Hazzard et al. (2002) found that online interactive health education opportunities to meet other hospitalized children with SCD were associated with an increase in perceived social support and a decrease in negative coping skills. Kaslow et al. (2000) reported a family psychoeducational intervention with improved disease-related knowledge but not psychological symptoms, family, or social functioning compared with the treatment-as-usual condition. On the other hand, Applegate et al.'s (2003) educational intervention that involved oral or written instructions to parents found no effect on the total number of questions that parents asked of their physicians.

Berkovitch et al. (1998) combined behavioral rewards (giving children a sticker for each day they took their antibiotic) with education about the risks of infection and benefits of antibiotics in SCD. Families who received the 8-week intervention had children whose adherence to antibiotic treatment improved pre- to postintervention. However, between-groups analyses did not find differences at posttreatment between the intervention group and a control group that received usual medical care.

Combined Behavioral–Psychopharmacological Approaches

Powers, Mitchell, Graumlich, Byars, and Kalinyak (2002) found that children who received integrated pharmacological and behavioral strategies of pain management, including a program that applied cognitive strategies (i.e., education and relaxation), demonstrated decreased negative thinking.

Social Support Approaches

Ireys, Chernoff, DeVet, and Kim (2001) described the positive effects of social support provided by mothers of children with clinical conditions, including SCD, to other mothers on children's and mothers' psychological adjustment.

School-Based Approaches

Koontz, Short, Kalinyak, and Noll (2004) tested the feasibility and efficacy of a randomized pilot study that compared routine services with a school intervention program for children with SCD intervention that involved information packets, teacher in-service, and peer in-service. Compared with children in the routine services intervention, children and teachers who received the school-based intervention demonstrated more accurate information about SCD. In addition, children with SCD whose teachers experienced the intervention had fewer school absences than the comparison group.

Recommendations for Future Research

Research concerning psychological interventions for children and adolescents with SCD is, with some notable exceptions, such as the programmatic research of Gil and colleagues (Gil et al., 1997, 2001), in a formative stage. This may reflect the difficulty of conducting research with this population. On the basis of their review, E. Chen et al. (2004) described a comprehensive set of research recommendations concerning psychological interventions in SCD, some of which are summarized here. First, researchers should clarify the extent and nature of the effects of cognitive–behavioral techniques (e.g., relaxation and imagery) that have been shown to be effective in pain management by testing variations in the length, timing, and content of interventions. Second, it will also be important to determine whether cognitive–behavioral techniques such as problem solving can modify daily behaviors that are necessary to promote adherence to treatment (E. Chen et al., 2004). In general, extending developing studies of psychological interventions to promote adherence to treatment for SCD is a priority area. Research is also needed to determine the extent to which adherence to recommended behavioral management approaches for pain is associated with changes in the psychological experience of pain and long-term functional outcomes of pain (E. Chen et al., 2004). Third, future studies of social support and family interventions for SCD are also needed. These studies should include control groups in which contact provided to families is regulated and should document a greater range of pain and health care utilization outcomes of intervention (E. Chen et al., 2004). Social support promotion interventions that have been shown to be effective with other populations (Ireys, Chernoff, Stein, DeVet, & Silver, 2001; Sahler et al., 2002) should also be tested with parents of children with SCD.

As noted by E. Chen et al. (2004), the majority of studies in SCD have been designed to manage pain crises when they occur and have been focused on pain outcomes such as severity, frequency, or emergency room visits and hospitalizations. However, national guidelines for preventive home care of SCD emphasize a wide range of ongoing, daily practices (e.g., drinking plenty of fluids, avoiding extreme temperatures) that may be important in managing SCD but have not been the focus of intervention. For this reason, psychological interventions targeted at facilitating such adherence behaviors could help to prevent future pain episodes and related complications (E. Chen et al., 2004). Individual differences in response to psychological intervention among children and adolescents with SCD and their parents should be studied in future research (E. Chen et al., 2004). Potential moderators of psychological interventions among children and adolescents with SCD include their age, developmental stage, and socioeconomic status as well as the therapist's race (Collins et al., 1998).

In addition to the recommendations noted by E. Chen et al. (2004), other areas in need of more extensive research with children with SCD include psychological interventions to enhance the psychological adjustment (e.g., reduce the level of psychological distress) of individual children. Family-centered interventions are also needed to reduce the level of psychological distress and burden experienced by parents of children with SCD. The problem-solving models of intervention that have been developed and tested by Sahler and colleagues (Sahler et al., 2002, 2005) with parents of children with cancer might be applicable to SCD. Given the importance of the extended family within African American culture, the evaluation of family-centered interventions, especially those that involve families, will be an important future research priority (Kaslow et al., 2000).

Finally, given the prevalence of neurocognitive deficits in this population (R. T. Brown et al., 1993), there is an important need to develop and evaluate school-based interventions to enhance the school attendance and school performance of children and adolescents with SCD, as Koontz et al. (2004) have done. Approaches to remediate the cognitive and academic achievement deficits associated with SCD either through direct remediation or through compensatory education and advocacy should be developed and studied (M. J. Bonner et al., 2004). The basic principles of such school-based interventions that have been developed for children with cancer who experience cognitive and academic deficits (Armstrong & Briery, 2004) should be applicable to children and adolescents with SCD.

Recommendations for Clinical Care and Research on Clinical Applications

One vital need for future research and clinical care in SCD is the evaluation of clinical effectiveness of comprehensive medical and psychological care for children and adolescents with SCD and their families. Such interventions might focus on increasing the access to psychological intervention services, including preventive intervention services and multidisciplinary models of care. The promotion of access to comprehensive clinical psychological care, including advocacy for necessary school-related accommodations for children with cognitive deficits, is important for a number of pediatric chronic illness populations (R. T. Brown, 2004) but may be especially important in SCD, which affects mainly African American children and adolescents. The combination of their minority status and economic disadvantage places many children and adolescents with SCD at special risk for a range of problems, including problematic access to care (R. T. Brown et al., 2003). To my knowledge, the most effective ways to enhance access to care for children and adolescents with SCD have not been documented but may involve greater use of staff-initiated contacts with families, including outreach.

Continuity of comprehensive care and integration of such care across multiple sites (e.g., emergency rooms, inpatient hospitals) may be particularly important in the effective management of pain crises and in the prevention of pain-related functional impairments. Some centers have integrated psychological services in comprehensive care, including standardized "care paths" for the management of pain. For example, Vichinsky, Johnson, and Lubin (1982) described the benefits (e.g., reduction in emergency room visits and hospital admissions) of a multidisciplinary approach for the management of SCD. This approach included the following elements: (a) adequate pain medications administered on a fixed-time schedule, (b) treatment planned in routine patient care conferences in which management plans were developed, and (c) reinforcement of positive coping efforts in children and their families that are based on the management plan. The benefits of comprehensive care on health care utilization, which were demonstrated with a small sample ($N = 10$), need to be extended with larger samples across a range of settings.

Similar to other pediatric chronic conditions, psychological intervention research concerning SCD will require multisite studies for optimal statistical power and generalizability. The National Cooperative Study of SCD, which provides a model for such studies, has generated important information about medical and psychological outcomes (R. J. Thompson et al., 2003).

Another relevant area for future development involves the implementation of and education about services designed to identify and manage the cognitive and psychoeducational problems experienced by children and adolescents with SCD. In this regard, C. C. Peterson, Palermo, Swift, Beebe, and Drotar's (2005) needs assessment found that although the majority of parents of children with SCD identified concerns about their children's learning, only a minority of children had actually received psychological testing for learning problems or had individualized education plans through the school system. This finding underscores the importance of ongoing academic needs assessment and educational advocacy for children and adolescents with SCD (M. J. Bonner et al., 2004). Research and clinical care programs that involve parents of children and adolescents with SCD in planning for priorities for psychological interventions may be particularly critical, given the wide range of stressors experienced by this population (Lemanek et al., 2003).

JUVENILE RHEUMATOID ARTHRITIS

Pediatric rheumatic diseases are chronic disorders that involve acute and chronic tissue inflammation of the musculoskeletal system, blood vessels, and skin, including sinusitis (inflammation of the sensorial membrane of a joint). The most common of pediatric rheumatic diseases, juvenile rheumatoid arthritis (JRA), is a significant cause of short- and long-term disability among chronic pediatric diseases (Cassidy & Petty, 2001). A wide range of factors such as genetic predisposition, unknown environmental triggers, and immune reactivity may be important in the etiology of JRA (Rapoff, McGrath, & Lindsley, 2003).

Systemic-onset JRA affects approximately 10% of children with JRA and is defined by the presence of a characteristic rash or high cyclic fevers, along with joint symptoms, either arthritis or arthralgias. Children with JRA often are hospitalized to establish a diagnosis and begin therapy. Although many children with systemic-onset JRA will respond to appropriate therapy, this subtype remains the most difficult group to treat, and up to 25% of children demonstrate a poor prognosis characterized by continually active and poorly responsive disease, generally in the hands, hips, and neck (Rapoff et al., 2003). Other subtypes of JRA are defined by the number of joints that are affected.

Medical Treatment

Once the diagnosis of JRA is established, most children require regular medical therapy. Specific regimens will depend on the age of the child and the severity of the arthritis. Nonsteroidal anti-inflammatory agents are the standard therapy. Naproxin and ibuprofen are used in young children. In addition, daily medications such as nambutome are often used in older children and adolescents (Rapoff et al., 2003). Intra-articular corticosteroids may be needed for joints that are unresponsive to the first-line medications, and occasionally second-line agents such as sulfasalzaine are also used. Low-dose short-term corticosteroid therapy may also be used to control symptoms. In addition to drug therapy, therapeutic exercise programs with professional supervision may be needed to maximize joint motion and minimize muscle atrophy. Children with JRA are also monitored for a range of physical problems (e.g., growth abnormalities, nutrition, and vision; Rapoff et al., 2003).

Psychological Impact of Juvenile Rheumatoid Arthritis on Children and Families

Most children and adolescents with JRA live with chronic pain (Varni et al., 1996). Moreover, for some children with JRA, this pain persists into adulthood and is associated with long-term disability (L. S. Peterson, Mason, Nelson, O'Fallon, & Gabriel, 1997). The most systematic evidence concerning the psychological adjustment of children and adolescents with JRA comes from LeBovidge et al.'s (2003) meta-analytic review of 21 studies that described psychological adjustment problems, internalizing symptoms, externalizing symptoms, and poor self-concept among youths with chronic arthritis. Children and adolescents with arthritis demonstrated increased risk for overall psychological adjustment problems, especially internalizing symptoms, but not for externalizing symptoms or poor self-concept compared with physically healthy controls (LeBovidge et al., 2003). Findings from this meta-analysis suggest internalizing symptoms might be targeted in psychological interventions for children with JRA.

In addition to experiencing psychological symptoms, children and adolescents with JRA may demonstrate functional limitations in their daily activities and school attendance, which need to be addressed in psychological interventions, including family-centered interventions. C. C. Peterson and Palermo (2004) found that the level of children's psychological distress may exacerbate the impact of parental solicitous behaviors to pain and affect functioning among children with recurrent pain, including those with JRA. These and other available data underscore the need to develop individual and family-centered psychological interventions to enhance the functioning of children and adolescents with JRA (Palermo, 2000; C. C. Peterson & Palermo, 2005).

The problems experienced by Tammy, an 11-year-old girl with a 4-year history of JRA, illustrate some of the psychological concerns associated with JRA that may require psychological intervention. From the outset of her illness, Tammy has always reacted negatively to her illness. She has felt singled out by her condition, which has caused her to limit her interactions with peers. However, she now feels bad about herself because she cannot keep up with her peers in activities. Tammy has become increasingly withdrawn, which in turn has further limited her capacity to engage in prescribed exercise. The combination of her activity limitations and concerns about her condition has been associated with increasing frequency of pain. Her parents feel bad about her distress. However, because they do not want to upset her, they have been reluctant to set limits on her behavior.

Given the demands of medical treatment and psychological management of JRA, caring for a child with this condition can pose a significant burden on families, especially mothers, who have reported significantly higher levels of emotional distress than mothers of physically healthy children (Manuel, 2001). Moreover, the level of depressed mood among mothers of children with JRA predicted more frequent adjustment problems in children with JRA (Manuel, 2001). Such findings suggest that psychological interventions are needed to provide support for mothers of children with JRA.

Adherence to Medical Regimens

Children with JRA and their parents are asked to consistently follow a wide range of prescribed regimens, most notably medications, therapeutic exercises, and splinting of joints over a long period of time (Rapoff et al., 2003). As is true for many pediatric chronic illnesses, beneficial effects of such treatments may not be immediately apparent and do not relieve all of the pain and dysfunction associated with JRA. Moreover, treatments such as medications cause side effects (e.g., gastrointestinal irritation). For these and other reasons, it may be difficult for children and adolescents with JRA and their families to adhere to recommended medical treatment. Kroll, Barlow, and Shaw's (1999) review of descriptive studies found rates of nonadherence to medication treatment from 55% to 96% and adherence to physiotherapy from 47% to 86% in JRA. A detailed series of studies by Rapoff and his colleagues at one center, which was based on adherence data from electronic monitoring of pill counts, have documented rates of baseline adherence with medications as assessed by parental observations or pill counts from 38% to 59% (Rapoff, Lindsley, & Christophersen, 1984; Rapoff, Purviance, & Lindsley, 1988a, 1988b). Moreover, adherence problems have been found to be more frequent for prescribed exercises than with prescribed medications or splint wearing (Hayford & Ross, 1988; Rapoff, Lindsley, & Christophersen, 1985). Taken together, data concerning the prevalence of treatment nonadherence in JRA underscore the need for psychological interventions to enhance rates of adherence to treatment, which may enhance long-term medical outcomes and quality of life.

Reviews of Psychological Interventions in Juvenile Rheumatoid Arthritis

Walco, Sterling, Conte, and Engel's (1999) review of three studies that focused on pain management in JRA (Lavigne et al., 1992; Walco & Ilowite, 1992; Walco, Varni, & Ilowite, 1992) found that behavioral interventions such as progressive muscle relaxation, electromyogram feedback and thermal feedback, and guided imagery were associated with improvements in pain as well as increase in functional status (e.g., activities of daily living, school and peer interaction). Lemanek et al.'s (2001) review identified four studies of adherence to treatment in JRA, all of which were single-subject designs with children who demonstrated less than 80% of adherence to treatment during a 1- to 2-month baseline period (Pieper, Rapoff, Purviance, & Lindsley, 1989; Rapoff et al., 1984, 1988a, 1988b). Empirical support was found for a range of behavioral intervention approaches (e.g., self and parent monitoring, positive verbal feedback, behavior reinforcement) with or without educational strategies (e.g., instruction concerning the importance of taking medications and potential side effects; Lemanek et al., 2001).

Examples of Psychological Interventions in Juvenile Rheumatoid Arthritis

Published reports of psychological interventions in JRA are summarized in Table 9.2.

Cognitive–Behavioral Approaches: Pain Management

In an RCT, Field et al. (1997) found that massage therapy compared with progressive muscle relaxation was associated with a decrease in anxiety and cortisol after each massage session and a decrease in the incidence and severity of pain and pain-limiting activities. Lavigne et al. (1992) tested the effects of relaxation and electromyogram thermal feedback and monitoring of physical therapy and school attendance and found that the parents reported a decrease in pain posttreatment and on 3- to 6-month follow-up in the intervention group but no difference in behavioral symptoms. Walco et al. (1992) found that cognitive–behavioral and self-regulatory methods, including progressive muscle relaxation, guided imagery, and meditative breathing, were associated with a reduction in pain intensity posttreatment and a decrease in child- and parent-reported pain at 6- and 12-month follow-up.

Several case series and intervention studies by Rapoff and his colleagues have demonstrated effects of various educational and behavioral interventions to promote adherence to various components of the treatment for JRA, including prednisone, anti-inflammatory medications, and splint wearing (Rapoff et al., 1984, 1988a, 1988b, 2002). Among these studies, the most extensive and well controlled was Rapoff et al.'s (2002) RCT that compared an educational and behavioral contingency-based intervention with a control. The experimental group demonstrated greater adherence to medication than the control group, but no differences were found in frequency of pain.

Educational and Support Approaches

Hagglund et al. (1996) found that an intervention that provided education and support concerning JRA and medical management in the context of a 3-day retreat improved children's internalizing symptoms and reduced children's pain intensity and strain on caregivers; however, the intervention did not improve children's externalizing symptoms or caregivers' psychological distress. Stefl, Shear, and Levinson (1989) noted that outdoor camping and education to improve JRA-related knowledge and illness management were associated with increased self-esteem but not locus of control.

TABLE 9.2
Psychosocial Interventions for Juvenile Rheumatoid Arthritis

Authors	Target population	Sample	Design and content	Sessions			Outcomes	Findings	
				No.	Length	Duration		+ Significant	− Nonsignificant
Cognitive–behavioral interventions for pain									
Field et al. (1997)	Parents and child	N = 20, mean age = 9.8 years	Massage therapy versus progressive muscle relaxation (RCT)	30	15 minutes/day	30 days	Anxiety, cortisol samples	Decrease in anxiety and stress hormones (salivary cortisol) after each massage; at 30 days; decrease in pain (incidence and severity) and activities limited by pain	
Lavigne et al. (1992)	Parents and child	N = 8, age = 9–17 years	Child: relaxation training, electromyogram, thermal feedback; parent: behavioral methods to monitor physical therapy and school attendance (wait-list control group)	6, bi-weekly	First = 90 minutes, second–sixth = 60 minutes	3-month and 6-month follow-ups	Pain (child, parent, doctor report); behavioral symptoms, CBCL	Parent reported decrease in pain and pain-related behavior posttreatment at follow-up	Behavioral symptoms
Walco et al. (1992)	Parents and child	N = 13	Cognitive–behavioral self-regulatory methods: progressive muscle relaxation, guided imagery, meditative breathing	8 (1/week)	Not specified	8-week and 6- and 12-month follow-ups	Chronic joint pain, pain intensity disease activity, level of functional disability	Reduction in child and parent pain intensity posttreatment and at 6-month follow-up, functional status improved	Disease activity

Educational and support interventions

Study	Population	N; age	Intervention	Sessions	Time	Follow-up	Measures	Results	
Hagglund et al. (1996)	Parents and child	N = 27, mean age = 10.4 years	Retreat/intervention: education concerning JRA and medical management; improve functional capacities, coping skills, and self-esteem; enhance family functioning; exercise therapy (uncontrolled study)	3	14 hours	3-day retreat, follow-up 6 months posttreat	CBCL, Pediatric Pain Questionnaire, caregivers' strain and caregivers' distress (SCL-90-R)	Improved internalizing symptoms, pain intensity (child report), strain on caregivers	Externalizing symptoms, pain intensity (parent report), caregivers' psychological distress
Stefl et al. (1989)	Child	N = 32; mean age = 12.5 years	Traditional outdoor camping and educational sessions to improve knowledge and illness management (uncontrolled study)	5	Evening at camp	5 days; 6-month follow-up	Self-concept, locus of control	Self-esteem	Locus of control

Social support: Parents

Study	Population	N; age	Intervention	Sessions	Time	Follow-up	Measures	Results	
Ireys et al. (1996)	Parents	N = 48, age (child) = 2–11 years; age (parent) = 24–55 years	Social support intervention (RCT): mothers of children with JRA paired with mentors who were mothers of adult children (ages 18–24 years) with JRA; telephone contact; individual meeting with mentor; special event (e.g., picnic, small group lunch)	Varied	Phone call ≥5 minutes every 2 weeks; individual meeting every 6 weeks	15 months	Mental health = psychiatric symptom index; social support: information support, affirmation support, emotional support; mental health symptoms	Anxiety decreased and number of persons perceived as source of support increased in experimental group	Social support

Behavioral–educational approaches to promote adherence to treatment

Study	Population	N; age	Intervention	Sessions	Time	Follow-up	Measures	Results	
Pieper et al. (1989)	Child	N = 3, age = 11–18 years	Multiple baseline across subjects (standardized education and behavioral intervention)	2	30 minutes	8–12-month follow-up	Adherence (pill count) to prednisone medication	Increased adherence posttreatment and follow-up	

(continued)

TABLE 9.2 (Continued)

Authors	Target population	Sample	Design and content	Sessions No.	Length	Duration	Outcomes	Findings + Significant	Findings - Nonsignificant
Rapoff et al. (1984)	Parents and child	N = 1, age = 7 years	Token economy	Daily		10 weeks	Adherence (parent observation of adherence to medication and splint wearing)	Increase in all three behaviors posttreatment and follow-up	
Behavioral-educational approaches to promote adherence to treatment									
Rapoff et al. (1988a)		N = 1, age = 14 years	Organizational strategy (simplified regimen) and token economy		1.5 hours	9 months	Adherence (pill count, parental ratings of symptoms), joint count	Increase in adherence and active joint counts; decreased symptoms	
Rapoff et al. (1988b)	Child	N = 3, age = 3–13 years	Multiple baseline across subjects; standardized educational versus behavioral intervention		1.5 hours	4 months	Adherence (pill counts, parental ratings)	Increase in adherence on both measures for 2 of 3 participants	
Rapoff et al. (1988b)	Parent and child	N = 1, age = 14 years, JRA	Organizational strategy (simplified regimen) and token economy	Baseline regimen, 41 weeks		45 weeks, 9-month follow-up	Adherence to tolmetin sodium (pill count, parental ratings), joint count; pain symptoms	Fewer active joints, similar trend for morning stiffness and activity level; decreased pain symptoms	
Rapoff et al. (2002)	Parents and child	N = 34, mean age = 8.44 years	Educational and behavioral (contingency-shaped behavioral) intervention (RCT)	1 session, nurse called family every 2 weeks for 2 months, then monthly for 10 months	1 clinic visit = 30 minutes	52 weeks	Adherence (electronic bottle cap), disease activity, functional limitations	Improved adherence in experimental groups	Disease activity, functional limitations

Note. Empty cells indicate that data were not available. RCT = randomized controlled trials; CBCL = Child Behavioral Checklist; JRA = juvenile rheumatoid arthritis; SCL-90-R = Symptom Checklist–90 Revised.

Social Support Approaches: Parents

Ireys et al. (1996) reported that maternal social support intervention was effective in reducing anxiety among mothers of children with a number of chronic illnesses, including JRA, but not in improving overall level of social support.

Behavioral Approaches to Enhance Treatment

Stark, Janicke, et al. (2005) tested the efficacy of a behavioral intervention that involved parents and children in behavioral management and reinforcement compared with an enhanced standard of care, including counseling to increase calcium intake in children with JRA. Children with JRA are at risk for low bone density and hence higher rates of fractures as adults and are in need of calcium supplementation (Zak & Pederson, 2000). Behavioral intervention was associated with a greater increase in average dietary calcium intake than enhanced standard of care. In addition, a significantly greater percentage of children who received behavioral intervention attained the goal of 1,500 mg of calcium at posttreatment compared with standard care.

Research Recommendations

Although the findings of a number of behavioral and educational interventions to enhance psychological adaptation and pain management in JRA have been positive, there are too few studies of psychological interventions to warrant firm conclusions concerning the efficacy of these approaches. To date, a number of studies have shown promising findings, but many of these have had small samples and no controls (Lavigne et al., 1992; Walco et al., 1992). For this reason, there is a serious need for well-controlled, psychological intervention studies with relatively large samples of children with JRA that are designed to reduce pain and enhance functioning.

Rapoff (2000) recommended a comprehensive research program concerning psychological intervention to promote adherence to treatment in pediatric chronic illness that is based on research with JRA. The recommended program includes (a) manipulations of specific variables to improve adherence to treatment, including single-subject designs, which can accommodate small sample sizes and allow for changes in intervention protocols to address variables that can affect the adherence of individual children and adolescents; and (b) randomized, between-groups studies to test the effects of psychological interventions on the adherence of children and adolescents with JRA (Rapoff et al., 2002). In addition to Rapoff's (2000) recommendations, it would be useful to study the effectiveness of psychological interventions that are provided to children and adolescents with JRA and their families in the context of comprehensive care. In particular, it would be helpful to determine the extent to which psychological interventions are associated with reduction in frequency and severity of pain as well as enhanced psychological adjustment and ability to function in activities. The next section on clinical applications describes additional recommendations for studies of clinical effectiveness.

Clinical Applications

On the basis of their review, Kroll et al. (1999) concluded that psychological interventions that focus only on enhancing the knowledge of the child and family about JRA and its treatment may not necessarily translate into action. For this reason, these authors recommend that family-centered behavior modification should be part of any comprehensive educational approach.

Rapoff et al. (2003) offered a number of cogent suggestions for psychological interventions to enhance pain management that should be tested in future research in clinical care settings with children and adolescents with JRA. For example, helping children to manage disease-related stressors (e.g., relaxation and problem-solving techniques) would be expected to reduce negative emotions and pain. In addition, cognitive restructuring may be useful in countering maladaptive thinking about pain by having children identify negative thoughts, challenge or question these thoughts, and substitute more helpful thoughts. Imagery techniques, combined with relaxation exercises, can help divert attention from pain (Rapoff et al., 2003). Finally, helping parents to use adaptive strategies for coping with pain so that they can model these strategies for their children and enlisting the social support and reinforcement of family and friends are potentially useful approaches.

With respect to treatment adherence problems, Rapoff (2000) proposed an innovative preventive intervention model for children with chronic illness, including JRA, who present with different levels of risk for nonadherence to medical treatment. This model is comparable in concept to the tiered intervention model described by Kazak et al. (2003) for pediatric cancer (see chap. 8). Intensive educational and behavioral strategies implemented by highly trained mental health practitioners are typically given to children and adolescents with serious treatment adherence problems in many settings. However, primary and secondary preventive approaches, which have the potential to prevent or minimize the deleterious effects of medical nonadherence on pain management and medical morbidity, need to be developed and implemented at many centers. It would be instructive to implement and evaluate the effectiveness of a prevention-based approach in clinical care of children and adolescents with JRA on frequency of pain medical morbidities and the costs of medical care. Tertiary prevention efforts should be provided and evaluated for those patients with JRA who demonstrate the most problematic psychological adjustment difficulties or patterns of adherence to treatment. In particular, the impact of such interventions on medical morbidity and children's functioning should be documented as well (Rapoff, 2000). Research and clinical applications of psychological interventions for children and adolescents with JRA present important opportunities for pediatric psychologists.

10

PSYCHOLOGICAL INTERVENTIONS: CYSTIC FIBROSIS

Cystic fibrosis (CF) is a genetically inherited disease that affects 25,000 to 30,000 individuals in the United States (P. B. Davis, Drumm, & Konstan, 1996; Stark, Mackner, Patton, & Action, 2003). This multifaceted chronic condition, which affects the secretory glands of major organs in the respiratory, gastrointestinal, and reproductive systems, is characterized by chronic progressive pulmonary disease and pancreatic insufficiency (Stark, Mackner, et al., 2003). The production of thick mucus that is a hallmark of the condition leaves the patient's lungs vulnerable to recurrent pulmonary infections. These infections can result in a continuing cycle of progressive vulnerability to pulmonary exacerbations and complications (e.g., symptoms of fatigue, reduced pulmonary function and appetite, weight loss, increased cough and sputum production, and fever), recurrent bronchial obstruction due to infection, inflammation, and eventually brochiectasis or lung damage (P. B. Davis et al., 1996). If these symptoms do not respond to first-line antibiotics, treatment with intravenous antibiotics during a hospitalization may be required (Cystic Fibrosis Foundation, 2001).

A second major medical problem associated with CF, pancreatic insufficiency, prevents the efficient digestion of fat, protein, and fat-soluble

Kathy Zebracki made significant contributions to the writing of this chapter and creation of the table.

vitamins and can also result in significant symptoms and complications. Such malabsorption coupled with the energy demands due to lung disease can result in inadequate nutrition and reduced physical growth (Stark, Mackner, et al., 2003).

Because CF is a progressive disease, some patients experience an increasing number and severity of complications as they become older, such as CF-related diabetes (Stark, Mackner, et al., 2003), liver disease (Cystic Fibrosis Foundation, 2001), and osteoporosis (Stark, Mackner, et al., 2003). The complications (primarily pulmonary) that are associated with CF result in early death as a result of cardiorespiratory failure. In addition, men with CF also experience fertility problems as a consequence of the disease. Women with CF are fertile and, although often advised not to become pregnant because of health risks, are giving birth in increasing numbers (Gilljam et al., 2000).

MEDICAL TREATMENT

Advances in medical treatment and management have resulted in an increase in the average life span of individuals with CF to 32 years (Cystic Fibrosis Foundation, 2001; Doershuk, 2001). Optimal medical management for CF involves a strenuous, multifaceted treatment regimen that focuses on assisting the patient in clearing the mucus from the lungs and treating infections, with the goal of lowering the risk of multiple infections. For example, to help the patient clear mucus from the lungs and reduce airway obstruction, chest physiotherapy (CPT) methods require a caregiver to clap on the patient's chest two to four times daily for up to 30 minutes each time. To assist in clearing the mucus prior to CPT, patients may also use inhaled or nebulized bronchodilators to open their airways and/or mucolytic agents to thin the mucus (Stark, Mackner, et al., 2003). Two devices, the Flutter and the high-frequency chest compression (HFCC) vest (ThAIRapy vest), are also available that give patients a way to do airway clearance without assistance from others (Stark, Mackner, et al., 2003). The Flutter is an inexpensive, small, plastic handheld device that loosens mucus and accelerates airflow in the mid and large airways by vibrating airway walls when the patient exhales into it. The HFCC vest loosens mucus by delivering sharp compression pulses to the entire chest via an inflatable vest worn by the patient. Although the HFCC vest is effective compared with standard CPT, it is expensive and is not always covered by health insurance. Another recent advance in airway clearance is the development of rhDNase to decrease the viscosity of lung secretions (Stark, Mackner, et al., 2003).

Antibiotics have been a critical component of treatment for bronchial infections associated with CF for many years. In addition to routine use of antibiotics, anti-inflammatory therapy, including steroids such as prednisone, and nonsteroidal anti-inflammatory agents, such as ibuprofen, are used in treatment. During episodes of pulmonary exacerbation, the antibiotic regimen is often intensified, as are airway clearance treatments (Stark, Mackner, et al., 2003).

Nutritional treatment is also important in the clinical management of CF, because it can offset the energy loss from malabsorption and the energy demands due to lung disease. Individuals with CF are advised to consume 120% to 150% of the recommended daily allowance of calories for healthy individuals and a regimen of fat-soluble vitamins (Ramsey, Farrell, & Pencharz, 1992). Finally, during the past decade, double lung transplantation has become a therapeutic option for patients with CF who have end-stage lung disease, although a shortage of donors has limited the number of patients with CF who can potentially benefit (P. B. Davis et al., 1996).

PSYCHOLOGICAL IMPACT OF CYSTIC FIBROSIS ON CHILDREN, ADOLESCENTS, AND YOUNG ADULTS

The physical symptoms, morbidity (including deterioration in functioning), and treatment-related demands associated with CF have significant psychological implications (Stark, Mackner, et al., 2003). A wide range of psychological adjustment problems in peer, family, and school situations have been described in children and adolescents with CF (Drotar, 1978; Stark, Mackner, et al., 2003). For example, controlled studies have described a higher than average risk for insecure attachment among young children with CF (Goldberg, Gotowiec, & Simmons, 1995) and less adaptive feeding behaviors, such as taking longer to eat and refusing food more frequently, than healthy children (Powers et al., 2002; Stark et al., 1996, 2005). In addition, school-age children with CF may be at risk for anxiety and behavioral problems, which may be potential targets for psychological interventions (R. J. Thompson et al., 1992, 1998).

On the other hand, studies of the psychological adjustment of school-age children with CF have shown varying findings concerning the frequency and severity of psychological symptoms (Stark, Mackner, et al., 2003). Controlled studies using objective methods have generally identified fewer adjustment problems than noncontrolled studies. Moreover, prospective studies have found that psychological symptoms lessen over time among school-age children with CF (R. J. Thompson et al., 1999).

The nature of psychological adjustment among adolescents and young adults with CF has not been well described in empirical research that has been based on controlled methods. However, clinical experiences indicate that some young adults with CF may experience increased painful psychological adjustments in response to deterioration in their physical condition that may require psychological intervention (Drotar, 1978). Adolescents and young adults with CF face significant psychological dilemmas related to the worsening of their symptoms, dealing with an increasing number of school and work absences related to their illness, physical appearance and body image problems such as delayed puberty and small physical stature, maintaining peer relationships, conflicts with their parents about adherence to medical treatment (DiGirolamo, Quittner, Ackerman, & Stevens, 1997), and problems developing intimate relationships (D'Auria, Christian, Henderson, & Haynes, 2000). However, these stressors do not inevitably result in adjustment problems or psychiatric diagnoses. Some studies have found that many adults with CF experience surprisingly good psychological adjustment (D. L. Anderson, Flume, & Hardy, 2001).

A number of adolescents and young adults with CF experience problems that require psychological intervention, such as Katelyn, a 19-year-old with CF. She had been a leader in her high school class and was doing well in college. Moreover, until recently, she had not had significant exacerbations of her condition. However, Katelyn developed an infection, which necessitated a 2-week hospitalization. She was informed that her pulmonary functioning (a measure of the overall capacity and functioning of her lungs) had decreased. She became depressed in response to her hospitalization. She also became increasingly concerned about the implications of her illness for her future and wondered whether she should drop out of school. She asked to see a psychologist to discuss her concerns.

As shown by Katelyn, the psychological functioning and quality of life (QOL) of adolescents and young adults with CF may depend on their level of physical functioning (Stark, Mackner, et al., 2003). For example, one would expect adults in the more advanced phases of illness to demonstrate higher levels of depression and anxiety and lower QOL than those with less advanced illness-related complications (D. L. Anderson et al., 2001). This group may benefit from psychological support and intervention.

Another set of important but unanswered questions that are highly relevant to potential psychological interventions for young adults with CF concerns the stressors associated with family formation among adults with CF. The fact that some young women are choosing to have children at a time when they face significant deterioration in their physical condition raises extraordinary challenges that need to be addressed in psychological interventions (Gilljam et al., 2000).

PSYCHOLOGICAL IMPACT OF CYSTIC FIBROSIS ON FAMILIES

The medical treatment of CF imposes extensive treatment demands on patients and their families that affect every aspect of their daily lives, including family interactions, peer relationships, school, and participation in sports and other activities (Quittner et al., 1996; Quittner, Opipari, Regoli, Jacobsen, & Eigen, 1992). A wide range of illness-related and non-illness-related demands have been described by parents of children and adolescents with CF (Ievers & Drotar, 1996; Quittner et al., 1996). On the basis of a detailed activity log, Quittner et al. (1992) found that mothers of infants with CF differed from mothers of healthy infants in time spent on family chores, child care, and medical care versus recreation but not on measures of general role strain. In addition, parents of children with CF have shown more conflict over child rearing and a greater burden of child care than parents of healthy children (Quittner et al., 1998).

Ievers and Drotar's (1996) review of family and parental functioning concluded that parents of children with CF experienced greater stress and burdens than parents of healthy children. On the other hand, parenting behavior and family functioning were comparable in CF and healthy controls. Higher levels of parental distress, an avoidant coping style, and low levels of family support were associated with more problematic psychological adjustment in children. Using observational methods of family intervention at mealtimes, Mitchell, Powers, Byars, Dickstein, and Stark (2004) found that the families of children with CF demonstrated lower functioning on a number of dimensions, such as communication, interpersonal involvement, behavioral control, affect management, and roles. These and other findings that underscore problems in the functioning among families of children with CF compared with healthy children (Spieth et al., 2001) highlight the need for psychological interventions that focus on helping parents and family members manage the burdens of the child's CF more effectively to reduce the level of family dysfunction. Moreover, enhancement of family functioning and interactions during mealtimes may improve the child's calorie intake (Mitchell, Powers, et al., 2004; Stark, Jelalian, et al., 2005).

ADHERENCE TO TREATMENT

Problems with adherence to the complex, multifaceted CF treatment regimen are often a primary focus of referrals for psychological intervention for children and adolescents with CF (Koocher et al., 1990). Czajkowski and Koocher's (1986) study of adherence in a controlled hospital setting found that more than one third of hospitalized adolescents had clinically significant levels of nonadherence to CPT. One would expect that the prevalence of adherence problems would be even higher among outpatients who must fit the demands of a complex treatment regimen, including CPT, diet, and antibiotic treatment, into their daily activities (Ricker, Delamater, & Hsu, 1998).

Adherence problems are important given the medical evidence that regular CPT along with other components of the medical treatment is effective in delaying the progression of lung disease in patients with CF (Patterson, Budd, Goetz, & Warwick, 1993; Reisman et al., 1988). In addition, treatment adherence problems are a major source of conflict for families of patients with CF, particularly during adolescence (DiGirolamo et al., 1997; Patterson et al., 1993; Quittner, Drotar, et al., 2000). On the basis of the above data, problems with adherence to treatment and family conflict concerning adherence to treatment are important potential targets of psychological interventions, as illustrated by Brad, a 17-year-old with CF, which was diagnosed in his 1st year of life. Brad's parents have been concerned that he has become increasingly nonadherent to his treatment for CF. In fact, Brad was outspoken about his nonadherence to treatment. He noted that the time that is taken up by his different treatments limited the time that he had for peer relationships, which were a priority for him. He also wondered what good his treatment was doing anyway because it was not going to cure his illness. His problems with adherence had increased after a recent hospitalization. Brad's refusal to complete his CF-related treatment caused increased conflict between him and his parents, who are worried about him and cannot understand why he does not want to be in better health. Brad and his family are in need of intervention to help them develop more effective strategies of communication and management of his adherence to treatment.

REVIEWS OF PSYCHOLOGICAL INTERVENTIONS TO PROMOTE ADJUSTMENT

The state of the art concerning the empirical support for psychological interventions for CF is less developed than it is for other chronic conditions such as diabetes and asthma. Glasscoe and Quittner's (2005) detailed search and review of psychological interventions for CF identified eight studies that conducted randomized controlled trials (RCTs) or quasi-randomized trials. Five of these studies included children and adolescents and were published (Delk, Gevirtz, Hicks, Carden, & Rucker, 1994; Grasso, Button, Allison, & Sawyer, 2000; Hernandez-Reif et al., 1999; Powers, 1999; Stark et al., 1996). However, no studies were identified that focused explicitly on interventions to promote adherence to medical treatment. Methodological limitations in this body of intervention research included the relative absence of RCTs, valid measures of outcome, and blinding of assessors in study methods. The heterogeneity of the studies reviewed made it impossible to combine the results into an overall effect size for the psychological interventions. Moreover, high-quality efficacy trials for psychological interventions with CF were rare. Studies were uncontrolled and had small samples. Finally, the findings were inconsistent (Glasscoe & Quittner, 2005).

A meta-analysis that compared the effects of behavioral interventions versus medical interventions to enhance parenteral and enteral nutrition for children with CF found that the gains associated with the behavioral treatment were comparable with that of medical interventions in promoting weight gain and caloric intake (Jelalian, Stark, Reynolds, & Seifer, 1998). These findings suggest that behavioral interventions that are targeted to enhance feeding behaviors and caloric intake are promising methods to enhance children's nutritional status but need to be studied in controlled trials with long-term follow-up.

EXAMPLES OF PSYCHOLOGICAL INTERVENTIONS

Specific examples of studies of psychoeducational interventions in CF are described in this section. A summary of the published empirical studies of interventions conducted to enhance the psychological adjustment and adaptation of children and adolescents is shown in Table 10.1. These interventions included the following content areas: psychoeducational, psychosocial, behavioral, cognitive–behavioral, and combined educational and behavioral approaches.

Psychoeducational Approaches

Using a pre–post study design, Bartholomew et al. (1997) evaluated a family-centered educational intervention that was conducted with parent–child dyads. Specific educational modules were given in respiratory care, nutrition, malabsorption, communication, and coping using behavioral methods such as goal setting, modeling, and skill training. The family education intervention was associated with an increase in knowledge of CF self-efficacy, self-management of CF by parents and children, and adherence in behavioral symptoms. On the other hand, no changes were obtained on parenting stress or well-being.

Using a similar design and a psychoeducational intervention with a smaller sample, Goldbeck and Babka (2001) found increases in children's competence and optimism but no difference in knowledge of or adherence to CF treatment as a function of intervention. Finally, M. A. Davis et al.'s

TABLE 10.1
Psychological Interventions for Children and Adolescents With Cystic Fibrosis (CF)

Authors	Target population	Sample	Design and content of intervention	Sessions No.	Sessions Length	Treatment duration and follow-up	Outcomes	Findings + Significant	Findings – Nonsignificant
Psychoeducational interventions									
Bartholomew et al. (1997)	Parent and child	N = 199 dyads, age = 1–18 years (M = 8.6)	Family Education Program: social cognitive theory methods (goal setting, reinforcement, modeling, skill training, self-monitoring); instructional modules (class management, care, communication, coping); pre–post design, nonrandomized design	1	Unknown	Post-intervention 1.5–2.5 years	Knowledge, self-efficacy, self-management behaviors, health, and impact on parent and family, QOL, and internalizing–externalizing symptoms, pulmonary function	Increase in knowledge (parent, adolescent, child), self-efficacy (parent, child), self-management (parent, adolescent), problem solving (parent)	Self-efficacy (adolescent), outcome expectations (parent, adolescent), problem solving (parent), pulmonary function, QOL, impact on family, Parenting Stress index
Goldbeck & Babka (2001)	Parents and child	N = 16, age = 0–12 years (M = 7); 2 groups: 0–6 and 7–12 years) SES: 50% middle class, 50% lower class	Psychoeducational concerning genetics, pulmonary symptoms and treatment	3–4	4 hours	Not specified	Parent and child decrease in coping, parental health beliefs, adherence to CPT	Child's competence, optimism, and knowledge of CF	Knowledge about CF, child's irritability, adherence to treatment
M. A. Davis et al. (2004)	Children and adolescents	N = 47, age 7–17 years	Viewing CD-ROM: *Fitting Cystic Fibrosis Into Your Life Every Day* (Starbright Foundation, 2003)	1	30 minutes	2–3 months	Knowledge of CF coping strategies	Knowledge; frequency of effective situations	Frequency or difficulty of problem situations

Social support interventions

Study	Population	N, age	Intervention	Sessions	Length	Duration	Measures	Results	
Ireys, Chernoff, DeVet, & Kim (2001)	Parents of children with CF, diabetes mellitus, sickle cell anemia, and asthma	$N = 139$ ($n = 13$ with CF), age = 7–11	FFN: enhancement of mothers' perceived availability of social support by linking mothers of school-aged children with "veteran" mothers whose similarly affected children were now young adults	7; biweekly telephone contact, 3 special events (e.g., bowling, lunch)	60–90 minutes; phone, 5 minutes	15 months; follow-ups at 4, 8, and 16 months	BDI, PSI	Maternal anxiety decreased; self-reported health improved	Depression, stressful life events
Chernoff et al. (2002)	Parents and children with CF, diabetes mellitus, sickle cell anemia, and asthma	$N = 136$ ($n = 13$ with CF), age = 7–11 years	KIDS: enhancement of the mental health, adjustment, and self-esteem of children; FFN: focus on mothers; discussed significant issues that arose during visits	KIDS: 7+ monthly phone calls to children; FFN: weekly	KIDS: 60–90 minutes	15 months	Adjustment (PARS), depression, anxiety, self-perception	PARS: hostility, anxiety, and depression decreased; physical self-esteem	PARS: dependency, withdrawal, productivity, peer relations; depression, self-esteem

Behavioral interventions

Study	Population	N, age	Intervention	Sessions	Length	Duration	Measures	Results	
Delk et al. (1994)	Children and adults	$N = 26$, age = 10–41 years	Biofeedback assisted breathing retraining (control): biofeedback assisted relaxation training)	8	Not specified	4 weeks	Lung function	Improvement in lung function, mean forced expiratory flow	

(continued)

TABLE 10.1 (Continued)

Authors	Target population	Sample	Design and content of intervention	No.	Length	Treatment duration and follow-up	Outcomes	+ Significant	– Nonsignificant
			Behavioral interventions						
Stark et al. (1987)	Child	N = 1, age = 11 years, female	Behavioral contracting (e.g., rewards, treats, privileges, activities)	50 (1–24 baseline, 25–50 behavioral contract)	20–30 minutes (for CPT)	3, 6, and 9 weeks	Adherence to CPT	Adherence, physiological measures, family functioning	
Hagopian & Thompson (1999)	Child	N = 1, age = 8 years	Shaping and cooperation	120	5–20 minutes	14 weeks	Adherence to respiratory treatment	Increase in adherence to respiratory treatment, decrease in problem behavior	
Singer et al. (1991)	Parents and children	N = 4, ages = 10–42 months	Behavioral management (e.g., use of range of reinforcers), contingency management	—	Daily during hospital-ization	Approximately 3–13 days; 3-year follow-up	Caloric intake	Increase mean % of caloric intake, persistent catch-up growth in some children	
Hernandez-Reif et al. (1999)	Parents and children	N = 20, age = 5–12 years (M = 9.9)	RCT of massage therapy: parents instructed on how to conduct massage; parents conducted 20-minute child massage at bedtime each night; reading control: parents read to child for 20 minutes	30	20 minutes	1 month	Parent and child anxiety; child's mood (POMS), peak air flow	Decrease in parent and child anxiety, improvement in child's mood and peak air flow	

Cognitive–behavioral interventions

Study	Age group	Sample	Intervention	Sessions	Length	Frequency	Measures	Results	Coping
Hains et al. (1997)	Adolescent	$N = 5$, age = 13–15 years, 60% male	Training in cognitive restructuring and problem-solving skills; no comparison group	9	1 hour	Weekly	Trait anxiety, coping, functional disability, psychological functioning (parent report)	Decrease in anxiety, maladaptive coping with CF-related problems, functional disability, increase in positive coping	Coping
Hains et al. (2001)	Young adult	$N = 4$, age = 22–27 years, 75% female, 100% Caucasian	Cognitive restructuring and problem solving; no comparison group	8	—	Weekly, 3-month follow-up	Anxiety, anger, perceptions of functional disability, coping	Decreased anxiety ($n = 1$), anger ($n = 1$), functional disability ($n = 2$), increase in approach and avoidant coping ($n = 2$)	Anxiety, anger ($n = 3$), functional disability ($n = 2$), approach–avoidant coping ($n = 2$)
Taylor et al. (2003)	Children and adults	$N = 39$, age = 15–37 years	Written self-disclosure: writing about an important emotionally distressing event of personal significance (control: standard care)	3	20 minutes	3–5 days; 2–3.7-month follow-up	Health care utilization, health status, psychological adjustment	Reduction in days in hospital over 3-month period	Outpatient utilization, physiological health status (FEV, BMI) or depression, anxiety, somatic complaints, stressful life events

(continued)

TABLE 10.1 (Continued)

Combined educational and behavioral interventions

Authors	Target population	Sample	Design and content of intervention	Sessions No.	Sessions Length	Treatment duration and follow-up	Outcomes	Findings + Significant	Findings − Nonsignificant
Stark et al. (1990)	Parents and children	$N = 5$, age = 5–12 years, 60% female	Nutritional education: behavioral management, contingency management strategies, and reward system	6	90 minutes	1-, 3-, 6-, and 9-month follow-ups	Caloric intake, weight gain	Caloric intake increased across meals; increase in weight and height maintained at follow-up	Proportion of food consumed as protein, carbo-hydrate, and fat
Stark et al. (1993)	Parents and children	$N = 3$, age = 3–8 years	Nutritional education: contingency management, relaxation training, rewards	7	1/week	7 weeks; follow-up: 4, 12, 24, 48, and 96 weeks	Caloric intake, weight gain	Caloric intake increased across meals; at posttreatment, maintained on follow-up; weight gain	
Stark et al. (2002)	Parents and children	$N = 44$, age = 3–12 years ($M = 7.5$)	Parent–child sessions: weigh and measure foods, strategies to boost caloric intake, differential attention, contingency management, and shaping	6–7	60–90 minutes	8–9 weeks, 12-month follow-up	Caloric intake and calcium intake	Increase in mean daily dietary calories posttest; especially older children increased calories more on 12-month follow-up ($n = 15$), maintained gains	
Stark et al. (1996)	Parents and children	$N = 9$, age = 5–10 years ($M = 7.3$)	Parents: nutritional education, behavioral management strategies aimed at mealtime behavior; children: relaxation techniques, nutritional education, and behavior	7	Not specified	6 weeks: 3- and 6-month follow-ups	Caloric intake (weight, height, skinfold), pulmonary functioning, resting energy expenditure, physical activity	Increased caloric intake, weight, catch-up growth maintained at follow-up	Pulmonary functioning, resting energy expenditure, activity level

Powers et al. (2003)	Parents	$N = 12$, age = 1–3 years	Nutrition intervention: nutrition education, review of education, physiology of CF, use of enzyme; nutrition + behavior intervention: same as above and behavioral management	8	60 minutes	1-year follow-up	Caloric intake, weight gain, height	Weight and height, caloric intake
Stark et al. (2003)	Parents and children	$N = 7$, age = 6–12 years	Nutrition education: behavioral intervention (differential attention, contingency privilege, sticker charts)	7	5 sessions = 90 minutes, 2 sessions = 90 minutes	Weekly for 9 weeks, follow-up at 6, 12, and 24 months	Caloric intake, weight gain	% fat intake; parent and child mealtime behaviors, family stress scale, adherence
Stark et al. (1994)	Parents	$N = 2$, age = 2–5 years; SES: middle/upper middle class; 100% male, 100% Caucasian	Behavioral parent training, didactic training, vignettes from videotapes, in vivo practice of differential attention, contingent privileges, setting limits	6–9	90 minutes/ week	6–9 weeks, follow-up at 3 and 8 months (Family 1) and 1 and 12 months (Family 2)	Parent–child mealtime interactions	Parental decrease in attention to disruptive behavior, increase in appropriate eating and parental control at meals, increase in children's appropriate behavior during mealtimes, caloric intake and weight

Note. Empty cells indicate no data were available. QOL = quality of life; SES = socioeconomic status; CPT = chest physiotherapy; FFN = Family to Family Network; BDI = Beck Depression Inventory; PSI = Psychiatric Symptom Inventory; KIDS = Kids Involved in Discovery and Sharing; PARS = Personal Adjustment and Roles Skill Scale; RCT = randomized controlled trial; POMS = Profile of Mood States; FEV = forced expiratory volume; BMI = body mass index.

(2004) RCT-based intervention evaluated the efficacy of the CD-ROM *Fitting Cystic Fibrosis Into Your Life Every Day* (Starbright Foundation, 2003). These investigators found that children's CF-related knowledge and coping strategies improved as a consequence of the intervention.

Social Support Approaches

Ireys, Chernoff, DeVet, and Kim (2001) tested the effects of a psychological intervention that was designed to enhance maternal social support by using a family-to-family support network. Support to mothers of children with CF was provided by mothers of children who also had a child with CF. The intervention was associated with improvements in maternal psychological distress. In a separate study, this intervention was found to be associated with decreased maternal anxiety (Ireys, Chernoff, DeVet, & Kim, 2001). This intervention also had a positive impact on children, because it reduced their levels of anxiety and depression (Ireys, Chernoff, DeVet, & Kim, 2001). However, because the research design involved families of children with diabetes and asthma in addition to CF, it was impossible to determine whether there were any unique effects for the small subgroup of children with CF and their families.

Behavioral Approaches

Several different methods of behavioral interventions with children and adolescents with CF have shown positive, short-term effects on psychological and physical functioning. For example, Delk et al. (1994) demonstrated that biofeedback-assisted breathing and retraining control resulted in enhanced pulmonary functioning in a sample of children, adolescents, and adults. Hernandez-Reif et al. (1999) found that massage therapy that was conducted by parents of children with CF was associated with a decrease in parent and child anxiety, improvement in mood, and peak air flow. Several case studies and series have also demonstrated the effectiveness of behavioral interventions (e.g., behavioral contracting, shaping, behavioral management) to improve adherence to CPT and children's caloric intake (Hagopian & Thompson, 1999; Singer, Nofer, Benson-Szekely, & Brooks, 1991; Stark, Miller, Plienes, & Drabman, 1987).

Cognitive–Behavioral Approaches

Hains and his colleagues conducted two detailed case series with adolescents (Hains, Davies, Behrens, & Bilber, 1997) and young adults (Hains, Davies, Behrens, Freeman, & Bilber, 2001) with CF that evaluated the effects of a cognitive–behavioral intervention that involved cognitive reframing and problem solving on psychological status (e.g., coping style, functional outcomes). This intervention was associated with a decrease in maladaptive coping with CF and functional disability, as well as an increase in positive coping (Hains et al., 1997). However, the strength of the intervention findings with young adults varied considerably across individuals (Hains et al., 2001). In a controlled study, L. A. Taylor, Wallander, Anderson, Beasley, and Brown (2003) found that written self-disclosure about an emotionally distressing event was associated with reduction in days of hospitalization but no change on a range of outcomes such as physical and mental health status among young adults.

Combined Educational and Behavioral Approaches

In a series of programmatic studies, Stark and her colleagues have tested the effects of combined nutrition education and behavioral interventions, including contingency management strategies and reward systems, on the caloric intake and weight gain of children with CF (Stark, Opipari, et al., 2003). One of the important features of this intervention approach was the involvement of parents and children. Two case series found that a combined intervention resulted in improved caloric intake and weight gain that was maintained at 6- to 9-month follow-up for school-age children (Stark, Bowen, Tyc, Evans, & Passero, 1990) and young children ages 3 to 8 years (Stark et al., 1993). Stark et al. (1996) added relaxation training to nutritional education, as well as behavioral management strategies directed at mealtime behaviors, and they found that this comprehensive evaluation was associated with increased caloric intake, weight gain, and catch-up growth. In a larger sample ($N = 44$), Stark, Mackner, Kessler, Opipari, and Quittner (2002) found that a manualized group behavioral intervention with separate but simultaneous parent–child sessions was associated with an increase in calcium intake.

In contrast, Powers et al. (2003) compared behavioral and nutrition education with nutrition education alone and found no differences in weight gain and caloric intake between the two groups. Finally, Stark, Opipari, et al. (2003) compared behavioral intervention with nutrition education. Both groups had an increase in weight gain and caloric intake, but the behavioral intervention had a greater increase including fat intake. No changes were found for adherence to treatment.

FUTURE DIRECTIONS IN INTERVENTION RESEARCH

As shown in Table 10.1, the science of psychological interventions for children and adolescents with CF and their families is in its early phases.

Two reviews of psychological intervention research in CF have generated recommendations for future research. With respect to developing the science of behavioral interventions to enhance nutrition in children with CF, Jelalian et al. (1998) recommended controlled clinical trials with larger sample sizes that have been studied to date. Moreover, these authors suggested that interventions should be administered uniformly to patients of similar age and disease severity and include frequent assessment periods during treatment coupled with long-term follow-up assessment. Studies of the costs, both economic and psychosocial, associated with various types of psychological interventions were also recommended. Jelalian et al. cautioned that in all likelihood, future studies of psychological intervention in CF will need to be multisite studies, owing to the limited availability of sufficient numbers of patients within restricted age ranges at single centers.

Glasscoe and Quittner's (2005) review underscored the following recommendations for future intervention research: (a) larger sample sizes and more rigorous research designs to replicate the promising findings of behavioral interventions; (b) studies of more complex interventions such as family therapy, psychotherapy, and cognitive–behavioral therapy and comprehensive behavioral interventions that focus on dietary management; and (c) more complete reporting of RCT design criteria in published articles and studies of interventions to promote adherence to medical treatment for CF (Glasscoe & Quittner, 2005).

One example of such research is Quittner, Drotar, et al.'s (2000) multisite RCT of psychological interventions that targeted adherence to treatment in adolescents with CF. Two structured 10-session interventions— the Family Learning Program, involving family-based education about CF and its management (Bartholomew et al., 1997), and behavioral family systems therapy, including problem solving, communication skills, cognitive restructuring, and functional–structural family issues—were compared with one another and standard psychosocial care. Preliminary analyses of the data have indicated that the behavioral family systems therapy intervention was associated with a reduction of family conflict as reported by the mother and adolescent, better communication, and fewer CF-specific problems (Quittner, Drotar, Ievers-Landis, & De Lambo, 2004).

In addition to the recommendations based on these research reviews, it would be useful to replicate and extend findings of innovative interventions (e.g., writing about emotional experiences) with larger populations at different sites (Taylor et al., 2003). Psychological interventions should also target potentially vulnerable subgroups such as adolescents and young adults who demonstrate deterioration in physical functioning and thus at are risk for increased psychological distress. Preventive interventions to provide support for young married individuals with CF, who face a unique set of stressors, should be developed and tested. Finally, a sufficient body of promising intervention findings have been gathered with children and adolescents with CF (e.g., M. A. Davis et al., 2004; Stark, Mackner, Patton, & Acton, 2003) to warrant studies examining the clinical effectiveness of psychological interventions that are delivered in the context of ongoing medical care.

RECOMMENDATIONS FOR CLINICAL CARE

One of the important future needs concerns the application of successful psychological interventions in ongoing clinical care with children, adolescents, and young adults with CF and their families. For example, the promising findings of behavioral and educational approaches to enhance nutritional management in preschool children with CF (Stark et al., 2002; Stark, Opipari, et al., 2003) should be extended to older children. It would also be useful to develop strategies to implement the principles of these behavioral–educational models in the comprehensive care of children with CF. On the basis of their research, Duff (2001) suggested that the following interventions be included in ongoing comprehensive care for CF: (a) more frequent use of cognitive–behavioral therapy for psychological distress in patients with CF; (b) greater patient access to psychological services early in the course of their medical care; (c) routine provision of support for parents and screening for psychological problems; (d) opportunities for Web-based support sites that allow children to express their emotions "safely," that is, without the pressure of face-to-face contact (e.g., http://www.tsa.uk.com; http://www.headroom.net.au); (e) CD-ROM–based educational approaches (M. A. Davis et al., 2004); and (f) psychological support to facilitate the transition to adolescents' management of their medical treatment and more independent functioning (Stark, Mackner, et al., 2003). It is clear that there is a wide range of important future clinical and research opportunities for psychologists who have an interest in helping children and adolescents with CF and their families.

IV

SUMMARY AND CONCLUSION

11

RECOMMENDATIONS TO ENHANCE SCIENCE, PRACTICE, AND POLICY

As described throughout this book, a great deal of progress has been made in developing and testing psychological intervention designs to enhance psychological adaptation and adherence to medical treatment of children and adolescents with various chronic health conditions. Nevertheless, much remains to be accomplished to develop the scientific knowledge of efficacious interventions and use these data to develop effective clinical applications. The purpose of this chapter is to summarize recommendations to enhance the development of science, practice, and policy concerning psychological interventions with children and adolescents with chronic health conditions.

GUIDING FRAMEWORK FOR RECOMMENDATIONS

The specific agenda to develop intervention research, clinical, or policy applications needs to be tailored to state-of-the-art of intervention science for individual chronic illness populations. For example, because of a longer, more extensive body of research, the state of the art concerning psychological intervention science is more well developed for conditions such as Type 1 diabetes mellitus (DM1) or asthma (see chaps. 6–7) than it is for conditions such as cystic fibrosis (CF) or sickle cell disease (SCD; see chaps. 9–10).

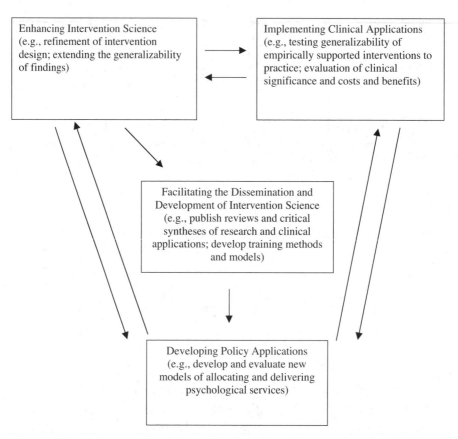

Figure 11.1. Conceptual framework for recommendations to enhance science, practice, and policy in psychological interventions.

For this reason, specific recommendations for research, clinical application, and policy cannot easily be generalized across different chronic pediatric illnesses. However, as shown in Figure 11.1, a general conceptual framework can be applied to psychological intervention research across different pediatric chronic illnesses to formulate recommendations.

This framework describes categories of recommendations in each of four key areas: (a) enhancing intervention science; (b) implementing clinical applications; (c) facilitating the dissemination and development of research findings of intervention science; and (d) developing policy applications. As shown in Figure 11.1, critical interrelationships among recommendations made in each of these critical areas should also be considered. For example, the need to use research findings to develop clinical applications of interventions is well recognized (Drotar, 2002). However, it must also be recognized that the influence of research and clinical practice is bidirectional. Consequently, findings from clinical application and observation of intervention effects (e.g., studies of clinical effectiveness) can and should be used to refine models of intervention that can be tested in controlled research studies.

Findings from both research and clinical application need to be synthesized, critically evaluated, and disseminated to researchers and practitioners. In addition, such findings should also be used to develop and guide training of practitioners as well as influence applications of policy such as the development of new models of allocation of services and comprehensive care. Finally, as shown in Figure 11.1, policy-related applications of psychological intervention science can suggest new clinical applications, models of service delivery, and research that can inform policy (e.g., research on program evaluation and cost-effectiveness).

STAGES OF INTERVENTION RESEARCH

In developing an agenda for intervention research, researchers should appreciate that the scientific state of the art is at different stages for different chronic conditions (see chaps. 6–10) as well as for different types or models of intervention. Exhibit 11.1 describes potential phases of psychological intervention research. It should be noted that this is intended as a guiding framework and not as a prescriptive one. Although research with pediatric chronic conditions does not necessarily proceed in discrete stages, this framework may help to determine benchmarks for the progress of psychological intervention research with specific chronic illness populations.

An initial phase of research concerns studies that provide the foundation for psychological intervention research (e.g., studies of prevalence and impact of specific target problems, description of risk and resilience factors that contribute to individual variation in clinical outcomes). Such data may be useful in determining targets of intervention and potential facilitators or barriers to change. Another phase of intervention research concerns pilot and feasibility studies that document the feasibility of the intervention, acceptability of the intervention to children and families, and preliminary evidence of intervention effects. A subsequent phase of intervention research focuses on establishing a sufficient body of scientific evidence for the intervention in controlled studies, randomized controlled trials (RCTs), and replications of interventions. Once an intervention model has been shown to be effective with a specific target problem in a specific chronic condition, the research emphasis shifts toward understanding why the intervention works and for whom. This phase of research involves studies of the efficacy of an intervention with different subgroups (e.g., analyses of moderators) and identification of the critical processes that underlie intervention effects through controlled studies and analyses of mediating processes. The final phase of intervention research concerns clinical application and policy to

EXHIBIT 11.1
Stages of Research in Psychological Interventions
in Pediatric Chronic Illness

1. Descriptive research that provides the foundation for intervention research
   - What are the prevalence and functional impact of target problems?
   - What are the risk factors that are potential barriers to change?
   - What are the resilience factors that facilitate change?

2. Pilot feasibility studies
   - Is the intervention feasible?
   - Can parents and children accept and manage the demands of the intervention?
   - Can the intervention be conducted in a realistic time frame?
   - Is there preliminary evidence of the interventions efficacy?

3. Efficacy studies
   - Is the intervention study effective in specific populations?
   - Is there sufficient evidence to consider the intervention empirically supported (e.g., randomized controlled trials and replication)?

4. Studies that analyze the source and power of intervention effects
   - Is the intervention more effective with some families than others (e.g., studies of moderators)?
   - What are the active ingredients in the intervention over and beyond support and contact?
   - By what process does the intervention affect outcomes (e.g., studies of mediators)?

5. Clinical application
   - Is the intervention model effective with clinical populations (studies of effectiveness)?
   - Does the intervention model result in clinically significant change?
   - Is the model effective with a range of populations in different settings?

promote clinical application. The primary data in this phase concern whether intervention models are effective with clinical populations in clinical settings and result in clinically significant change. The relevant policy-related questions and implementing strategies to develop the necessary resources to promote access concern the degree to which various empirically supported interventions are available and accessible to children and families in different settings.

ENHANCING THE SCIENCE
OF PSYCHOLOGICAL INTERVENTIONS

Specific recommendations to develop research, clinical applications, dissemination, and policy are summarized in Exhibit 11.2 and are now

EXHIBIT 11.2
Recommendations to Enhance the Science and Practice of
Psychological Interventions for Childhood Chronic Illness

1. Strategies to enhance the science of psychological interventions
   - Conduct case studies and case series that document feasibility and preliminary evidence for efficacy.
   - Conduct controlled studies including randomized controlled trials and replicate successful interventions with larger samples.
   - Determine why interventions work when they work (e.g., identify mediators and critical components of intervention effects).
   - Generalize intervention principles across different chronic conditions.
   - Conduct analyses of moderators of intervention effects.

2. Strategies to enhance clinical significance
   - Describe participants.
   - Include measures of functional impact.
   - Describe context of research.

3. Strategies to enhance clinical applications
   - Research and develop interventions in practice settings before testing them; produce case studies and case series.
   - Test the generalizability of empirically supported interventions to clinical populations.
   - Evaluate the effectiveness of tailoring psychological interventions to specific clinically relevant problems.
   - Study costs–benefits and offset of intervention.
   - Conduct program evaluations and monitor outcomes of comprehensive care.
   - Evaluate the implementation of interventions in practice settings.

4. Facilitating the dissemination and development of intervention science
   - Disseminate information on empirically supported interventions.
   - Synthesize the clinical significance of intervention research findings.
   - Publish reports on translating intervention research practice.
   - Develop new training methods and models for psychological intervention research.
   - Develop collaborations among intervention researchers.

5. Developing policy applications
   - Develop funding to support intervention services for children with chronic conditions.
   - Document allocation and funding of intervention services.
   - Create system-level change to reduce disparity in access and enhance prevention.

discussed. To develop the science of psychological interventions for pediatric chronic conditions, there is a continuing need for controlled studies, including RCTs. With a number of pediatric chronic conditions, there is a need to extend the findings of successful case studies and case series to controlled studies and RCTs (see chaps. 6–10). Well-executed and documented case studies and case series provide a scientifically valid and clinically relevant method of extending the state of the art in intervention research (Drotar, LaGreca, et al., 1995). Nevertheless, the transition from research that focuses on case studies and series to controlled trials is a challenge that requires considerable resources from grant funding. The degree to which grant funding can be obtained to fund controlled research studies often depends on the quality and demonstrated feasibility of the previous research.

Investigators who conduct RCTs of psychological intervention should follow recommendations based on the consolidated standards of reporting trials (CONSORT; Begg et al., 1996) statement for reporting the results of RCTs in journal articles (Altman et al., 2001; Stinson, McGrath, & Yamada, 2003). The recommendations cover the following parts of a typical journal article: title and abstract (e.g., how participants were allocated to interventions), introduction and background (e.g., scientific background and explanation of rationale), method and results (see below), and discussion (e.g., interpretation of results in the context of current evidence, generalizability of findings; Altman et al., 2001). Recommendations for inclusion of information are especially detailed for the method and results sections. For example, the method section should include eligibility criteria for participants; settings and locations where data were collected; how, when, and where interventions were administered; clearly defined primary and secondary outcomes; how the sample size was determined; randomization (including generation of the random allocation sequence and implementation); blinding or masking of participants and investigators; and statistical methods for primary and secondary analyses (Altman et al., 2001). Finally, the CONSORT statement recommends that the results section specify the flow of participants through each stage of protocol with a diagram, define the time periods of recruitment, describe the baseline demographic and clinical characteristics of each group, list the number of participants in each group, summarize results for each group for primary and secondary outcomes, present ancillary analyses, estimate effect size, and document adverse or side effects in each intervention group.

In some areas of research (e.g., psychological interventions to reduce procedure-related distress in pediatric cancer; Kuppenheimer & Brown, 2002), the most compelling research questions have moved beyond demonstrating whether psychological interventions work to determining why interventions work when they work and with whom they work most effectively. Nevertheless, obtaining the answers to these important but difficult questions poses challenges. Successful psychological interventions with pediatric chronic illness populations have included both general (e.g., psychological support, education) and specific (e.g., problem solving methods; see chaps. 6–10) components. Consequently, it is difficult to identify the most active ingredients of an intervention that accounted for efficacy in promoting behavior change and influencing relevant psychological outcomes. However, identification of the active ingredients of psychological intervention models is potentially important. Such research may lead to the development of psychological interventions that are more powerful, efficient, and potentially cost-effective because they target critical processes that are generalizable across specific samples and settings.

Analysis of Mediators of Intervention Effects

Identification of the active ingredients of psychological intervention models can also be accomplished by evaluating the processes that mediate the effects of successful interventions (Holmbeck, 1997; Kraemer et al., 2002; Rose, Holmbeck, Coakley, & Franks, 2004). Figure 11.2 depicts a general model for mediation effects.

Although analyses of mediation effects have not been conducted often in psychological intervention research with pediatric chronic illness, they can be instructive. Consider the example of an investigator who is interested in testing a cognitive–behavioral intervention to reduce psychological distress in children with cancer. In addition to documenting whether the intervention worked, the investigator wants to identify the mechanism or process by which the intervention worked. To accomplish this aim, he or she will need to develop a hypothesis concerning the factors that might account for a reduction in psychological distress. Potential mediating processes could involve practice in changing maladaptive cognitions about chronic illness or reducing maladaptive coping strategies (e.g., avoidance of distress) in favor of active coping strategies. Let us assume that change in maladaptive cognitions is hypothesized to be the primary mediator of the intervention effects. In this case, the study might be designed to test whether (a) the intervention resulted in changes in maladaptive cognitions and (b) these changes in maladaptive cognitions mediated or accounted for the changes in distress based on statistical analyses of mediation (Holmbeck, 1997). To test for mediation, the study will need to include reliable and valid measures of mediation. Investigators will need to plan their research design and measurement strategies accordingly (see chap. 3).

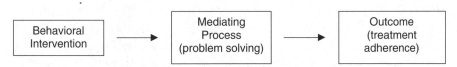

Figure 11.2. Illustration of mediating effect in an intervention study (problem-solving mediates the intervention effect on treatment adherence).

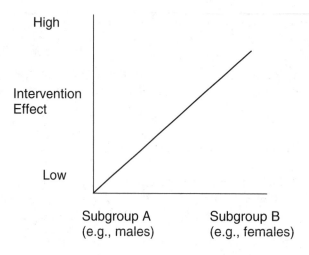

High

Intervention
Effect

Low

Subgroup A   Subgroup B
(e.g., males)   (e.g., females)

Figure 11.3. Illustration of moderating effect of gender in an intervention study (moderating effect is greater in females).

Identifying Moderators of Interventions

As noted in chapter 1, children and adolescents with chronic illness represent heterogeneous populations that vary considerably in age, socioeconomic status, family resources, and individual psychological functioning. Such variation poses significant challenges to the analysis and generalizability of effects of psychological interventions. For example, suppose that a particular psychological intervention is very effective for subgroups of children (e.g., younger but not older children) and families (those with moderate but not high levels of conflict). An analysis of intervention effects for the sample as a whole would obscure powerful interactions with age and family conflict. Consequently, an analysis of the intervention effects for the sample as a whole would lead to the faulty conclusion that the intervention was not effective. For this reason, an analysis of moderators of intervention effects as depicted in Figure 11.3 should be considered (Kraemer et al., 2000). To identify potential moderators of intervention effects, investigators should carefully consider previous research, clinical experience, and theoretical models. Study designs should include sufficient sample size so that there is adequate power to detect moderators of intervention effects. This is a difficult challenge, given the increased power that is needed to detect intervention effects (Aiken & West, 1991) and the limited sample sizes of children and adolescents with chronic illness at single sites.

Generalizability of Interventions

As increasing research documents the efficacy of specific psychological interventions with specific chronic conditions, this will set the stage for evaluating whether successful psychological intervention models can generalize across a range of settings and a range of chronic conditions. Generalizable models of psychological intervention are important from a public health perspective because they have the potential of improving the health and psychological adaptation of large numbers of children who share the stressors of chronic illness (Glasgow, Kleges, Dzewaltowski, Bull, & Estabrooks, 2004; R. E. K. Stein & Jessop, 1982). Intervention models that have been shown to be effective with heterogeneous chronic conditions include social support for parents (Ireys, Chernoff, Stein, DeVet, & Silver, 2001) and parent-centered psychological support and education models (Stein, 2001).

On the other hand, the scientific and public health importance of such noncategorical and potentially generalizable models of psychological interventions in pediatric chronic illness need to be balanced against the significant challenges posed by their implementation. One such challenge is that psychological intervention models that have been shown to be effective in work with children with one chronic condition need to be adapted to the specific illness-related stressors or illness management challenges that are characteristic of other conditions. For example, assume an investigator has successfully tested a problem-solving model of intervention to promote adherence to medical treatment among parents and adolescents with DM1 (see chap. 7). Key elements of this problem-solving intervention model as applied to adherence to treatment in DM1 (Wysocki, Harris, et al., 2000) included (a) enhancing parent–adolescent communication, (b) generating alternative ways of managing adherence-related challenges in DM1 (e.g., managing insulin, diet, etc.), (c) trying the strategies out, and (d) modifying them on the basis of experience. Such principles can be applied to any number of other chronic pediatric conditions (e.g., asthma) but would need to focus on adherence-related challenges specific to that particular condition that are quite different. For example, the specific adherence-related challenges in pediatric asthma would involve managing the symptoms of an asthma attack, preventing the triggers of an asthma attack, managing daily treatments such as daily steroidal medications, and so on (see chap. 6).

CHALLENGES TO ENHANCING CLINICAL SIGNIFICANCE OF INTERVENTION RESEARCH

As an increasing number of psychological interventions are documented to be effective in controlled studies (see chaps. 6–10), the need to test such interventions in clinical settings and to integrate successful interventions into clinical care is heightened. To accomplish such clinical applications, investigators need to consider several challenges that relate to the considerable differences in the nature of research-based interventions versus clinical services. For example, salient challenges are presented by the following issues: (a) the differences in participants in research versus clinical care, (b) differences in the structure and focus of research-based intervention versus clinical care, and (c) limited consideration of clinical significance in available studies of psychological intervention. Each of these challenges is now considered.

To reduce variability in target problems, maximize the internal validity of study findings, and enhance feasibility of study implementation, many intervention studies with children with chronic illness include relatively homogeneous samples. Complex problems such as serious family dysfunction or children with comorbid mental health problems may be excluded from such samples (Drotar & Lemanek, 2001). In contrast, children and adolescents with complex and comorbid clinical problems may often be those who are most likely to be referred for psychological intervention in clinical settings and are seen by practicing pediatric psychologists. For this reason, data that are generated from some psychological intervention studies may have limited applicability to clinical populations of children with chronic illness.

Other differences in research versus clinical samples, which are not directly under investigators' direct control, may also limit the generalizability of findings from research on psychological interventions to clinical care. For example, family decisions to either not participate in or drop out of intervention studies may limit generalizability of findings to clinical settings (Riekert & Drotar, 1999). Moreover, nonparticipation or dropout in intervention studies may be more common among children with chronic illness who have more serious mental health or adherence-related problems (Zebracki et al., 2003). Participants in research-based intervention studies may not resemble children and adolescents who receive clinical services. For this reason, it is important to describe how the participants in intervention research either resemble or differ from children who are referred for psychological services in practice settings on such dimensions as those of the *Diagnostic and Statistical Manual of Mental Disorders* (4th ed. [DSM–IV]; American Psychiatric Association, 1994) diagnoses, comorbid psychological problems, health status, and so on.

A second set of challenges relates to the differences in the structure and focus of research-based versus clinical intervention. Psychological practitioners tend to work with children and adolescents with chronic illness with complex clusters of problems. For this reason, it is not uncommon for practitioners to target multiple problems in their interventions. In contrast, research-based interventions tend to be more focused and targeted toward fewer and more specific problems because they are easier to manualize, implement, and replicate. This is another reason why it may be difficult to apply the results of highly structured and focused research-based interventions to the broad range of children with chronic illness who are seen in clinical practice.

The degree to which the intervention is delivered under conditions that are similar to practice is another important aspect of clinical significance. In fact, there are often substantial differences in the resources that are typically available for funded intervention research versus clinical psychological care for children with chronic illness. For example, significant resources for intervention staff are necessary to facilitate manageable caseloads and incentives for families to enhance their participation and adherence to interventions. Such resources are available to facilitate psychological intervention research, especially studies funded by the National Institutes of Health (NIH). However, under the current constraints imposed by managed care, the level of resources and support for families that are available in research studies is much greater than what is available to fund clinical practice (Walders & Drotar, 1999). For this reason, it may not be feasible or realistic to implement some empirically supported psychological interventions in the context of clinical care for children with chronic illness unless some support from other sources (e.g., hospitals, foundations) is available. Owing to research-related resources, children's access to preventive interventions designed to prevent psychological adjustment problems or adherence problems before they become serious may be greater in research-based interventions than in clinical practice. One reason for this is that insurance reimbursement for clinical practice with pediatric chronic conditions has been tied to diagnosis of a mental disorder based on the *DSM–IV* system, at least until the recent advent of the Health and Behavior Codes (Noll & Fischer, 2004).

Another challenge to clinical applications of psychological intervention research concerns the lack of information on the clinical significance of intervention effects. Clinical significance is complex and multifaceted and has not been well described in most research reports of psychological interventions with pediatric chronic conditions (Drotar, 2002). Relevant dimensions of the clinical significance of psychological intervention studies include (a) the clinical significance of the intervention effects that are obtained in the research, (b) the degree to which the intervention that is tested is delivered under conditions that are similar to those in practice, (c) the degree to which the sample that is studied in the research-based intervention resembles clinical populations, and (d) the functional impact of changes in target outcomes (e.g., psychological symptoms; Kazdin, 2000). Unfortunately, research in pediatric chronic illness has not routinely assessed clinical significance of intervention effects on clinically relevant outcomes (e.g., adherence to treatment, illness-related morbidity such as symptoms and hospitalizations; or functioning and quality of life). Consequently, documentation of clinical significance remains an important challenge for the future.

STRATEGIES TO ENHANCE CLINICAL APPLICATIONS

A comprehensive set of strategies will be needed to meet the considerable challenges of enhancing clinical applications of research-based psychological interventions (Drotar & Lemanek, 2001). These include the following: (a) research and develop interventions in practice settings before testing them, (b) test the generalizability of empirically supported interventions with clinical populations, (c) evaluate the effectiveness of tailoring psychological interventions to clinically relevant problems, (d) conduct program evaluations and monitor the outcomes of comprehensive care, (e) study the costs versus benefits of intervention, and (f) evaluate the implementation of interventions in clinical settings.

Given the considerable agenda for potential clinical applications described above, one question that arises is what strategy should be considered first. Individual investigators will generally want to consider alternative strategies based on the resources that are available to them for their research, the stage of their research program, and the stage of psychological intervention research in the specific chronic condition of interest (see previous section on stages of intervention research). Investigators will also want to consider alternative strategies depending on the purpose of their research. For example, studies of program evaluation, including comprehensive psychological care, may be important to demonstrate efficacy of services with a specific clinical population and may also be useful in developing funding for services in a particular setting. Studies of the costs versus benefits of psychological interventions may be important to inform decisions about allocation of services in settings where such decisions are necessary for the next steps in program development in a particular setting.

Research and Develop Interventions in Practice Settings Before Testing Them

To reduce the gap between research- and practice-based interventions, Weisz (2000) recommended that the development and testing of psychological interventions take place in clinical practice settings. Although this innovative approach has not been used often in intervention research with pediatric populations, there is considerable potential for such research. In many instances, it may be premature to conduct an RCT of psychological intervention with a specific chronic illness population because there is insufficient empirical evidence concerning a particular intervention model to warrant the investment of time, energy, and funds in an RCT. For this reason, it may be most advantageous to gather data concerning the feasibility and preliminary results of interventions in clinical settings prior to a controlled test.

Another important but relatively little-used research-related strategy to facilitate the evaluation of interventions in practice settings is the use of case studies and series (Drotar, La Greca, Lemanek, & Kazak, 1995). Case studies and series can be used to illustrate the impact of a new intervention or to extend the generalizability of an empirically supported intervention to larger samples or a new population or setting. Rapoff and his colleagues' series of case studies that have demonstrated the impact of behavioral interventions to enhance adherence to medical treatment for juvenile rheumatoid arthritis (see chap. 9) are an excellent example of such research that led to the development of an RCT for this population (see Rapoff et al., 2002).

Test Generalizability of Empirically Supported Interventions to Clinical Populations

One of the important next steps in psychological intervention research in a number of chronic conditions is to apply the models that have been demonstrated as effective in RCTs to practice settings. Harris and Mertlich (2003) described a clinically relevant example of this approach in their adaptation of a home-based version of behavioral family systems therapy (BFST) for adolescents with diabetes with chronically poor blood sugar control, which is a serious clinical problem. The BFST model has been shown to be effective with adolescents with conduct problems (Robin & Foster, 1989) and has also been applied to adolescents with diabetes to promote their adherence to treatment (Wysocki, Harris, et al., 2000). Harris and Mertlich (2003) used a within-subject design to test the effectiveness of ten 1.5-hour sessions of home-based BFST with adolescents that focused on parental conflict and school expulsion, which were sources of distress for adolescents recruited for their study. The posttreatment evaluation indicated that participants showed pre- to posttreatment decreases in general family conflict, diabetes-related family conflict, behavioral problems, and self-reported adherence to treatment but not in metabolic control.

Another example of a relevant application of an empirically supported intervention is the RCT conducted by Ellis and colleagues (Ellis, Frey, et al., 2005; Ellis, Naar-King, et al., 2005; Ellis, Naar-King, Frey, Rowland, & Greger, 2003) of a multisystemic therapy (MST), an intensive home-based psychotherapy (Henggeler, 1999; Henggeler, Schoenwald, Borduin, Rowland, & Cunningham, 1998) with adolescents with poorly controlled diabetes. Compared with adolescents who received standard care, those who received the MST treatment had a decreasing number of inpatient hospitalizations from baseline to 9-month follow-up (Ellis, Frey, et al., 2005; Ellis, Naar-King, et al., 2005).

Evaluate the Efficacy of Tailoring Interventions

In clinical practice, children and adolescents with chronic illness who are referred for psychological intervention have multiple problems that may involve different domains of psychological adaptation or adherence to treatment (see chaps. 1, 6–10). For example, problems in adherence to medical treatment are heterogeneous and may include various domains of recommended treatment (e.g., medication, dietary intervention, exercise), each of which may have very different causes (Koocher, McGrath, & Gudas, 1990). Given the specificity of behavioral change that is required to modify adherence to treatment, tailoring intervention approaches to the specific problems or barriers identified in each of these areas of nonadherence may be more effective than a general intervention approach. Such tailored interventions have the potential advantage of involving children and parents in the process of identifying problem areas, setting goals, and priorities for intervention.

Although tailoring of psychological interventions in pediatric chronic illness has not been extensively investigated, some initial positive results have been described. For example, Quittner, Drotar, Ievers-Landis, and De Lambo (2004) performed an RCT-based application of a BFST-based approach that was tailored to specific adherence-related barriers identified by adolescents with CF and their parents on the basis of objective assessment of CF- and non-CF-related problems. Their study was associated with a reduction in family conflict. In addition, Walders et al. (in press) demonstrated that a one-session problem-solving intervention that was tailored to the barriers to adherence to asthma treatment for children and adolescents with symptomatic asthma was associated with a reduction in hospitalizations compared with an educational intervention.

Study Costs–Benefits and Offset of Interventions

Research concerning the cost-effectiveness and cost-offset of psychological interventions with various pediatric chronic illness populations is another understudied area but one that is critical for future research and clinical application. *Cost-effectiveness* refers to a detailed evaluation of the economic costs versus benefits of psychological intervention on health and psychological outcomes. *Cost-offset* refers to the total economic costs of health and mental health care that are saved by a psychological intervention, especially with respect to health care costs (Petitti, 1994). Data concerning cost-effectiveness and cost-offset are potentially important in developing clinical applications of psychological interventions on a large scale. For example, some psychological intervention models may be found to be efficacious and powerful on the basis of research results but may be too intensive and hence costly to be used in widespread clinical applications.

On the other hand, it is important to recognize that some effective psychological interventions that are relatively expensive compared with traditional mental health services (Geist, 1995) may result in significant offsets in health care costs for subgroups of children with chronic conditions (Walders & Drotar, 1999). For example, a home-based model of psychological intervention, MST has been shown to be effective in improving adherence to treatment for adolescents with diabetes who are consistently and significantly nonadherent to diabetes management (Ellis, Frey, et al., 2005; Ellis, Naar-King, et al., 2005). Such serious problems in treatment adherence are generally difficult to manage with traditional mental health intervention. Although MST is expensive in relation to available outpatient mental health interventions, the cost savings of this intervention, as shown by reduction of emergency room visits and hospitalizations for diabetic ketoacidosis, may be significant (Ellis, Frey, et al., 2005; Ellis, Naar-King, et al., 2005).

Koocher et al. (2001) have published what is to my knowledge the only demonstration of the cost-effectiveness of a preventive psychological intervention for individuals with chronic illness. This RCT evaluated the impact of medical crisis counseling, a short-term intervention that addressed illness-related psychosocial problems for patients with newly diagnosed cancer, first heart attacks, or adult onset diabetes. The intervention resulted in reduced psychological distress and utilization of mental health services and costs in some patient groups compared with a control group that received standard care in a health maintenance organization (Koocher et al., 2001).

Although this study was conducted with adults, the principles of the intervention model may be applicable to children and adolescents with chronic illness and should be tested in pediatric care. There are other examples of psychological interventions for children and adolescents with chronic illness that are potentially cost-effective that need to be documented with more detailed analyses of costs versus benefits. These include Ellis and colleagues' (Ellis, Frey, et al., 2005; Ellis, Naar-King, et al., 2005) research on MST with adolescents with diabetes and Cuttler et al.'s (2004) research on the impact of an outpatient (including psychological support) versus inpatient model of care on control of diabetes and a wide range of psychological and family outcomes (see chap. 7).

Conduct Program Evaluations and Monitor the Outcomes of Comprehensive Care

In some settings, psychological services and comprehensive psychological care are already being provided to pediatric populations, and it may not be feasible to implement a controlled intervention study. Process and program evaluations provide an alternative method for intervention research in such circumstances. Program evaluations include a description of the participants in a program, the specific intervention delivered, and an evaluation of outcomes (C. Weiss, 1998). Such evaluations are used to document the feasibility and acceptability of interventions and to describe the impact of an intervention in changing psychological problems or medical symptoms from pretreatment to posttreatment levels.

Naar-King, Siegel, Smythe, and Simpson (2000) proposed a detailed model that can be used to evaluate comprehensive health care and mental health service programs for children with chronic conditions. This model includes two major components: an evaluation of the process components of the program and an outcome evaluation. The *process* components can include the following information: (a) the number of visits, including utilization of services by children and families; (b) accountability or documentation of services that were provided; (c) continuity of service; and (d) coordination, or the degree to which the team communicates with other caregivers. The *outcome* evaluation includes such data as the following: (a) parent, staff, and child satisfaction with the services provided; (b) level of teamwork in the service; (c) medical outcomes (e.g., visits to the emergency room or inpatient hospitalization); and (d) psychosocial outcomes (e.g., behavioral adjustment or adherence to medical treatment; Naar-King et al., 2000).

A key aspect of such program evaluations is the development of a comprehensive database that routinely monitors the process and outcomes of services. At a minimum, such a database might include, first, the nature of services provided and, second, measures of the proximal impact of comprehensive care or psychological interventions (e.g., illness-related morbidity such as recurrent symptoms leading to emergency room visits and hospitalization in pediatric asthma, or episodes of serious hypoglycemia or recurrent ketoacidosis in diabetes; Drotar et al., 2001). Detailed evaluations of clinical programs for children with chronic illness are uncommon but are nonetheless significant. One example of a program evaluation is Kelley, Van Horn, and DeMaso's (2001) description of the development and feasibility of a hospital-based mental health clinic for children coping with medical stressors. These authors documented a clinical need for such a service as shown by 356 referrals in a 21-month period (Kelley et al., 2001).

Evaluate the Level of Implementation of Interventions in Clinical Settings

One key area of future clinical application will be documenting the degree to which psychological interventions, including empirically supported interventions, have been implemented in various clinical settings with different chronic illness populations. Such data will provide a much-needed benchmark of how many children and their families are receiving specific empirically supported psychological interventions. Glasgow, McKay, Piette, and Reynolds (2001) proposed the "RE-AIM" model as a template for the degree to which psychological interventions have been implemented in practice settings. The model includes the following components:

Reach: the percentage and representativeness of patients who are willing to participate in a given program (percentage of eligible participants).

Efficacy or *effectiveness*: the impact of an intervention on important outcomes.

Adoption: the percentage and representativeness of settings that adopt these interventions.

Implementation: to what extent the various intervention components were delivered as intended, especially when conducted by different nonresearch staff members in an applied setting.

Maintenance: long-term effects and attrition rate; to what extent different intervention components were continued versus modified or abandoned.

In their review of psychological interventions with children, adolescents, and adults in health care settings, Glasgow, Bull, Gillette, Kleges, and Dzewaltowski (2002) found that internal validity criteria were reported more than external validity in published work. Moreover, data on representativeness of individual participants or settings were conspicuously absent in published reports.

Improving the generalizability of empirically supported psychological interventions is not an easy task and will take sustained efforts on the part of individual researchers and efforts from funders. Glasgow et al. (2004) suggested a number of specific strategies to enhance the translation of psychological intervention to practice settings. These include the following (among others): (a) involve target audience in the decision and implementation of studies; (b) design interventions so that they can reach larger numbers of patients and families; (c) investigate recruitment methods to reach large populations; (d) replicate interventions across heterogeneous settings and persons; (e) study the consistency of implementation and outcomes across a range of intervention modalities, settings, and intervention delivery agents; and (f) develop a plan for a clinical application phase to follow research studies once they are completed.

Glasgow et al. (2004) also recommended increasing research and funding support for research on real-world practice issues, organizational issues, and health care policies to facilitate systems-based support for the implementation of psychological interventions. Recommendations that are applicable to pediatric populations include research to describe optimal and effective ways of interdisciplinary management of chronic illness and evaluation of behavioral intervention strategies to provide feedback to patients and providers.

ENHANCING THE CLINICAL SIGNIFICANCE OF RESEARCH AND PUBLISHED REPORTS

The sparse amount of data concerning the clinical significance of psychological interventions in published reports has limited the potential clinical application (Drotar, 2002). Consequently, an important recommendation for the design and reporting of future research is to describe the clinical significance of the effects of psychological interventions. Kazdin's (1995, 2000) framework for the description of clinical significance in intervention studies, which is applicable to studies of children with chronic conditions, includes four primary methods of evaluating clinical significance of intervention change. Such methods include the following: (a) the comparison method (e.g., test similarity to normative samples or dissimilarity, such as statistical departure from a dysfunctional sample on a measure of behavioral symptoms), (b) absolute change (e.g., assess the amount of change an individual makes from pre- to posttreatment, such as no longer meeting criteria for psychiatric diagnosis or elimination of problems or symptoms), (c) subjective evaluation (e.g., whether the change or changes produced by the intervention continue to be evident or to affect functioning as judged by parents, physicians, or teachers), and (d) social impact (e.g., change on measures that are recognized as being considered critically important to society such as school attendance, hospitalizations, doctors' visits, emergency room visits, and costs of care). Kazdin's framework should be used in future studies of psychological intervention research.

In addition to using traditional measures of statistical significance, it will also be important to document the clinical significance of intervention effects by including statistics such as effect size, odds ratio, and risk ratio statistics. The clinical significance of reports of intervention findings would also be enhanced by including measures of functional outcomes such as health-related quality of life, morbidity of chronic illness, and family members' perceptions of the impact of intervention. Such measures would complement and add clinical significance to typical measures of outcomes. Measures of functional outcomes should be included in psychological intervention research for a number of reasons. One is that some children with chronic conditions who are included in preventive intervention studies may not demonstrate clinically significant psychological symptoms. This limits the degree to which conventional methods of evaluating clinical significance (e.g., reliable change index; Jacobson & Truax, 1991) can be used with pediatric chronic illness populations. Another reason is that psychological interventions may result in improvements in functional outcomes that have great value for children and adolescents, parents, and providers. For example, Olness (1981) described a reduction in pain frequency and number of medications required to manage pain as a consequence of imagery and hypnosis in children with cancer. Another example is Varni, Gilbert, and Dietrich's (1981) demonstration that imagery increased activity and reduced mediations and hospitalizations for a child with hemophilia.

In addition to the strategies for evaluating the clinical significance of intervention research recommended by Kazdin (2000), other strategies are relevant to pediatric populations. For example, one strategy is to provide a detailed description of the sample that is included in an intervention study on clinical parameters such as psychological symptoms and comorbid problems. Such descriptions will help practitioners determine how closely the sample of participants in an intervention study resembles children and adolescents who are seen in practice. Moreover, the similarities and differences of children and families who refused participation as well as those who dropped out versus those who participated in interventions should be described (Drotar & Riekert, 2000). Finally, the context in which the interventions take place as well as the resources that support them should be described in some depth so that the potential applicability to practice settings can be ascertained.

One essential future direction will be to facilitate the dissemination and development of psychological intervention science and practice. Several strategies will be needed to accomplish this task. These include the following: (a) disseminate information concerning empirically supported interventions; (b) publish critical reviews of intervention research, especially meta-analyses; (c) synthesize the clinical significance of intervention research; (d) develop new training methods and models for the conduct of intervention research; and (e) facilitate collaborations among intervention researchers, including multisite collaboration.

Disseminate Information Concerning Empirically Supported Interventions

As new intervention models for children with chronic illness are developed, tested, and supported by research, researchers will need to inform practitioners about them and their potential relevance to practice. The interchange between researchers and practitioners concerning psychological interventions should be reciprocal: Practitioners who develop new ideas about potentially effective interventions forged in the experiences of clinical practice need to communicate with researchers to test the validity of their ideas (Weisz, 2000).

To facilitate such information exchange, pediatric psychology researchers and practitioners can make empirically supported treatments more available to their colleagues through presentations and workshops, publications, and expert consultation. In this regard, Henggeler and colleagues' continuing work (see Henggeler & Randall, 2000) implementing MST in multiple sites through formal training and consultation in local communities is an example of generalizing a model of empirically supported intervention to different settings and populations (Ellis et al., 2003). The recent *Journal of Pediatric Psychology* section on RCTs is another example (Drotar, 2005). This section was developed to feature the results of RCTs with pediatric populations, including chronic illness populations, and contains commentaries that describe the methodological issues related to RCTs (see Drotar, 2005; Stark, Janicke, et al., 2005). Another good example of dissemination involves detailed summaries of the content and process of psychological interventions. In this regard, Spirito and Kazak (2006) have published a volume that describes examples of interventions and manuals and provide readers with access to manuals for various research-based interventions for children with different chronic conditions.

Because psychological intervention research often takes a long time to implement and complete, it may be years before researchers learn about one another's work. However, there is a need to share ongoing experiences, manuals, and outcome measures with interested colleagues sooner, prior to publication. For this reason, investigators who share an interest in intervention methods might wish to make their materials and experiences available to other researchers via the Internet, for example, with suitable caveats concerning the level of development of their research and empirical support for their work.

Publish Critical Reviews and Meta-Analyses of Intervention Research

As the findings from studies of psychological interventions with different chronic illnesses accumulate, there will be an increasing need to synthesize and critically review this research (Drotar & Lemanek, 2001). Such reviews provide a way to describe the benchmarks for the current state of the art in intervention research with various conditions and make recommendations for next steps in intervention research. The series on empirically supported interventions developed by the *Journal of Pediatric Psychology* is a step in this direction. However, this series should be extended by meta-analyses of psychological intervention findings with specific conditions or specific intervention models (e.g., cognitive–behavioral methods) that have been applied across different chronic conditions. Meta-analyses have critical methodological advantages, such as the systematic evaluation of data from interventions using the single metric of effect size, that should be exploited by intervention researchers who are interested in pediatric chronic conditions (Drotar & Lemanek, 2001).

Synthesize the Clinical Significance of Intervention Research Findings

Syntheses of research and research reviews also need to evaluate the clinical significance of intervention research and consider the policy-related implications of such research. Examples of such syntheses include meta-analyses, in which effect sizes of psychological intervention are related to benchmarks of clinical morbidity (e.g., symptom control, hospitalizations) and functional outcomes, and critical reviews that describe the level of application and translation of psychological interventions to practice settings (Glasgow et al., 2004). With respect to this latter recommendation, Glasgow et al.'s (2004) guidelines for translation of research to practice are potentially applicable to pediatric chronic illness populations and should be considered in reporting individual studies as well as synthesizing the findings from psychological intervention studies with specific chronic conditions. These include the following: (a) describe results on reach, adoption, implementation, and maintenance as well as effectiveness in standardized ways; (b) report distribution of targeted population, compare characteristics of participants and nonparticipants, and document attrition or dropout; (c) describe the context of the intervention, including specific recruitment methods and program features as they relate to program participation, as well as intervention agents and modalities of intervention delivery; (d) document maintenance of individual behavior change over time (e.g., 6 months); (e) present costs of intervention materials, training, and delivery; and (f) describe the continuance or modification of the program in clinical settings.

Develop New Training Methods and Models for Psychological Intervention Research

Intervention research raises many difficult decisions as well as formidable methodological and pragmatic problems (see chaps. 1–5). Specialized didactic training and experiences with a range of methods (e.g., training in single case study designs, program evaluation research, and methods related to RCTs of intervention) are needed at all levels of training to enhance the training of researchers who are interested in pursuing careers as intervention researchers.

Graduate and postgraduate training programs can facilitate the training and career development of researchers, enhancing their ability to make significant contributions to intervention science at a graduate and postgraduate level. However, there are challenges for the training of intervention researchers that need to be met in training, including the need to finish a graduate or fellowship training program within a reasonable time frame and the lack of mentored opportunities to conduct intervention research for master's and doctoral research. Such opportunities may involve work with established datasets concerning psychological interventions, participation in ongoing psychological intervention studies, and independent student-initiated research on psychological interventions.

Comprehensive and focused training models that involve didactic and experiential components will be needed to provide opportunities for the career development of intervention researchers. Didactic training should include formal courses that describe the critical issues in the design and implementation of interventions (e.g., RCTs, alternative research designs, sampling issues, measurement, statistical analysis, ethical issues in the conduct of interventions, and theoretical models; see chaps. 1–5). Experiential learning related to intervention research is also a cornerstone of training in psychological intervention.

One way to facilitate this training is to provide opportunities for students and fellows to join teams that are conducting intervention research; participate in team meetings; and help with data collection, implementation of the intervention, data management, or analysis. Another way that students and fellows can gain valuable experience is in working on analyses of datasets that have been gathered by faculty's psychological intervention research. In addition, the opportunity for mentored, student-initiated research on the development and testing of new intervention models is critical.

To implement these recommendations, graduate and postdoctoral training programs need to be led by mentors who are experienced in psychological intervention research, are currently conducting psychological intervention research, or have datasets concerning psychological intervention research that can be accessed by students or fellows for their research. Training experiences in intervention research are best accomplished in those settings in which a critical mass of faculty researchers, including interdisciplinary teams, have ongoing research programs. Such resources are not available in each and every setting. However, our experiences with trainees indicate that with suitable mentorship support and availability of populations, trainees can participate in and initiate independent research concerning psychological interventions (Drotar, Palermo, & Landis, 2003; Palermo & Drotar, 1999; Schwartz & Drotar, 2004; Walders et al., in press).

On a national level, faculty intervention researchers are clearly needed to provide support and structure for trainees to learn skills in intervention research as well as training and mentoring experiences to promote their career development. The career development series of training grants sponsored by NIH provides a mechanism for researchers who are interested in careers in intervention research to obtain such a mentored experience. In addition, NIH also sponsors an intensive summer training institute providing specialized training in the design and evaluation of RCTs that is designed for fellows or junior faculty. In addition to these efforts, pediatric psychologists need to provide support for intervention research at local, regional, and national levels.

Develop Collaborations Among Intervention Researchers

Sample size and other methodological challenges will require researchers to work collaboratively to design and implement psychological interventions to advance the state of the art in intervention science. There is a considerable agenda for such collaboration, including (a) sharing information about methods of psychological intervention that have been shown to be feasible and applicable in one setting to other settings, (b) providing technical assistance and advice about funding to other investigators, and (c) developing collaborative groups of researchers to implement intervention studies across sites. Such collaboration can occur at many levels at different sites in the same community, at a regional level, and in multisite collaborations at sites in different regions. Multisite psychological intervention studies that have been conducted in pediatric cancer (Armstrong & Drotar, 2000), including maternal problem-solving interventions (Sahler et al., 2002, 2005), provide outstanding models for the field. Future progress in psychological intervention research in pediatric chronic illness will depend in no small measure on the collaborative and logistical skills of psychologists, physicians, and other professionals to develop and manage multisite intervention studies (Armstrong & Drotar, 2000).

POLICY APPLICATIONS

One important area for the future concerns the development of policy that will support the development of research concerning psychological interventions and services with pediatric populations. Policy-related applications of psychological intervention research in pediatric chronic illness include developing funding for psychological intervention services, documenting the allocation and funding of intervention services in clinical settings, and creating systems change to reduce disparity and enhance prevention models (Stein & Brooks, 1997).

Develop Funding to Support Psychological Intervention Services

Data from studies of costs, benefits, and cost offsets have a potential role to play in the development of policy for the funding of psychological intervention services for children with chronic health conditions and their families. The services that are necessary for optimal care of children and adolescents with chronic health conditions are very time consuming and involve nonreimbursable services such as collaboration with physicians, nurses, social workers, teachers, and advocacy. Intervention research can help further the development of services in pediatric settings by documenting the efficacy, clinical effectiveness, significance, and costs versus benefits of such interventions (see Figure 11.1).

Over and beyond empirical support, a multifaceted strategy of resource development will be needed to develop psychological services for children and adolescents with chronic health conditions (Drotar, 2004). Such strategies include securing funding from hospital resources, obtaining foundation support for innovative services, and using creative strategies of reimbursement for comprehensive care of chronic illness that pushes the current limits of managed care (Walders & Drotar, 1999). For example, one strategy used in some settings is to "bundle" psychological services, that is, deliver them with medical care that is reimbursed by health insurers as a comprehensive package.

A significant new development with respect to reimbursement of psychological assessment and intervention services is the Health and Behavior CPT Codes (Noll & Fischer, 2004). In contrast to the *DSM*-based codes, which focus on traditional procedures such as psychotherapy that are tied to a diagnosis of a mental disorder, the Health and Behavior codes focus on health and behavior assessment and intervention. Such procedures encompass a wide range of procedures in response to a range of health-related problems, including chronic illness. Moreover, they permit pediatric psychologists to describe and code psychological services using a system that matches the services being provided with a focus on psychological health-related services to children with a medical diagnosis (Noll & Fischer, 2004). Data need to be gathered concerning the use of these codes and their success in facilitating reimbursement in different settings. Although the development of health and behavior codes is important, the use of these codes will not solve the problems of reimbursement of psychological intervention services. One reason is that there is extraordinary variation in the level of reimbursement in different settings owing to differences in local insurance markets and companies.

Document Allocation and Funding of Intervention Services

There is well-recognized empirical support for psychological services in the management of pediatric chronic illness (Drotar, 1999). Nevertheless, there is extraordinary variation from center to center in the provision and allocation of these services (Drotar & Zagorski, 2001). They can vary from setting to setting in specific content, focus, and intensity of services (e.g., whether in response to referral only or more integrated); access or availability of services (e.g., how soon services can be provided to various populations of children with chronic illness and their families); and the level of integration of psychological services with medical care (Drotar, 2001). Psychological services that may be offered to children and adolescents with specific chronic conditions include a wide range. For example, they encompass services that are provided on the basis of referral only to patients who have significant psychological problems as well as programs that reflect a high level of integration of medical and psychological services, including proactive primary and secondary prevention services, delivered to populations of children and their families. (See chaps. 6–10 for information about clinical services for specific chronic conditions.) The availability and success of such services in specific settings may depend on situational considerations, such as the history of collaboration (including shared resource development) between psychologists and the comprehensive care teams in individual settings, as well as economic issues.

Given such individual variation across settings, it will be important to document how psychological services to children with chronic illness are provided and reimbursed in various settings and how service allocation and deployment are decided on. In particular, it will be important to document which particular empirically supported interventions for children with chronic conditions are implemented in different settings and the barriers and facilitators of such development (see Kazak, 2001; Kazak, Blackall, et al., 1996). As an example of such research, Drotar et al. (1997) surveyed 21 providers (social workers, nurses, and psychologists) at 53 hemophilia treatment centers that received funding from the Bureau of Maternal and Child Health concerning their patient populations, types of problems encountered, types of psychosocial services provided, and obstacles to service delivery (Drotar et al., 1997). Respondents spent more time providing direct services for illness-related problems (e.g., child or parent adjustment to hemophilia) compared with general psychological problems and utilized a wide range or services to address clinical problems. Distance from family home to the center was rated as the most significant obstacle to delivery of psychosocial services. However, this study did not describe the total sources of funding for these services or setting-based differences in allocation of services.

Create System-Level Change to Reduce Disparity in Access and Enhance Prevention

One of the most critical policy-related issues in psychological interventions for children with chronic health conditions concerns disparities in access to care (R. T. Brown et al., 2003). Economic issues, such as insurance coverage, and other issues, such as parent–provider communication, result in differential access to care for children with chronic illness who are of ethnic and minority status. For this reason, psychological interventions will need to be developed that reduce the disparities in access to health services and psychological interventions, which is at least one factor that accounts for morbidity in chronic conditions such as asthma (McQuaid & Walders, 2003). Psychological interventions for minority and economically disadvantaged children with chronic illness need to address special barriers to care experienced by this population, which is one reason that NIH has solicited research proposals on this topic (NIH, 2001).

Related is development of a public-health-focused, preventive model to implement psychological interventions in primary pediatric as well as specialized comprehensive care. Toward this end, Glasgow and colleagues (Glasgow et al., 2001, 2004) have described an innovative proactive service delivery model for chronic disease. At a program level, this model includes the use of a population-based approach, proactive contracts, surveillance and reminders in follow-up procedures including patients and families as active participants, focus on responsibilities and activities of important nonphysician team members such as nurses, planning and focusing office visits on key clinical outcomes, and the use of information systems such as electronic medical records to improve quality of care.

Although Glasgow et al.'s (2001) recommendations for a population-based primary focus of care are innovative, it is not clear how they would be implemented with children and adolescents with chronic health conditions whose care is much more likely to be delivered by subspecialists compared with adults with chronic disease, perhaps with the exception of asthma. The American Academy of Pediatrics (1992) has recognized the concept of "medical home" (i.e., the necessity for one caregiver in primary care to organize the care of children with chronic illness). However, factors such as wide individual variation in different structures of care delivery, inconsistent training of primary care physicians in the care of chronic illness, and problems in resources for primary care and unresolved issues in care coordination between primary versus specialty care practitioners with chronic illness have limited the widespread application of the medical home (American Academy of Pediatrics, 1999). For the foreseeable future, the care of children with chronic health conditions will be delivered by subspecialists. Nevertheless, pediatric psychologists who provide interventions for children and adolescents with chronic illness can certainly facilitate communication among primary care providers and subspecialists in their provision of services and research.

Another preventive approach is to develop proactive services for children and adolescents with chronic health conditions that address individual needs and level of risk. To address the need for such targeted approaches to psychological service allocation, Kazak et al. (2003) have been testing a method that can be used to assess family risk and to tailor the deployment of resources for psychosocial interventions for children with cancer and their families (see chap. 8). Rapoff et al. (2000) described a similar framework for interventions that can address individual differences in adherence to treatment in chronic conditions such as juvenile rheumatoid arthritis (see chap. 9). The effectiveness of the application of such models, including data on costs, to clinical practice needs to be documented. However, these models provide logical frameworks on which to plan allocation of psychological services to children and adolescents with chronic illness and to evaluate the impact of this allocation.

The formidable agenda for research, clinical care, training, and policy described here will challenge pediatric psychologists and their colleagues who work with children and adolescents with chronic illness. The considerable progress that has been made concerning the development, implementation, and evaluation of psychological interventions with this population in a relatively short period of time underscores a bright outlook for the future. However, there is much more to be learned and done to ensure that empirically supported psychological intervention services reach a broader population of children and adolescents who need these services. The work described in this book, which details the current state of the art in psychological intervention science and practice, is at best a summary of the first chapter of this work. The final chapters will be written by others who will, it is hoped, find both utility and inspiration in this work.

REFERENCES

Abramovitch, R., Freedman, J. L., Henry, K. L., & Van Brunschot, M. (1995). Children's capacity to agree to psychological research: Knowledge of risks and benefits and voluntariness. *Ethics and Behavior, 5,* 25–48.

Achenbach, T. M. (1991). *Manual for the Child Behavior Checklist and 1991 Profile.* Burlington: University of Vermont, Department of Psychiatry.

Aiken, L. S., & West, S. G. (1991). *Multiple regression: Testing and interpreting interactions.* Newbury Park, CA: Sage.

Alderfer, M., Labay, L., & Kazak, A. (2003). Brief report: Does posttraumatic stress apply to siblings of childhood cancer survivors? *Journal of Pediatric Psychology, 28,* 281–286.

Altman, D. C. (1996). Better reporting of randomized controlled trials: The CONSORT statement. *British Medical Journal, 313,* 570–571.

Altman, D. C., Schulz, K. F., Moher, D., Egger, M., Davidoff, F., Elbourne, D., et al. (2001). The revised CONSORT statement for reporting randomized trials: Explanation and elaboration. *Annals of Internal Medicine, 134,* 663–694.

Alvirdrez, J., & Arean, P. A. (2002). Psychosocial treatment research with ethnic minority populations: Ethical considerations in conducting clinical trials. *Ethics and Behavior, 12,* 103–116.

American Academy of Pediatrics. (1992). The medical home. *Pediatrics, 90,* 774.

American Academy of Pediatrics. (1999). Care coordination: Integrating health and related systems of care for children with special health care needs. *Pediatrics, 104,* 978–981.

American Diabetes Association. (2000). Type 2 diabetes in children and adolescents (consensus statement). *Diabetes Care, 23,* 739–743.

American Lung Association. (2000). *Trends in asthma morbidity and mortality: Epidemiology and statistics unit.* New York: Author.

American Psychiatric Association. (1994). *Diagnostic and statistical manual of mental disorders* (4th ed.). Washington, DC: Author.

American Psychological Association. (2002). Ethical principles of psychologists and codes of conduct. *American Psychologist, 57,* 1024–1040.

Anderson, B. J. (2002). Involving family members in diabetes treatment. In B. J. Anderson & R. R. Rubin (Eds.), *Practical psychology for diabetes clinicians* (pp. 199–208). Alexandria, VA: American Diabetes Association.

Anderson, B. J., Brackett, J., Ho, J., & Laffel, L. (1999). An office-based intervention to maintain parent–adolescent teamwork in diabetes management: Impact on parent involvement, family conflict, and subsequent glycemic control. *Diabetes Care, 22,* 713–721.

Anderson, B. J., Brackett, J., Ho, J., & Laffel, L. M. B. (2000). An intervention to promote family teamwork in diabetes management tasks: Relationships among parental involvement, adherence to blood glucose monitoring, and glycemic control in young adolescents with Type 1 diabetes. In D. Drotar (Ed.), *Promoting adherence to medical treatment in chronic childhood illness: Concepts, methods, and intervention* (pp. 347–366). Mahwah, NJ: Erlbaum.

Anderson, B. J., & Coyne, J. C. (1991). "Miscarried helping" in the families of children and adolescents with chronic disease. In J. H. Johnson & S. B. Johnson (Eds.), *Advances in child health psychology* (pp. 166–177). Gainesville: University of Florida Press.

Anderson, B. J., Ho, J., Brackett, J., Finkelstein, D., & Laffel, L. (1997). Parental involvement in diabetes management tasks: Relationships to blood glucose monitoring adherence and metabolic control in young adolescents with insulin-dependent diabetes mellitus. *Journal of Pediatrics, 130,* 257–265.

Anderson, B., Loughlin, C., Goldberg, E., & Laffel, L. (2001). Comprehensive, family-focused outpatient care for the very young children living with chronic disease: Lessons from a program in pediatric diabetes. *Children's Services: Social Policy, Research, and Practice, 4,* 235–250.

Anderson, B. J., & Rubin, R. R. (Eds.). (2002). *Practical psychology for diabetes clinicians.* Alexandria, VA: American Diabetes Association.

Anderson, B. J., Wolf, F. M., Burkhart, M. T., Cornell, R. G., & Bacon, G. E. (1989). Effects of peer-group intervention on metabolic control of adolescents with IDDM: Randomized outpatient study. *Diabetes Care, 12,* 179–184.

Anderson, D. L., Flume, P. A., & Hardy, K. K. (2001). Psychological functioning of adults with cystic fibrosis. *Chest, 119,* 1079–1084.

Antisdel, J. E., & Chrisler, J. C. (2000). Comparison of eating attitudes and behaviors among adolescent and young women with Type 1 diabetes mellitus and phenylketonuria. *Journal of Developmental and Behavioral Pediatrics, 21,* 81–86.

Applegate, H., Webb, P. M., Elkin, T. D., Neul, S. K., Drabman, R. S., Moll, G. W., Jr., et al. (2003). Improving parent participation at pediatric diabetes and sickle cell appointments using a brief intervention. *Children's Health Care, 32,* 125–136.

Armstrong, F. D., & Briery, B. C. (2004). Childhood cancer and the school. In R. T. Brown (Ed.), *Handbook of pediatric psychology in school settings* (pp. 263–282). Mahwah, NJ: Erlbaum.

Armstrong, F. D., & Drotar, D. (2000). Multi-institutional and multi-disciplinary research collaboration: Strategies and lessons from cooperative trials. In D. Drotar (Ed.), *Handbook of research methods in clinical child and pediatric psychology* (pp. 281–304). New York: Kluwer Academic/Plenum Publishers.

Armstrong, F. D., & Reaman, G. H. (2005). Psychological research in childhood cancer: The children's oncology group perspective. *Journal of Pediatric Psychology, 30,* 89–97.

Bandura, A. (1997) *Self-efficacy: The exercise of control.* New York: Freeman.

Barakat, L. P., Hetzke, J., Foley, B., Carey, M. E., Gyato, K., & Phillips, P. C. (2003). Evaluation of a social-skills training group intervention with children treated for brain tumors: A pilot study. *Journal of Pediatric Psychology, 28,* 299–307.

Barakat, L. P., Smith-Whitley, K., & Ohene-Frempong, K. (2002). Treatment adherence in children with sickle cell disease: Disease-related risk and psychosocial resistance factors. *Journal of Clinical Psychology in Medical Settings, 9,* 201–209.

Bartholome, W. G. (1989). A new understanding of consent in pediatric practice. Consent, parental permission, and child assent. *Pediatric Annals, 18,* 262–265.

Bartholomew, L. K., Czyzewski, D. I., Parcel, G. S., Swank, P. R., Sockrider, M. M., & Mariotto, M. J. (1997). Self-management of cystic fibrosis: Short-term outcomes of the Cystic Fibrosis Family Education Program. *Health Education and Behavior, 24,* 652–666.

Bartsch, C., Barnes, B., Jarrett, L., & Lindsey, R. (1989). Where did they go? Life after teen diabetes clinic [Abstract]. *Diabetes, 38*(Suppl. 2), 40A.

Baum, D., & Creer, T. L. (1986). Medication compliance in children with asthma. *Journal of Asthma, 23,* 49–59.

Bauman, L. J. (2000). A patient-centered approach to adherence: Risks for nonadherence. In D. Drotar (Ed.), *Promoting adherence to medical treatment in chronic childhood illness: Concepts, methods, and interventions* (pp. 71–94). Mahwah, NJ: Erlbaum.

Bauman, L. J., Drotar, D., Leventhal, J. M., Perrin, E. C., & Pless, I. B. (1997). A review of psychosocial interventions for children with chronic health conditions. *Pediatrics, 100,* 244–251.

Begg, C., Cho, M., Eastwood, S., Horton, R., Mhoer, D., Olkin, I., et al. (1996). Improving the quality of reporting of randomized clinical trials. The CONSORT statement. *Journal of the American Medical Association, 276,* 637–639.

Bellg, A. J., Resnick, B., Minicucci, D. S., Ogedegbe, G., Ernst, D., Borrelli, B., et al. (2004). Enhancing treatment fidelity in health behavior change studies: Best practices and recommendations from the NIH Behavior Change Consortium. *Health Psychology, 23,* 443–451.

Bennett, D. S. (1994). Depression among children with chronic medical problems: A meta-analysis. *Journal of Pediatric Psychology, 19,* 149–169.

Berkovitch, M., Papadouris, D., Shaw, D., Onnaka, N., Dias, C., & Oliver, N. F. (1998). Trying to improve compliance with prophylactic penicillin therapy in children with sickle cell disease. *British Journal of Clinical Pharmacology, 45,* 605–607.

Bernard-Bonnin, A. C., Stachenko, S., Bonin, D., Charette, C., & Rousseau, E. (1995). Self-management teaching programs and morbidity of pediatric asthma: A meta-analysis. *Journal of Allergy and Clinical Immunology, 95,* 34–41.

Betan, E. J., Roberts, M. C., & McCluskey-Fawcett, K. (1995). Rates of participation for clinical child and pediatric psychology research issues in methodology. *Journal of Clinical Child Psychology, 24,* 227–236.

Birkhead, B., Olfaway, N. J., Strunk, R. C., Townsend, M. C., & Teutsch, S. (1989). Investigation of a cluster of deaths of adolescents with asthma: Evidence implicating inadequate treatment and poor patient adherence to medications. *Journal of Allergy and Clinical Immunology, 84,* 484–491.

Blechman, E. A., & Delamater, A. M. (1993). Family communication and Type 1 diabetes: A window on the social environment of chronically ill children. In R. Cole & D. Reiss (Eds.), *How do families cope with chronic illness?* (pp. 1–24). Hillsdale, NJ: Erlbaum.

Blount, R. L., Piira, T., & Cohen, L. L. (2003). Management of pediatric pain and distress due to medical procedures. In M. C. Roberts (Ed.), *Handbook of pediatric psychology* (3rd. ed., pp. 211–233). New York: Guilford Press.

Boardway, R. H., Delamater, A. M., Tomakowsky, J., & Gutai, J. P. (1993). Stress management training for adolescents with diabetes. *Journal of Pediatric Psychology, 18,* 29–45.

Boer, H., & Seydel, E. R. (1996). Protection motivation theory. In M. Conner & P. Norman (Eds.), *Predicting health behaviors* (pp. 95–120). Philadelphia: Open University Press.

Boland, E. A., Grey, M., Oesterle, A., Fredrickson, L., & Tamborlane, W. V. (1999). Continuous subcutaneous insulin infusion: A new way to lower risk of severe hyperglycemia, improve metabolic control, and enhance coping in adolescents with Type 1 diabetes. *Diabetes Care, 22,* 1779–1784.

Bollen, K. A. (1989). *Structural equations with content variables.* New York: Wiley.

Bonner, M. J., Gustafson, K. E., Schumacher, E., & Thompson, R. J., Jr. (1999). The impact of sickle cell disease on cognitive functioning and learning. *School Psychology Review, 28,* 102–193.

Bonner, M. J., Hardy, K. K., Ezell, E., & Ware, R. (2004). Hematological disorders: Sickle cell disease and hemophilia. In R. T. Brown (Ed.), *Handbook of pediatric psychology in school settings* (pp. 241–262). Mahwah, NJ: Erlbaum.

Bonner, S., Zimmerman, B. J., Evans, D., Irogoyen, M., Resnick, D., & Mellins, R. B. (2002). An individualized intervention to improve asthma management among urban Latino and African-American families. *Journal of Asthma, 39,* 167–179.

Bradshaw, B. (2002). The role of the family in managing therapy in minority children with Type 2 diabetes mellitus. *Journal of Pediatric Endocrinology & Metabolism, 15,* 547–551.

Bratton, D. L., Price, M., Gavin, L., Glenn, K., Brenner, M., Gelfand, E. W., & Klinnert, M. D. (2001). Impact of a multidisciplinary day program on disease and healthcare costs in children and adolescents with severe asthma: A two-year follow-up study. *Pediatric Pulmonology, 31,* 177–189.

Bronfenbrenner, V. C. (1979). *The ecology of human development.* Cambridge, MA: Harvard University Press.

Brooks-Gunn, J., & Rotheram-Borus, M. (1994). Rights to privacy in research: Adolescents versus parents. *Ethics and Behavior, 4,* 109–121.

Broome, M. E., Maikler, V., Kelber, S., Bailey, P., & Lea, G. (2001). An intervention to increase coping and reduce health care utilization for school-age children and adolescents with sickle cell disease. *Journal of National Black Nurses Association, 12,* 6–14.

Brown, J. V., Bakeman, R., Celano, M. P., Demi, A. S., Kobrynski, L., & Wilson, S. R. (2002). Home-based asthma education of young low-income children and their families. *Journal of Pediatric Psychology, 27,* 677–688.

Brown, R. T. (Ed.). (1999). *Cognitive aspects of chronic illness in children.* New York: Guilford Press.

Brown, R. T. (Ed.). (2004). *Handbook of pediatric psychology in school settings.* Mahwah, NJ: Erlbaum.

Brown, R. T., Armstrong, F. D., & Eckman, J. R. (1993). Neurocognitive aspects of pediatric sickle cell disease. *Journal of Learning Disabilities, 26,* 33–45.

Brown, R. T., Davis, P. C., Lambert, R., Hsu, L., Hopkins, K., & Eckman, J. (2000). Neurocognitive functioning and magnetic resonance imaging in children with sickle cell disease. *Journal of Pediatric Psychology, 25,* 503–513.

Brown, R. T., Fuemmeler, B., & Forti, E. (2003). Racial and ethnic health disparity and access to care. In M. C. Roberts (Ed.), *Handbook of pediatric psychology* (3rd ed., pp. 683–695). New York: Guilford Press.

Brownlee-Duffeck, M., Peterson, L., Simonds, J. F., Goldstein, D., Kilo, C., & Hoette, S. (1987). The role of health beliefs in the regimen adherence and metabolic control of adolescents and adults with diabetes mellitus. *Journal of Consulting and Clinical Psychology, 55,* 139–144.

Bussell, D. A. (1994). Ethical issues in observational family research. *Family Process, 33,* 361–376.

Butler, R. W. (1998). Attentional processes and their remediation in childhood cancer. *Medical and Pediatric Oncology, 30*(Suppl. 1), 75–78.

Butler, R. W., & Copeland, D. R. (2002). Attentional processes and their remediation in children treated for cancer: A literature review and the development of a therapeutic approach. *Journal of the International Neuropsychological Society, 8,* 113–124.

Butler, R. W., & Mulhern, R. K. (2005). Neurocognitive interventions for children and adolescents surviving cancer. *Journal of Pediatric Psychology, 30,* 65–78.

Cadman, D., Boyle, M. L., & Offord, D. R. (1988). The Ontario Child Health Study: Social adjustment and mental health of siblings of children with chronic health problems. *Journal of Developmental and Behavioral Pediatrics, 9,* 117–121.

Cadman, D., Boyle, M., Szatmari, P., & Offord, D. R. (1987). Chronic illness, disability, and mental and social well-being: Findings of the Ontario Child Health Study. *Pediatrics, 79,* 805–812.

Caplan, G. (1964). *Principles of preventive psychiatry.* New York: Basic Books.

Carey, M. E., Barakat, L. P., Foley, B., Gyato, K., & Phillips, P. C. (2001). Neuropsychological functioning and social functioning of survivors of pediatric brain tumors: Evidence of nonverbal learning disability. *Child Neuropsychology, 7*, 265–272.

Caskey, J. D., & Rosenthal, S. L. (2005). Conducting research on sensitive topics with adolescents: Ethical and developmental considerations. *Journal of Developmental and Behavioral Pediatrics, 26*, 61–67.

Cassidy, J. T., & Petty, R. E. (2001). *Textbook of pediatric rheumatology* (4th ed.). Philadelphia: Saunders.

Celano, M., & Geller, R. J. (1993). Learning, school performance, and children with asthma: How much at risk? *Journal of Learning Disabilities, 26*, 23–32.

Celano, M., Geller, R. J., Phillips, K. M., & Zimen, R. (1998). Treatment adherence among low-income children with asthma. *Journal of Pediatric Psychology, 23*, 345–349.

Centers for Disease Control and Prevention. (1996, May 3). Asthma mortality and hospitalization among children and young adults: United States, 1980–1993. *Morbidity and Mortality Weekly Report, 45*, 350–353.

Chalmers, T. C., Smith, H., & Blackburn, B. (1981). A method for assessing the quality of a randomized control trial. *Controlled Clinical Trials, 2*, 31–49.

Chambless, D. L., Baker, M. J., Baucom, D. H., Beutler, L. E., Calhoun, K. S., Crits-Christoph, P., et al. (1998). Update on empirically validated therapies: II. *Clinical Psychologist, 51*, 3–16.

Chambless, D. L., & Hollon, S. D. (1998). Defining empirically supported therapies. *Journal of Consulting and Clinical Psychology, 66*, 7–18.

Chambless, D. L., Sanderson, W. C., Shoham, V., Bennet-Johnson, S., Pope, K. S., Crits-Christoph, P., et al. (1996). An update on empirically validated therapies. *Clinical Psychologist, 49*, 5–18.

Charache, S., Terrin, M. L., Moore, R. D., Dover, G. J., Barton, F. B., Eckert, S. V., et al. (1995). Effect of hydroxyurea on the frequency of painful crises in sickle cell anemia. *New England Journal of Medicine, 332*, 1317–1322.

Charron-Prochownik, C., Becker, M. H., Brown, M. B., Liang, W. M., & Bennett, S. (1993). Understanding young children's health beliefs and diabetes regimen adherence. *Diabetes Educator, 19*, 409–418.

Chen, E., Cole, S. W., & Kato, P. M. (2004). A review of empirically supported intervention for pain and adherence outcomes in sickle cell disease. *Journal of Pediatric Psychology, 29*, 197–209.

Chen, H. T. (1990). *The only driven evaluations.* Newbury Park, CA: Sage.

Chernoff, R. G., Ireys, H. T., DeVet, K. A., & Kim, Y. J. (2002). A randomized controlled trial of a community-based support program for families of children with chronic illnesses: Pediatric outcomes. *Archives of Pediatrics and Adolescent Medicine, 156*, 533–539.

Child Abuse Prevention and Treatment and Adoption Reform Act, Public Law No. 102-295, 42 U.S.C.A. 5101 *et seq.* (1999).

Clark, N. M., Feldman, C. H., Evans, D., Levison, M. J., Wasilewski, Y., & Mellins, R. B. (1986). The impact of health education on frequency and cost of health care use by low income children with asthma. *Journal of Allergy and Clinical Immunology, 78*, 108–15.

Clark, N. M., Rosenstock, I. M., Hassan, H., Evans, D., Wasilewski, Y., Feldman, C., & Mellins, R. B. (1988). The effect of health beliefs and feelings of self-efficacy on self-management behavior of children with a chronic disease. *Patient Education and Counseling, 11*, 131–139.

Clay, D. L. (2004). *Helping schoolchildren with chronic health conditions*. New York: Guilford Press.

Clement, S. (1995). Diabetes self-management education. *Diabetes Care, 18*, 1204–1214.

Clingempeel, W. G., & Henggeler, S. W. (2002). Randomized clinical trials, developmental theory and antisocial youth: Guidelines for research. *Development and Psychopathology, 14*, 695–711.

Coakley, R. M., Holmbeck, G. N., Friedman, D., Greenley, R. N., & Thill, A. W. (2002). A longitudinal study of pubertal timing, parent–child conflict, and cohesion in families of young adolescents with spina bifida. *Journal of Pediatric Psychology, 27*, 461–473.

Cohen, J. (1988). *Statistical power analyses for the behavioral sciences* (2nd ed.). Hillsdale, NJ: Erlbaum.

Cohen, J. (1992). A power primer. *Psychological Bulletin, 112*, 155–159.

Cohen, M. J., Branch, W. B., McKie, V. C., & Adams, R. J. (1997). Neuropsychological impairment in children with sickle cell anemia and cerebrovascular accidents. *Clinical Pediatrics, 33*, 517–524.

Cohen, S. Y., & Wamboldt, F. S. (2000). The parent–physician relationship in pediatric asthma care. *Journal of Pediatric Psychology, 25*, 69–77.

Collins, M., Kaslow, N., Doepke, K., Eckman, J., & Johnson, M. (1998). Psychosocial interventions for children and adolescents with sickle cell disease (SCD). *Journal of Black Psychology, 24*, 432–454.

Colton, P. A., Rodin, G. M., Olmsted, M. P., & Daneman, D. (1999). Eating disturbances in young women with Type 1 diabetes mellitus: Mechanisms and consequences. *Psychiatric Annals, 29*, 213–218.

Conrad, P. C. (1985). The meaning of medications: Another look at compliance. *Social Science and Medicine, 20*, 29–37.

Cook, T. D., & Campbell, D. T. (1979). *Quasi-experimentation: Design and analysis issues for field settings*. Chicago: Rand McNally.

Coyne, J. C., & Anderson, B. J. (1988). The "psychosomatic" family reconsidered: Diabetes in context. *Journal of Marital and Family Therapy, 114*, 113–123.

Coyne, J. C., & Anderson, B. J. (1989). The "psychosomatic" family reconsidered: II. Recalling a defective model and looking ahead. *Journal of Marital and Family Therapy*, 25–30.

Crain, E. F., Kercsmar, C., Weiss, K. B., Mitchell, H., & Lynn, H. (1998). Reported difficulties in access to quality care for children with asthma in the inner city. *Archives of Pediatric and Adolescent Medicine, 151*, 333–339.

Creer, T. L. (1998). The complexity of treating asthma. *Journal of Asthma, 35,* 451–458.

Creer, T. L. (2000). Self-management and the control of chronic pediatric illness. In D. Drotar (Ed.), *Promoting adherence to medical treatment in chronic childhood illness: Concepts, methods, and interventions* (pp. 95–130). Mahwah, NJ: Erlbaum.

Creer, T. L. (2001). Asthma, disease management, and research: Attempting to unravel a Gordian knot. *Journal of Asthma, 38,* 289–297.

Creer, T. L., Backial, M., Burns, K. L., Leung, P., Marion, R. J., Miklich, D. R., et al. (1988). Living with asthma. *Journal of Asthma, 25,* 335–362.

Creer, T. L., & Bender, B. (1995). Pediatric asthma. In M. C. Roberts (Ed.), *Handbook of pediatric psychology* (2nd ed., pp. 219–240). New York: Guilford Press.

Cuttler, L., Drotar, D., Singer, M., Dahms, W. T., Kerr, D. S., Palmert, M. R., et al. (2004, May). *A randomized controlled trial of outpatient vs. inpatient management of new onset Type I diabetes mellitus.* Paper presented at the meeting of the Society for Pediatric Research, San Francisco, CA.

Cystic Fibrosis Foundation. (2001, September). *Patient registry 2000 annual data report.* Bethesda, MD: Author.

Czajkowski, D. R., & Koocher, G. P. (1986). Predicting medical compliance among adolescents with cystic fibrosis. *Health Psychology, 5,* 297–305.

Czajkowski, D. R., & Koocher, G. P. (1987). Medical compliance and coping with cystic fibrosis. *Journal of Child Psychology and Psychiatry, 28,* 311–319.

da Costa, I. G., Rapoff, M. A., Lemanek, K., & Goldstein, G. L. (1997). Improving adherence to medication regimens for children with asthma and its effect on clinical outcome. *Journal of Applied Behavioral Analysis, 30,* 687–691.

Dahlquist, L. M., & Switkin, M. C. (2003). Chronic and recurrent pain. In M. C. Roberts (Ed.), *Handbook of pediatric psychology* (3rd ed., pp. 198–215). New York: Guilford Press.

D'Auria, J. P., Christian, B. J., Henderson, Z. G., & Haynes, B. (2000). The company they keep: The influence of peer relationships on adjustment to cystic fibrosis during adolescence. *Journal of Pediatric Nursing, 15,* 175–182.

Davies, H. A., & Lilleyman, J. (1995). Compliance with oral chemotherapy in childhood lymphoblastic leukemia. *Cancer Treatment Reviews, 21,* 93–103.

Davis, M. A., Quittner, A. L., Stack, C. M., & Yang, M. C. K. (2004). Controlled evaluation of the STARBRIGHT CD-ROM program for children and adolescents with cystic fibrosis. *Journal of Pediatric Psychology, 29,* 259–267.

Davis, P. B., Drumm, M., & Konstan, M. W. (1996). Cystic fibrosis. *American Journal of Respiratory Critical Care and Medicine,* 1229–1256.

De Civita, M., & Dobkin, P. (2004). Pediatric adherence as a multidimensional and dynamic construct, involving a triadic partnership. *Journal of Pediatric Psychology, 29,* 157–170.

Delamater, A. M. (2002). Working with children who have Type 1 diabetes. In B. J. Anderson & R. R. Rubin (Eds.), *Practical psychology for diabetes clinicians* (pp. 127–137). Alexandria, VA: American Diabetes Association.

Delamater, A. M., Bubb, J., Davis, S. G., Smith, J. A. , Schmidt, L., White, N. A., & Santiago, J. V. (1990). A randomized prospective study of self-management training with newly diagnosed diabetic children. *Diabetes Care, 13*, 492–498.

Delamater, A. M., Jacobsen, M. D., Anderson, B., Cox, D., Fisher, L., Lustman, P., et al. (2001). Psychosocial therapies in diabetes: Report of the Psychosocial Therapies Working Group. *Diabetes Care, 24*, 1286–1292.

Delk, K. K., Gevirtz, R., Hicks, D. A., Carden, F., & Rucker, R. (1994). The effects of biofeedback assisted breathing retraining on lung functions in patients with cystic fibrosis. *Chest, 105*, 23–28.

Diabetes Control and Complications Trial Research Group. (1993). The effect of intensive treatment of diabetes on the development and progression of long-term complications in insulin-dependent diabetes mellitus. *New England Journal of Medicine, 329*, 977–986.

Diabetes Control and Complications Trial Research Group. (1994). Effect of intensive diabetes treatment on the development and progression of long term complications in adolescents with insulin-dependent diabetes mellitus. *Journal of Pediatrics, 125*, 177–188.

DiGirolamo, A. M., Quittner, A. L., Ackerman, V., & Stevens, J. (1997). Identification and assessment of ongoing stressors in adolescents with a chronic illness: An application of the behavior-analytic model. *Journal of Clinical Child Psychology, 26*, 53–66.

Doershuk, C. F. (Ed.). (2001). *Cystic fibrosis in the 20th century: People, events, and progress.* Cleveland, OH: AM Publishing.

Dongen-Melman, J. E. W. M., Van Pruyn, J. F. A., DeGroot, A., Koot, H. M., Hahlen, K., & Verhulst, F. C. (1995). Late consequences for parents of children who survived cancer. *Journal of Pediatric Psychology, 20*, 567–586.

Dougherty, G. E., Soderstrom, L., & Schiffrin, A. (1998). An economic evaluation of home care for children with newly diagnosed diabetes: Results from a randomized controlled trial. *Medical Care, 36*, 586–598.

Drotar, D. (1978). Adaptational problems of children and adolescents with cystic fibrosis. *Journal of Pediatric Psychology, 3*, 45–50.

Drotar, D. (1981). Psychological perspectives in childhood chronic illness. *Journal of Pediatric Psychology, 6*, 211–228.

Drotar, D. (1989). Psychological research in pediatric settings: Lessons from the field. *Journal of Pediatric Psychology, 14*, 63–74.

Drotar, D. (1992). Integrating theory and practice in psychological interventions with children with a chronic illness. In T. J. Akamatsu, M. A. P. Stephens, S. E. Hobfoll, & J. H. Crowther (Eds.), *Family health psychology* (pp. 175–192). Washington, DC: Hemisphere.

Drotar, D. (1995). *Consulting with pediatricians: Psychological perspectives.* New York: Guilford Press.

Drotar, D. (1997a). Intervention research: Pushing back the frontiers of pediatric psychology. *Journal of Neuropsychological Society, 22,* 415–424.

Drotar, D. (1997b). Relating parent and family functioning to the psychological adjustment of children with chronic health conditions: What have we learned? What do we need to know? *Journal of Pediatric Psychology, 22,* 149–165.

Drotar, D. (1999). Psychological interventions for children with chronic physical illness and their families. Toward integration of research and practice. In M. J. Russ & T. Ollendick (Eds.), *Handbook of psychotherapies with children and families* (pp. 447–462). New York: Plenum Press.

Drotar, D. (Ed.). (2000a). *Handbook of research in pediatric and clinical child psychology: Practical strategies and methods.* New York: Kluwer Academic/ Plenum Publishers.

Drotar, D. (2000b). Managing research in pediatric and child clinical psychology. In D. Drotar (Ed.), *Handbook of research in pediatric and clinical child psychology: Practical strategies and methods* (pp. 245–260). New York: Kluwer Academic/ Plenum Publishers.

Drotar, D. (Ed.). (2000c). *Promoting adherence to treatment in childhood chronic illness: Concepts, methods, and interventions.* Mahwah, NJ: Erlbaum.

Drotar, D. (2001). Promoting comprehensive care for children with chronic health conditions and their families. *Children's Services: Social Policy, Research, and Practice, 4,* 157–166.

Drotar, D. (2002). Enhancing reviews of psychological interventions with pediatric populations: Thoughts on next steps. *Journal of Pediatric Psychology, 27,* 167–176.

Drotar, D. (2004). Commentary: We can make our own dime or two, help children and their families, and advance science while doing so. *Journal of Pediatric Psychology, 29,* 61–63.

Drotar, D. (2005). Commentary: Randomized controlled trials of psychological interventions with pediatric populations: The time has come and the *Journal of Pediatric Psychology* is ready. *Journal of Pediatric Psychology, 30,* 409–412.

Drotar, D., & Bush, M. (1985). Mental health issues and services. In N. Hobbs & J. H. Ferrin (Eds.), *Issues in the care of children with chronic illness* (pp. 514–550). San Francisco: Jossey-Bass.

Drotar, D., Crawford, P., & Bush, M. (1984). The family context of childhood chronic illness: Implications for psychosocial intervention. In M. G. Eisenberg, L. C. Sutkin, & M. A. Jansen (Eds.), *Chronic illness and disability through the life span: Effects on self and family* (pp. 103–132). New York: Springer Publishing Company.

Drotar, D., Crawford, P., & Ganofsky, M. A. (1984). Prevention with chronically ill children. In M. C. Roberts & L. Peterson (Eds.), *Prevention of problems in childhood: Psychological research and applications* (pp. 232–265). New York: Wiley.

Drotar, D., Eckl, C. L., Beitzl, M., Gil, E., Kocik, S., Kuekes, K., et al. (1997). Psychosocial services for children and adolescents with hemophilia and their families: Results of a national survey. *Children's Health Care, 26,* 137–150.

Drotar, D., La Greca, A. M., Lemanek, K. L., & Kazak, A. E. (1995). Case reports in pediatric psychology: Uses and guidelines for authors and reviewers. *Journal of Pediatric Psychology, 20,* 549–565.

Drotar, D., & Lemanek, K. (2001). Steps toward a clinically relevant science of interventions in pediatric settings. *Journal of Pediatric Psychology, 26,* 385–394.

Drotar, D., Malone, C. A., Nowak, M., Elamin, D., & Eckerle, D. (1985). Early preventive intervention in failure to thrive: Methods and early outcome. In D. Drotar (Ed.), *New directions in failure to thrive: Implications for research and practice* (pp. 119–138). New York: Plenum Press.

Drotar, D., Miller, V., Willard, V., Anthony, K., & Kodish, E. (2004). Correlates of parental participation during informed consent for randomized clinical trials in the treatment of childhood leukemia. *Ethics and Behavior, 14,* 1–15.

Drotar, D., Overholser, J. C., Levi, R., Walders. N., Robinson, J. R., Palermo, T. M., & Riekert, K. A. (2000). Ethical issues in conducting research with pediatric and clinical child populations in applied settings. In D. Drotar (Ed.), *Handbook of research methods in clinical child and pediatric psychology* (pp. 305–326). New York: Kluwer Academic/Plenum Publishers.

Drotar, D., Palermo, T. M., & Barry, C. (2003). Collaboration with schools: Models and methods in pediatric psychology and pediatrics. In R. T. Brown (Ed.), *Handbook of pediatric psychology in school settings* (pp. 21–36). Mahwah, NJ: Erlbaum.

Drotar, D., Palermo, T., & Landis, C. E. (2003). Training graduate level pediatric psychology researchers at Case Western Reserve University: Meeting the needs, challenges, and options for the new millenium. *Journal of Pediatric Psychology, 28,* 123–135.

Drotar, D., Perrin, E. C., & Stein, R. E. K. (1995). Methodological issues in using the Child Behavior Checklist and its related instruments in clinical child psychology research. *Journal of Clinical Child Psychology, 24,* 184–192.

Drotar, D., & Riekert, K. A. (2000). Understanding and managing sampling issues in research with children. In D. Drotar (Ed.), *Handbook of research in pediatric and clinical child psychology: Practical strategies and methods* (pp. 77–96). New York: Kluwer Academic.

Drotar, D., & Robinson, J. (1999). Researching failure to thrive: Progress, problems and recommendations. In D. Kessler & P. Dawson (Eds.), *Failure to thrive in infants and children: A transdisciplinary approach to nutritional adequacy in children* (pp. 97–98). Baltimore: Paul H. Brooks.

Drotar, D., Timmons-Mitchell, J., Williams, L. L., Palermo, T. M., Levi, R., Robinson, J. R., et al. (2000). Conducting research with children and adolescents in clinical and applied settings: Practical lessons from the field. In D. Drotar

(Ed.), *Handbook of research methods in clinical child and pediatric psychology* (pp. 261–280). New York: Kluwer Academic/Plenum Publishers.

Drotar, D., Walders, N., Burgess, E., Nobile, C., Dasari, M., Kahana, S., et al. (2001). Recommendations to enhance comprehensive care for children with chronic health conditions and their families. *Children's Services: Social Policy, Research, and Practice, 4,* 251–264.

Drotar, D., & Zagorski, L. (2001). Providing psychological services in pediatric settings in an era of managed care: Challenges and opportunities. In J. N. Hughes, A. M. La Greca, & J. C. Conoley (Eds.). *Handbook of psychological services for children and adolescents* (pp. 89–107). New York: Oxford University Press.

Duff, A. J. A. (2001). Psychological interventions in cystic fibrosis and asthma. *Paediatric Respiratory Reviews, 2,* 350–357.

DuHamel, K. N., Redd, W. H., & Vickberg-Johnson, S. M. (1999). Behavioral interventions in the diagnosis, treatment, and rehabilitation of children with cancer. *Acta Oncologica, 38,* 719–734.

Eiser, C. (1990). *Chronic childhood illness: An introduction to psychological theory and research.* New York: Cambridge University Press.

Ellis, D. A., Frey, M. A., Naar-King, S., Templin, T., Cunningham, P., & Cakan, N. (2005). Use of multisystemic therapy to improve regimen adherence among adolescents with Type 1 diabetes in chronic poor metabolic control: A randomized controlled trial. *Diabetes Care, 28,* 1604–1610.

Ellis, D. A., Naar-King, S., Frey, M., Rowland, M., & Greger, N. (2003). Case study: Feasibility of multisystemic therapy as a treatment for urban adolescents with poorly controlled Type 1 diabetes. *Journal of Pediatric Psychology, 28,* 287–293.

Ellis, D. A., Naar-King, S., Frey, M., Templin, T., Rowland, M., & Cakan, N. (2005). Multisystemic treatment of poorly controlled Type 1 diabetes: Effects on medical resource utilization. *Journal of Pediatric Psychology, 30,* 656–666.

Eney, R. D., & Goldstein, E. O. (1976). Compliance of chronic asthmatics with oral administration of theophylline as measured by serum and salivary levels. *Pediatrics, 57,* 513–517.

Erickson, S. R., Ascione, F. J., Kirking, D. M., & Johnson, C. E. (1998). Use of a paging system to improve medication self-management in patients with asthma. *Journal of the American Pharmaceutical Association, 38,* 767–769.

Evans, D., Clark, N. M., Feldman, C. H., Rips, J., Kaplan, D., Levison, M. J., et al. (1987). A school health education program for children with asthma aged 8–11 years. *Health Education Quarterly, 14,* 267–279.

Evans, R. (1992). Asthma among minority children: A growing problem. *Chest, 101,* 368S–371S.

Evans, R., Gergen, P. J., Mitchell, H., Kattan, M., Kercsmar, C., Crain, E., et al. (1999). A randomized clinical trial to reduce asthma morbidity among inner-city children: Results of the National Cooperative Inner City Asthma Study. *Journal of Pediatrics, 135,* 332–38.

Farber, H. J., Capra, A., Finkelstein, J. A., Lozano, P., Quesenberry, C. P., Jensvold, N. G., et al. (2003). Misunderstanding of asthma controller medications: Association with nonadherence. *Journal of Asthma, 40*, 17–25.

Festa, R. S., Tamaroff, M. H., Chasalow, F., & Lanzkowsky, P. (1992). Therapeutic adherence to oral medication regimens by adolescents with cancer: I. Laboratory assessment. *Journal of Pediatrics, 120*, 807–811.

Field, T., Hernandez-Reif, M., Seligman, S., Krasnegor, J., Sunshine, W., Rivas-Chacon, R., et al. (1997). Juvenile rheumatoid arthritis: Benefits from massage therapy. *Journal of Pediatric Psychology, 22*, 607–617.

Fiese, B. H., Wilder, J., & Bickham, N. L. (2000). The family context in developmental psychopathology. In A. J. Sameroff, M. Lewis, & S. M. Miller (Eds.), *Handbook of developmental psychopathology* (2nd ed., pp. 116–136). New York: Kluwer Academic/Plenum Publishers.

Fisher, C. B. (2004). Informed consent and clinical research involving children and adolescents: Implications of the revised APA ethics code and HIPAA. *Journal of Clinical Child and Adolescent Psychology, 33*, 832–839.

Fisher, C. B., & Fried, A. L. (2003). Psychological services and the Internet-mediated American Psychological Association ethics code. *Psychotherapy: Theory, Research, Practice, and Training, 40*, 103–111.

Fisher, C. B., Hoagwood, K., Boyce, C., Duster, T., Frank, D. A., Grisso, T., et al. (2002). Research ethics for mental health science involving ethnic minority children and youths. *American Psychologist, 57*, 1024–1040.

Forrest, C. B., Starfield, B., Riley, A. W., & Kang, M. (1997). The impact of asthma on the health status of adolescents. *Pediatrics, 99*, E1.

Frank, R. G., Thayer, J. F., & Hoaglund, K. J. (1998). Trajectories of adaptation in pediatric chronic illness: The importance of the individual. *Journal of Consulting and Clinical Psychology, 66*, 521–532.

Fritz, G. K., & McQuaid, E. L. (2000). Chronic medical conditions: Impact on development. In A. J. Sameroff, M. Lewis, & S. M. Miller (Eds.), *Handbook of developmental psychopathology* (2nd ed., pp. 277–289). New York: Kluwer Academic.

Garmezy, N., Masten, J., & Tellegen, A. (1984). The study of stress and competence in children: A building block for developmental psychopathology. *Child Development, 55*, 97–111.

Garrison, W. T., & McQuiston, S. (1989). *Chronic illness during childhood and adolescence: Psychological aspects.* Newbury Park, CA: Sage.

Gartstein, M. A., Short, A. D., Vannatta, K., & Noll, R. B. (1999). Psychosocial adjustment of children with chronic illness: An evaluation of three models. *Journal of Developmental and Behavioral Pediatrics, 20*, 157–163.

Geist, R. (1995). Psychosocial care in the pediatric hospital: The need for scientific validation of clinical and cost effectiveness. *General Hospital Psychiatry, 17*, 228–234.

Gerhardt, C. A., Walders, N., Rosenthal, S. L., & Drotar, D. (2003). Children and families coping with pediatric chronic illnesses. In K. I. Maton, C. J. Schellenbach, B. J. Leadbeater, & A. L. Solarz (Eds.), *Investing in children, youth, families, and communities: Strengths-based research and policy* (pp. 173–199). Washington, DC: American Psychological Association.

Gil, K. M., Anthony, K. K., Carson, J. W., Redding-Lallinger, R., Daeschner, C. W., & Ware, R. E. (2001). Daily coping practice predicts treatment effects in children with sickle cell disease. *Journal of Pediatric Psychology, 26,* 163–173.

Gil, K. M., Carson, J. W., Sedway, J. A., Porter, L. S., Schaeffer, J. J. W., & Orringer, E. (2000). Follow-up of coping skills training in adults with sickle cell disease: Analysis of daily pain and coping practice diaries. *Health Psychology, 19,* 85–90.

Gil, K. M., Porter, L., Ready, J., Workman, E., Sedway, J., & Anthony, K. K. (2000). Pain in children and adolescents with sickle cell disease: An analysis of daily pain diaries. *Children's Health Care, 29,* 225–241.

Gil, K. M., Williams, D. A., Thompson, R. J., Jr., & Kinney, T. R. (1991). Sickle cell disease in children and adolescents: The relation of child and parent pain coping strategies to adjustment. *Journal of Pediatric Psychology, 16,* 643–663.

Gil, K. M., Wilson, J. J., Edens, J. L., Workman, E., Ready, Y., Sedway, J., et al. (1997). Cognitive coping skills training in children with sickle cell disease. *International Journal of Behavioral Medicine, 4,* 364–377.

Gilljam, M., Antoniou, M., Shin, J., Dupuis, A., Corey, M., & Tullis, D. E. (2000). Pregnancy in cystic fibrosis. *Chest, 118,* 85–92.

Glantz, L. (1996). Conducting research with children: Legal and ethical issues. *Journal of the American Academy of Child and Adolescent Psychiatry, 34,* 1283–1291.

Glasgow, R. E., Bull, S. S., Gillette, C., Klesges, L. M., & Dzewaltowski, D. A. (2002). Behavior change intervention research in health care settings: A review of recent reports with emphasis on external validity. *American Journal of Preventive Medicine, 23,* 62–69.

Glasgow, R. E., Hiss, R. G., Anderson, R. M., Friedman, N. M., Hayward, R. A., Marrero, D. G., et al. (2001). Report of the health care delivery work group: Behavioral research related to the establishment of a chronic disease model for diabetes care. *Diabetes Care, 24,* 124–130.

Glasgow, R. E., Klesges, L. M., Dzewaltowski, D. A., Bull, S. S., & Estabrooks, P. (2004). The future of health behavior change research: What is needed to improve translation of research into health promotion practice? *Annals of Behavioral Medicine, 27,* 3–12.

Glasgow, R. E., McKay, H. G., Piette, J. D., & Reynolds, K. D. (2001). The RE-AIM framework for evaluating interventions: What can it tell us about approaches to chronic illness management? *Patient Education and Counseling, 44,* 119–127.

Glasgow, R. E., Vogt, T. M., & Boles, S. M. (1999). Evaluating the public health impact of health promotion interventions: The RE-AIM framework. *American Journal of Public Health, 89,* 1322–1327.

Glasscoe, C. A., & Quittner, A. L. (2005). Psychological interventions for cystic fibrosis. In *The Cochrane Database of Systematic Reviews, The Cochrane Library, The Cochrane Collaboration, 3,* 1–118. Retrieved October 6, 2005, from http://gateway.ut.ovid.com/gwl/ovidweb.cgi

Goldbeck, L., & Babka, C. (2001). Development and evaluation of a multi-family psychoeducational program for cystic fibrosis. *Patient Education and Counseling, 44,* 187–192.

Goldberg, S., Gotowiec, A., & Simmons, R. J. (1995). Infant–mother attachment and behavior problems in healthy and chronically ill preschoolers. *Development and Psychopathology, 7,* 267–282.

Goldberg, S., Morris, P., Simmons, R. J., Fowler, R. S., & Levison, H. (1990). Chronic illness in infancy and parenting stress: A comparison of three groups of parents. *Journal of Pediatric Psychology, 15,* 347–358.

Gonzalez, S., Steinglass, P., & Reiss, D. (1989). Putting the illness in its place. Discussion groups for families with chronic medical illnesses. *Family Process, 28,* 69–87.

Goodman, J. E., & McGrath, P. J. (1991). The epidemiology of pain in children and adolescents: A review. *Pain, 46,* 247–264.

Gordon, R. S., Jr. (1983). An operational classification of disease prevention. *Public Health Reports, 98,* 107–109.

Gortmaker, S. L., Walker, D. K., Weitzman, M., & Sobol, A. M. (1990). Chronic conditions, socioeconomic risks, and behavioral problems in children and adolescents. *Pediatrics, 85,* 267–276.

Gottman, J. M., & Fainsilber-Katz, L. (1989). Effects of marital disorder on young children's peer interaction and health. *Developmental Psychology, 25,* 373–381.

Grasso, M. C., Button, B. M., Allison, D. J., & Sawyer, S. M. (2000). Benefits of music therapy as an adjunct to chest physiotherapy in infants and toddlers with cystic fibrosis. *Pediatric Pulmonology, 29,* 371–381.

Gray, D. L., Marrero, D. G., Godfrey, C., Orr, D. P., & Golden, M. P. (1988). Chronic poor metabolic control in the pediatric population: A stepwise intervention program. *Diabetes Education, 14,* 516–520.

Greco, P., Shroff-Pendley, J. S., McDonell, K., & Reeves, G. (2001). A peer group intervention for adolescents with Type 1 diabetes and their best friends. *Journal of Pediatric Psychology, 26,* 485–490.

Greenberg, W. S., & Meadows, A. T. (1992). Psychological impact of cancer survival on school-age children and their parents. *Journal of Psychosocial Oncology, 9,* 43–56.

Greene, T., & Ernhart, C. B. (1991). Adjustment for cofactors in pediatric research. *Developmental and Behavioral Pediatrics, 12,* 378–385.

Greineider, D. K., Loane, K. C., & Parks, P. C. (1995). Reduction in resource utilization by an asthma outreach program. *Archives of Pediatric and Adolescent Medicine, 149,* 415–420.

Grey, M., Boland, E. A., Davidson, M., Li, J., & Tamborlane, W. V. (2000). Coping skills training for youth with poorly controlled diabetes mellitus has long-lasting effects on metabolic control and quality of life. *Journal of Pediatrics, 137,* 107–113.

Grey, M., Boland, E. A., Davidson, M., Yu, C., Sullivan-Bolyai, S., & Tamborlane, W. V. (1998). Short-term effects of coping skills training as adjunct to intensive therapy in adolescents. *Diabetes Care, 21,* 902–908.

Grey, M., Boland, E. A., Davidson, M., Yu, C., & Tamborlane, W. V. (1999). Coping skills training for youths with diabetes on intensive therapy. *Applied Nursing Research, 12,* 3–12.

Grodin, M. A., & Glantz, C. H. (Eds.). (1994). *Children as research subjects.* New York: Oxford University Press.

Guendelman, S., Meade, K., Benson, M., Chen, Y. Q., & Samuels, S. (2002). Improving asthma outcomes and self-management behaviors of inner-city children. *Archives of Pediatric and Adolescent Medicine, 156,* 114–120.

Haby, M. M., Waters, E., Robertson, C. F., Gibson, P. G., & Ducharme, F. M. (2005). Interventions for educating children who have attended the emergency room for asthma. *The Cochrane Database of Systematic Reviews, The Cochrane Library, The Cochrane Collaboration, 3,* 1–45. Retrieved October 6, 2005, from http://gateway.ut.ovid.com/gwl/ovidweb.cgi

Hagglund, K. J., Doyle, N. M., Clay, D. L., Frank, R. G., Johnson, J. C., & Pressly, T. A. (1996). A family retreat as a comprehensive intervention for children with arthritis and their families. *Arthritis Care & Research, 9,* 35–41.

Hagopian, L. P., & Thompson, R. H. (1999). Reinforcement of compliance with respiratory treatment in a child with cystic fibrosis. *Journal of Applied Behavior Analysis, 32,* 233–236.

Hains, A. A., Davies, W. H., Behrens, D., & Bilber, J. A. (1997). Cognitive behavioral interventions for adolescents with cystic fibrosis. *Journal of Pediatric Psychology, 22,* 669–687.

Hains, A. A., Davies, W. H., Behrens, D., Freeman, M. E., & Bilber, J. A. (2001). Effectiveness of a cognitive behavioral intervention for young adults with cystic fibrosis. *Journal of Clinical Psychology in Medical Settings, 8,* 325–336.

Hallstand, T. S., Curtis, T. R., Aitken, M. L., & Sullivan, S. D. (2003). Quality of life in adolescents with mild asthma. *Pediatric Pulmonology, 36,* 536–543.

Halterman, J. S., Aligne, C. A., Auinger, P., McBride, J. T., & Szilagyi, P. G. (2000). Inadequate therapy for asthma among children in the United States. *Pediatrics, 105,* 272–276.

Hampson, S. E., Skinner, T. C., Hart, J., Storey, L., Gage, H., Foxcroft, D., et al. (2000). Behavioral interventions with adolescents with Type 1 diabetes. *Diabetes Care, 23,* 1416–1422.

Hampson, S. E., Skinner, T. C., Hart, J., Storey, L., Gage, H., Foxcroft, D., et al. (2001). Effects of educational and psychosocial interventions for adolescents with diabetes mellitus: A systematic review. *Health Technology Assessment, 5,* 1–78.

Hanson, C. L. (1992). Developing systemic models of the adaptation of youths with diabetes. In A. M. La Greca, L. J. Siegel, J. L. Wallander, & C. E. Walker (Eds.), *Stress and coping in child health* (pp. 212–241). New York: Guilford Press.

Hanson, C. L., Henggeler, S. W., & Burghen, G. A. (1987a). Model of associations between psychological variables and health outcome measures of adolescents with IDDM. *Diabetes Care, 10,* 752–758.

Hanson, C. L., Henggeler, S. W., & Burghen, G. A. (1987b). Social competence and parental support as mediators of the link between stress and metabolic control in adolescents with insulin-dependent diabetes mellitus. *Journal of Consulting and Clinical Psychology, 55,* 529–533.

Harris, M. A., Harris, B. S., & Mertlich, D. (2005). Brief report: In-home therapy for adolescents with poorly controlled diabetes: Failure to maintain benefits at 6-month follow-up. *Journal of Pediatric Psychology, 30,* 683–688.

Harris, M. A., & Mertlich, D. (2003). Piloting home-based behavioral family systems therapy for adolescents with poorly controlled diabetes. *Children's Health Care, 32,* 65–79.

Hausenstein, E. J. (1990). The experience of distress in parents of chronically ill children: Potential or likely outcome? *Journal of Clinical Child Psychology, 19,* 356–364.

Hauser, S., Jacobson, A. M., Lavori, P., Wolfsdorf, J., Herskowitz, R., Milley, J., et al. (1990). Adherence among children and adolescents with insulin-dependent diabetes mellitus over a four-year longitudinal follow-up: Immediate and long-term linkages with the family milieu. *Journal of Pediatric Psychology, 15,* 527–542.

Hayford, J. R., & Ross, C. K. (1988). Medical compliance in juvenile rheumatoid arthritis. *Arthritis Care and Research, 1,* 190–197.

Hazzard, A., Celano, M., Collins, M., & Markov, Y. (2002). Effects of Starbright World on knowledge, social support, and coping in hospitalized children with sickle cell disease and asthma. *Children's Health Care, 31,* 69–86.

Health Insurance Portability and Accountability Act (HIPAA), Public Law 104-191, § 262 and § 42, U.S.C. § 1320 *et seq.* (1996).

Henggeler, S. W. (1999). Multisystemic therapy: An overview of clinical procedures, outcomes, and policy implications. *Child Psychology and Psychiatry Review, 4,* 2–10.

Henggeler, S. W., & Randall, J. (2000). Conducting randomized treatment studies in real-world settings. In D. Drotar (Ed.), *Handbook of research in pediatric and clinical child psychology: Practical strategies and methods* (pp. 447–462). New York: Kluwer Academic.

Henggeler, S. W., Schoenwald, S. K., Borduin, C. M., Rowland, M. D., & Cunningham, P. B. (1998). *Multisystemic treatment of antisocial behavior in children and adolescents*. New York: Guilford Press.

Hermanns, J., Florin, I., Dietrich, M., Rieger, C., & Hahlweg, K. (1989). Maternal criticism, mother–child interaction, and bronchial asthma. *Journal of Psychosomatic Research, 33,* 469–476.

Hernandez-Reif, M., Field, T., Krasnegor, J., Martinez, E., Schwartzmann, M., & Mavunda, K. (1999). Children with cystic fibrosis benefit from massage therapy. *Journal of Pediatric Psychology, 24,* 175–181.

Hill, R. (1958). Generic features of families under stress. *Social Case Work, 39,* 139–150.

Hill-Briggs, F. (2003). Problem solving in diabetes self-management: A model of chronic illness self-management behavior. *Annals of Behavioral Medicine, 25,* 182–193.

Hoagwood, K. (2003). Ethical issues in child and adolescent psychosocial treatment research. In A. E. Kazdin & J. R. Weisz (Eds.), *Evidence-based psychotherapies for children and adolescents* (pp. 60–79). New York: Guilford Press.

Hoagwood, K., Jensen, P. S., & Fisher, C. B. (1996). *Ethical issues in mental health research with children and adolescents.* Mahwah, NJ: Erlbaum.

Hobbs, H., & Perrin, J. M. (Eds.). (1985). *Issues in the care of children with chronic illness.* San Francisco: Jossey Bass.

Hobfoll, S. E. (1988). *The ecology of stress.* Washington, DC: Hemisphere.

Hobfoll, S. E. (1989). Conservation of resources: A new attempt at conceptualizing stress. *American Psychologist, 44,* 513–524.

Hoekstra-Weebers, W. E. H. M., Heuvel, F., Jaspers, J. P. L., Kamps, W. A., & Klip, E. L. (1998). Brief report: An intervention program for pediatric cancer patients: A randomized controlled trial. *Journal of Pediatric Psychology, 23,* 207–214.

Hoff, A. L. (2003). *An intervention to decrease illness uncertainty and psychological distress among parents of children newly diagnosed with Type 1 diabetes: A randomized clinical trial.* Unpublished doctoral dissertation, Oklahoma State University, Stillwater.

Holmbeck, G. N. (1997). Toward terminological, conceptual, and statistical clarity in the study of mediators and moderators: Examples from the child-clinical and pediatric psychology literatures. *Journal of Consulting and Clinical Psychology, 65,* 599–610.

Holmbeck, G. N., Li, S. T., Schurman, T. V., Friedman, D., & Coakley, R. M. (2002). Collecting and managing multisource and multimethod data in studies of pediatric populations. *Journal of Pediatric Psychology, 27,* 5–18.

Holzheimer, L., Mohay, H., & Masters, I. B. (1998). Educating young children about asthma: Comparing the effectiveness of a developmentally appropriate asthma education videotape and picture book. *Child: Care, Health, and Development, 24,* 85–99.

Howells, L., Wilson, A. C., Skinner, T. C., Newton, R., Morris, A. D., & Greene, S. A. (2002). A randomized control trial of the effect of negotiated telephone support on glycaemic control in young people with Type 1 diabetes. *Diabetic Medicine, 19,* 643–648.

Hudson, M. M., Tyc, V. L., Srivastava, D. K., Gattuso, J., Quargnenti, A., Crom, D. B., & Hinds, P. (2002). Multi-component behavioral intervention to promote health protective behaviors in childhood cancer survivors: The Protect Study. *Medical Pediatric Oncology, 39,* 2–11.

Ievers, C. E., & Drotar, D. (1996). Family and parent functioning in cystic fibrosis. *Journal of Behavioral and Developmental Pediatrics, 17,* 48–55.

Ievers-Landis, C. E., Brown, R. T., Drotar, D., Bunke, V., Lambert, R. G., & Walker, A. A. (2001). Situational analysis of parenting problems for caregivers of children with sickle cell symptoms. *Journal of Developmental and Behavioral Pediatrics, 22,* 1–10.

Individuals With Disabilities Education Act, 20 U.S.C., ch. 33, § 1400 (1997).

Ireys, H. T., Chernoff, R. G., DeVet, K. A., & Kim, Y. J. (2001). Maternal outcomes of a randomized controlled trial of a community-based support program for families of children with chronic illnesses. *Archives of Pediatric and Adolescent Medicine, 155,* 771–777.

Ireys, H. T., Chernoff, R. G., Stein, R. E. K., DeVet, K. A., & Silver, E. J. (2001). Outcomes of community-based family-family support: Lessons learned from a decade of randomized trials. *Children's Services: Social Policy, Research and Practice, 4,* 203–216.

Ireys, H. T., Sills, E. M., Kolodner, K. B., & Walsh, B. R. (1996). A social support intervention for parents of children with juvenile rheumatoid arthritis: Results of a randomized trial. *Journal of Pediatric Psychology, 21,* 633–641.

Jacobson, A., & Truax, P. (1991). Clinical significance: A statistical approach to defining meaningful change in psychotherapy research. *Journal of Consulting and Clinical Psychology, 59,* 12–19.

Janz, N. K., & Becker M. H. (1984). The health belief model: A decade later. *Health Education Quarterly, 11,* 1–47.

Jay, S. M., Elliott, C. H., Katz, E., & Siegel, S. E. (1987). Cognitive–behavioral and pharmacological interventions for children's distress during painful medical procedures. *Journal of Consulting and Clinical Psychology, 55,* 860–865.

Jay, S. M., Elliott, C. H., Ozolins, M., Olson, R. A., & Pruitt, S. D. (1985). Behavioral management of children's distress during painful medical procedures. *Behaviour Research and Therapy, 23,* 513–520.

Jelalian, E., Stark, L. J., Reynolds, L., & Seifer, R. (1998). Nutrition intervention for weight gain in cystic fibrosis: A meta-analysis. *Journal of Pediatrics, 132,* 486–492.

Jessop, D. J., Riessman, L. K., & Stein, R. E. K. (1989). Chronic childhood illness and maternal mental health. *Journal of Developmental and Behavioral Pediatrics, 9,* 147–158.

Johnson, S. B. (1995). Insulin dependent diabetes mellitus in childhood. In M. C. Roberts (Ed.), *Handbook of pediatric psychology* (2nd ed., pp. 263–285). New York: Guilford Press.

Kaplan, R. M., Chadwick, M. W., & Schimmel, L. E. (1985). Social learning intervention to promote metabolic control in Type 1 diabetes mellitus: Pilot experiment results. *Diabetes Care, 8,* 152–155.

Kaslow, N. J., Collins, M. H., Rashid, F. L., Baskin, M. L., Griffith, J. R., Hollins, L., & Eckman, J. E. (2000). The efficacy of a pilot family psychoeducational intervention for pediatric sickle cell disease (SCD). *Families, Systems & Health, 18,* 381–404.

Katz, E. R., Rubenstein, C. L., Hubert, N. C., & Blew, A. (1988). School and social reintegration of children with cancer. *Journal of Psychosocial Oncology, 6,* 123–140.

Katz, E. R., Varni, J. W., Rubenstein, C. L., Blew, A., & Hubert, N. (1992). Teacher, parent, and child evaluative ratings of a school reintegration for children with newly diagnosed cancer. *Children's Health Care, 21,* 69–75.

Kazak, A. E. (1989). Families of chronically ill children: A systems and social–ecological model of adaptation and challenge. *Journal of Consulting and Clinical Psychology, 57,* 25–30.

Kazak, A. E. (1998). Editorial: Change and continuity in the *Journal of Pediatric Psychology. Journal of Pediatric Psychology, 23,* 1–3.

Kazak, A. E. (2001). Comprehensive care for children with cancer and their families: A social ecological framework guiding research, practice, and policy. *Children's Services: Social Policy, Research, and Practice, 4,* 217–233.

Kazak, A. E. (2005). Evidence-based interventions for survivors of childhood cancer and their families. *Journal of Pediatric Psychology, 30,* 29–39.

Kazak, A. E., Alderfer, M. E., & Rodriguez, A. (in press). Psychological issues in cancer survival in pediatric populations. In S. Miller, D. Bowen, R. Croyle, & J. Rowland (Eds.), *Handbook of behavioral science and cancer.* New York: Guilford Press.

Kazak, A. E., Alderfer, M. E., Streisand, R., Simms, S., & Rourke, M. T. (in press). Treatment of posttraumatic stress symptoms in adolescent survivors of childhood cancer and their families: A randomized clinical trial. *Journal of Family Psychology.*

Kazak, A. E., Blackall, G., Boyer, B., Brophy, P., Buzaglo, J., Penati, B., & Himelstein, B. (1996). Implementing a pediatric leukemia intervention for procedural pain: The impact on staff. *Families, Systems and Health, 14,* 43–56.

Kazak, A. E., Cant, M. C., Jensen, M. M., McSherry, M., Rourke, M. T., Hwang, W., et al. (2003). Identifying psychosocial risk indicative of subsequent resource use in families of newly diagnosed pediatric oncology patients. *Journal of Clinical Oncology, 21,* 3220–3225.

Kazak, A. E., McClure, K. S., Alderfer, M. A., Hwang, W. T., Crump, T. A., Le, L. T., et al. (2004). Cancer-related parental beliefs: The Family Illness Beliefs Inventory (FIBI). *Journal of Pediatric Psychology, 29,* 531–542.

Kazak, A. E., & Meadows, A. T. (2000). Integrating psychosocial research and practice in a pediatric hospital. In D. Drotar (Ed.), *Handbook of research in pediatric and child clinical psychology* (pp. 511–528). New York: Kluwer Academic/Plenum Publishers.

Kazak, A. E., Meeske, K., Penati, B., Barakat, L. P., Christakis, D., Meadows, A. T., et al. (1997). Posttraumatic stress, family functioning, and social support in survivors of childhood leukemia and their mothers and fathers. *Journal of Consulting and Clinical Psychology, 65,* 120–129.

Kazak, A. E., & Noll, R. B. (2004). Child death from pediatric illness: Conceptualizing intervention from a family systems and public health perspective. *Professional Psychology: Research and Practice, 35,* 219–226.

Kazak, A. E., Penati, B., Boyer, B. A., Himelstein, B., Brophy, P., Waibel, M. K., et al. (1996). A randomized controlled prospective outcome study of psychological and pharmacological intervention protocol for reducing distress in pediatric leukemia. *Journal of Pediatric Psychology, 21,* 615–632.

Kazak, A., Prusak, A., McSherry, M., Simms, S., Beele, D., Rourke, M. T., et al. (2001). Psychosocial Assessment Tool (PAT): Pilot data on a brief screening instrument for identifying high risk families in pediatric oncology. *Families, Systems, and Health, 19,* 303–317.

Kazak, A. E., Simms, S., Alderfer, M. A., Rourke, M. T., Crump, T., McClure, K., et al. (2005). Feasibility and preliminary outcomes from a pilot study of a brief psychological intervention for families of children newly diagnosed with cancer. *Journal of Pediatric Psychology, 30,* 644–655.

Kazak, A. E., Simms, S., Barakat, L., Hobbie, W., Foley, B., Golomb, V., & Best, M. (1999). Surviving Cancer Competently Intervention Program (SCCIP): A cognitive–behavioral and family therapy intervention for adolescent survivors of childhood cancer and their families. *Family Process, 38,* 175–191.

Kazak, A. E., Stuber, M. C., Barakat, L. P., Mecsue, K., Guthrie, D., & Meadows, A. (1998). Predicting posttraumatic stress symptoms in mothers and fathers of survivors of childhood cancer. *Journal of the American Academy of Child and Adolescent Psychiatry, 37,* 823–831.

Kazdin, A. E. (1980). *Research design in clinical psychology.* New York: Harper & Row.

Kazdin, A. E. (Ed.). (1992). *Methodological issues and strategies in clinical research.* Washington, DC: American Psychological Association.

Kazdin, A. E. (1995). Scope of child and adolescent psychotherapy research: Limited sampling of dysfunctions, treatments, and client characteristics. *Journal of Clinical Child Psychology, 24,* 125–146.

Kazdin, A. E. (2000). *Psychotherapy for children and adolescents: Directions for research and practice.* New York: Oxford University Press.

Kazdin, A. E. (Ed.). (2003). *Methodological issues and strategies in clinical research* (3rd ed.). Washington, DC: American Psychological Association.

Kelley, S. D., Van Horn, M., & DeMaso, D. R. (2001). Using process evaluation to describe a hospital-based clinic for children coping with medical stressors. *Journal of Pediatric Psychology, 26,* 407–416.

Kelly, C. S., Morrow, A. L., Skults, J., Nakas, N., Stopis, G. C., & Adelman, R. D. (2000). Outcomes evaluation of comprehensive intervention program for asthmatic children enrolled in Medicaid. *Pediatrics, 105*, 1029–1035.

Kendall, P. C. (1993). Cognitive–behavioral therapies with youth: Guiding theory, current status, and emerging developments. *Journal of Consulting and Clinical Psychology, 61*, 235–247.

Kennard, B. D., Stewart, S. M., Olvera, R., Bawdon, R. E., OhAilin, A., Lewis, C. P., & Winick, N. J. (2004). Nonadherence in adolescent oncology patients: Preliminary data on psychological risk factors and relationships to outcome. *Journal of Clinical Psychology in Medical Settings, 11*, 30–39.

Kibby, M. Y., Tyc, V. L., & Mulhern, R. K. (1998). Effectiveness of psychological intervention for children and adolescents with chronic medical illness: A meta-analysis. *Clinical Psychology Review, 18*, 103–117.

Kirkpatrick, M. B., & Bass, J. B. (1989). Pulmonary complications in adults with sickle cell disease. *Pulmonary Perspectives, 6*, 6–10.

Klinnert, M. D., McQuaid, E. L., McCormick, D., Adinoff, A. D., & Bryant, N. E. (2000). A multimethod assessment of behavioral and emotional adjustment in children with asthma. *Journal of Pediatric Psychology, 25*, 35–46.

Kodish, E., Eder, M., Ruccione, K., Lange, B., Angiolillo, A., Pentz, R., et al. (2004). Communication of randomization in childhood leukemia trials. *Journal of the American Medical Association, 291*, 470–75.

Kodish, E., Lantos, J. D., & Siegler, M. (1990). Ethical considerations in randomized trials. *Cancer, 65*, 2400–2404.

Koocher, G. P. (2002). Using the CABLES model to assess and minimize risk in research: Control group hazards. *Ethics and Behavior, 12*, 75–86.

Koocher, G. P., Curtiss, E. K., Polin, I. S., & Patton, K. E. (2001). Medical crisis counseling in a health maintenance organization: Preventive intervention. *Professional Psychology Research and Practice, 32*, 52–58.

Koocher, G. P., & Keith-Spiegel, P. (1998). *Ethics in psychology: Professional standards and cases*. New York: Oxford University Press.

Koocher, G. P., McGrath, M. L., & Gudas, L. J. (1990). Typologies of nonadherence in cystic fibrosis. *Journal of Developmental and Behavioral Pediatrics, 11*, 353–358.

Koocher, G. P., & O'Malley, J. E. (1981). *The Damocles syndrome: Psychosocial consequences of surviving childhood cancer*. New York: McGraw Hill.

Koontz, K., Short, A. D., Kalinyak, K., & Noll, R. B. (2004). A randomized, controlled pilot trial of a school intervention for children with sickle cell anemia. *Journal of Pediatric Psychology, 29*, 7–17.

Kopta, S. M., Leuger, R. J., Saunders, S. S. M., & Howard, R. I. (1999). Individual psychotherapy outcome and progress research. *Annual Review of Psychology, 50*, 441–69.

Kovacs, M., Goldston, D., Obrosky, D. S., & Bonar, L. K. (1997). Psychiatric disorders in youths with IDDM: Rates and risk factors. *Diabetes Care, 20*, 36–44.

Kovatchev, B., Cox, D., Gonder-Frederick, L., Schlundt, G., & Clarke, W. (1998). Stochastic model of self-regulation decision making exemplified by decisions concerning hypoglycemia. *Health Psychology, 17,* 277–284.

Kraemer, H. C., Wilson, T. B., Fairburn, C. G., & Agras, W. S. (2002). Mediators and moderators of treatment effects in randomized clinical trials. *Archives of General Psychiatry, 59,* 877–883.

Kroll, T., Barlow, J. H., & Shaw, K. (1999). Treatment adherence in juvenile rheumatoid arthritis: A review. *Scandinavian Journal of Rheumatology, 28,* 10–18.

Kuppenheimer, W. G., & Brown, R. T. (2002). Painful procedures in pediatric cancer: A comparison of interventions. *Clinical Psychology Review, 22,* 753–786.

Kupst, M. J., Natta, M. B., Richardson, C. C., Schulman, J. L., Lavigne, J. V., & Das, L. (1995). Family coping with pediatric leukemia: Ten years after treatment. *Journal of Pediatric Psychology, 20,* 601–617.

Laffel, L. M. B., Fangsness, L., Connell, A., Goebel-Fabbri, A., Butler, D., & Anderson, B. J. (2003). Impact of ambulatory, family-focused teamwork intervention on glycemic control in youth with Type 1 diabetes. *Journal of Pediatrics, 142,* 409–16.

La Greca, A. M. (1990). Social consequences of pediatric conditions: Fertile area for future investigation and intervention. *Journal of Pediatric Psychology, 15,* 285–307.

La Greca, A. M., & Bearman, K. J. (2003). Adherence to pediatric treatment regimens. In M. C. Roberts (Ed.), *Handbook of pediatric psychology* (3rd ed., pp. 119–140). New York: Guilford Press.

La Greca, A. M., & Schuman, W. B. (1995). Adherence to prescribed medical regimens. In M. C. Roberts (Ed.), *Handbook of pediatric psychology* (2nd ed., pp. 65–83). New York: Guilford Press.

La Greca, A. M., & Varni, J. W. (1993). Editorial: Interventions in pediatric psychology. A look toward the future. *Journal of Pediatric Psychology, 18,* 687–697.

Lau, R. C. W., Matsui, D., Greenberg, M., & Koren, G. (1998). Electronic measurement of compliance with mercaptopurine in pediatric patients with acute lymphoblastic leukemia. *Medical and Pediatric Oncology, 30,* 85–90.

Lavigne, J. V. L., & Faier-Routman, J. (1992). Psychological adjustment to pediatric physical disorders: A meta-analytic review. *Journal of Pediatric Psychology, 17,* 133–157.

Lavigne, J. V., Ross, C. K., Berry, S. L., Hayford, J. R., & Pachman, L. M. (1992). Evaluation of a psychological treatment package for treating pain in juvenile rheumatoid arthritis. *Arthritis Care and Research, 5,* 101–110.

Lazarus, R. S., & Folkman, S. (1984). *Stress, appraisal, and coping.* New York: Springer Publishing Company.

LeBaron, S., Zeltzer, L. K., Ratner, P., & Kniker, W. T. (1985). A controlled study of education for improving compliance with cromolyn sodium: The importance of physician–patient communication. *Annals of Allergy, 55,* 811–818.

LeBovidge, J. S., Lavigne, J. V., Donenberg, G. R., & Miller, M. L. (2003). Psychological adjustment of children and adolescents with chronic arthritis: A meta-analytic review. *Journal of Pediatric Psychology, 28,* 29–39.

Lehrer, P., Feldman, J., Giardino, N., Song, H., & Schmaling, K. (2002). Psychological aspects of asthma. *Journal of Consulting and Clinical Psychology, 70,* 691–711.

Lemanek, K. L., Buckloh, L. M., Woods, G., & Butler, R. (1995). Diseases in the circulatory system: Sickle cell disease and hemophilia. In M. C. Roberts (Ed.), *Handbook of pediatric psychology* (2nd ed., pp. 286–309). New York: Guilford Press.

Lemanek, K. L., Kamps, J., & Chung, N. B. (2001). Empirically supported treatments in pediatric psychology: Regimen adherence. *Journal of Pediatric Psychology, 26,* 253–275.

Lemanek, K. L., Ranalli, M. A., Green, K., Biega, C., & Lupia, L. (2003). Diseases of the blood: Sickle cell disease and hemophilia. In M. C. Roberts (Ed.), *Handbook of pediatric psychology* (3rd ed., pp. 321–341). New York: Guilford Press.

Levi, R. B., Marsick, M. A., Drotar, D., & Kodish, E. D. (2000). Diagnosis disclosure and informed consent: Learning from parents of children with cancer. *Journal of Pediatric Hematology/Oncology, 22,* 3–12.

Lewis, M. A., Hatton, C. L., Salas, I., Leake, B., & Chiofalo, N. (1991). Impact of the children's epilepsy program on parents. *Epilepsia, 32,* 365–374.

Lidz, C. W., Appelbaum, P. S., Grisso, T., & Renaud, M. (2004). Therapeutic misconception and the appreciation of risks in clinical trials. *Social Science and Medicine, 58,* 1689–1697.

Linscheid, T. R. (2000). Case studies and case series. In D. Drotar (Ed.), *Handbook of research in pediatric and clinical child psychology: Practical strategies and methods* (pp. 429–446). New York: Kluwer Academic.

Littlefield, C. H., Daneman, D., Craven, J. L., Murray, M. A., Rodin, G. M., & Rydall, A. C. (1992). Relationship of self-efficacy and binging to adherence to diabetes regimen among adolescents. *Diabetes Care, 15,* 90–94.

Lobato, D. J., & Kao, B. T. (2002). Integrated sibling–parent group intervention to improve sibling knowledge and adjustment to chronic illness and disability. *Journal of Pediatric Psychology, 27,* 711–716.

Mackner, L. M., McGrath, A. M., & Stark, L. J. (2001). Dietary recommendations to prevent and manage chronic pediatric health conditions: Adherence, intervention, and future direction. *Journal of Developmental and Behavioral Pediatrics, 22,* 130–143.

Maddux, J. E., & DuCharme, K. A. (1997). Behavioral intentions in theories of health behavior. In D. S. Gochman (Ed.), *Handbook of health behavior research: I. Personal and social determinants* (pp. 133–152). New York: Plenum Press.

Maloney, R., Clay, D. L., & Robinson, J. (2005). Sociocultural issues in pediatric transplantation: A conceptual model. *Journal of Pediatric Psychology, 30,* 235–246.

Manne, S. L., DuHamel, K., Gallelli, K., Sorgen, K., & Redd, W. H. (1998). Posttraumatic stress disorder among mothers of pediatric cancer survivors: Diagnosis, comorbidity, and utility of the PTSD checklist as a screening instrument. *Journal of Pediatric Psychology, 23*, 357–366.

Mansour, M. E., Lanphear, B. P., & DeWitt, T. G. (2000). Barriers to asthma care in urban children: Parent perspectives. *Pediatrics, 106*, 512–519.

Manuel, J. C. (2001). Risk and resistance factors in the adaptation in mothers of children with juvenile rheumatoid arthritis. *Journal of Pediatric Psychology, 26*, 237–246.

McCarthy, A. M., Williams, J., & Plumer, C. (1998). Evaluation of a school re-entry nursing intervention for children with cancer. *Journal of Pediatric Oncology Nursing, 15*, 143–152.

McCubbin, H. L., & Patterson, J. M. (1982). Family adaptation to crises. In H. L. McCubbin, A. E. Cauble, & J. M. Patterson (Eds.), *Family coping and social support* (pp. 96–115). Springfield, IL: Charles C Thomas.

McFadden, E. T., LoPresti, F., Bailey, L. R., Clarke, E., & Wilkins, P. C. (1995). Approaches to data management. *Controlled Clinical Trials, 16*, 30S–65S.

McGrath, P. J., & Finley, G. A. (Eds.). (1999). *Progress in pain research and management: Vol. 13. Chronic and recurrent pain in children and adolescents.* Seattle, WA: IASP Press.

McGrath, P. J., Finley, G. A., & Turner, C. J. (1992). *Making cancer less painful: A handbook for parents.* Halifax, Nova Scotia, Canada: Izmak Wilton Killam Children's Hospital Oncology Unit.

McGrath, P. J., Stinson, J., & Davidson, K., (2003). Commentary: The *Journal of Pediatric Psychology* should adopt the CONSORT statement as a way of improving the evidence base in pediatric psychology. *Journal of Pediatric Psychology, 28*, 169–171.

McQuaid, E. L., Kopel, S. J., & Nassau, J. H. (2001). Behavioral adjustment in children with asthma: A meta-analysis. *Journal of Developmental and Behavioral Pediatrics, 22*, 430–439.

McQuaid, E. L., & Nassau, J. H. (1999). Empirically supported treatments of disease-related symptoms in pediatric psychology: Asthma, diabetes, and cancer. *Journal of Pediatric Psychology, 24*, 305–328.

McQuaid, E. L., & Walders, N. (2003). Pediatric asthma. In M. C. Roberts (Ed.), *Handbook of pediatric psychology* (3rd ed., pp. 269–285). New York: Guilford Press.

Mellin, A. E., Neumark-Sztainer, D., & Patterson, J. M. (2004). Parenting adolescent girls with Type 1 diabetes: Parents' perspectives. *Journal of Pediatric Psychology, 29*, 221–230.

Mendez, F., & Belendez, M. (1997). Effects of a behavioral intervention on treatment adherence and stress management in adolescents with IDDM. *Diabetes Care, 20*, 1370–1375.

Milgrom, H., & Bender, B. (1997). Nonadherence to treatment and failure of therapy. *Current Opinion in Pediatrics, 9,* 590–595.

Milgrom, H., Bender, B., Ackerson, L., Bowry, P., Smith, B., & Rand, C. (1996). Noncompliance and treatment failure in children with asthma. *Journal of Allergy & Clinical Immunology, 98,* 1051–1057.

Miller, B. D., & Wood, B. L. (1997). Influence of specific emotional states on autonomic reactivity and pulmonary function in asthmatic children. *Journal of the American Academy of Child and Adolescent Psychiatry, 36,* 669–677.

Miller, V. A., Drotar, D., Burant, C., & Kodish, E. (2005). Clinician–parent communication during informed consent for pediatric leukemia trials. *Journal of Pediatric Psychology, 30,* 219–229.

Miller, V. A., Drotar, D., & Kodish, E. (2004). Children's competence for assent and consent: A review of empirical findings. *Ethics and Behavior, 14,* 255–295.

Miller, W. R., & Rollnick, S. (2002). *Motivational interviewing: Preparing people for change* (2nd ed.). New York: Guilford Press.

Minuchin, S., Baker, L., Rosman, B. L., Liebman, R., Milman, L., & Todd, T. C. (1975). The conceptual model of psychosomatic illness in children: Family organization and family therapy. *Archives of General Psychiatry, 32,* 1031–1038.

Mishel, M. H. (1988). Uncertainty in illness. *Image: Journal of Nursing Scholarship, 20,* 225–232.

Mitchell, M. J., Kawchak, D. A., Stark, L. J., Zemel, B. S., Ohene-Frempong, K., & Stallings, V. A. (2004). Brief report: Parent perspectives of nutritional status and mealtime behaviors in children with sickle cell disease. *Journal of Pediatric Psychology, 29,* 315–320.

Mitchell, M. J., Powers, S. W., Byars, K. C., Dickstein, S., & Stark, L. J. (2004). Family functioning in young children with cystic fibrosis: Observations of interactions at mealtime. *Journal of Developmental and Behavioral Pediatrics, 25,* 335–346.

Moore, B. D. (2005). Neurocognitive outcomes in survivors of childhood cancer. *Journal of Pediatric Psychology, 30,* 51–63.

Moos, R. H., & Moos, B. S. (1981). *Family Environment Scale manual.* Palo Alto, CA: Consulting Psychologists Press.

Mrazek, P. G., & Haggerty, R. J. (Eds.). (1994). *Reducing risks for mental disorders: Frontiers for preventive intervention research.* Washington, DC: National Academy Press.

Mulhern, R. K., Hancock, J., Fairclough, D., & Run, L. (1992). Neuropsychological status of children treated for brain tumors: A critical review and integrative analysis. *Medical and Pediatric Oncology, 20,* 181–192.

Naar-King, S., Siegel, P. J., Smythe, M., & Simpson, P. (2000). A model for evaluating collaborative health care programs for children with special needs. *Children's Services: Social Policy, Research and Practice, 3,* 233–245.

Nachman, J., Sather, H., & Buckley, J. (1993). Young adults 16–21 years of age at diagnosis entered on Children's Cancer Group acute lymphoblastic leukemia and acute myeloblastic leukemia protocols. *Cancer, 71,* 3377–3385.

National Heart, Lung, and Blood Institute. (1996). *Sickle cell anemia* (NIH Publication No. 96-4057). Washington, DC: U.S. Government Printing Office.

National Institute of Diabetes and Digestive and Kidney Diseases. (2003). *Prevention and treatment of Type 2 diabetes in children and adolescents* (No. 5VO1 DKOG1230-03). Bethesda, MD: Author.

National Institute of Mental Health. (1998). *Priorities for prevention research: A National Advisory Mental Health Council work group on mental disorders prevention research.* Bethesda, MD: Author.

National Institutes of Health. (1991). *National Asthma Education Program Expert Panel: Guidelines for the diagnosis and management of asthma* (DHHS Publication No. 91-3042). Washington, DC: US Government Printing Office.

National Institutes of Health. (1997). *National Asthma Education and Prevention Program (National Heart, Lung, and Blood Institute) Second Expert Panel on the Management of Asthma—Expert Panel Report 2: Guidelines for the diagnosis and management of asthma* (DHHS Publication No. 97-4051). Bethesda, MD: Author.

National Institutes of Health. (2001). *Request for applications: 58555. Overcoming barriers to treatment adherence in minorities and persons living in poverty.* Bethesda, MD: Author.

Newacheck, P. W. (1994). Poverty and childhood chronic illness. *Archives of Pediatric Adolescent Medicine, 148,* 1143–1149.

Newacheck, P. W., McManus, M., Fox, H. B., Hung, Y., & Halfon, N. (2000). Access to health care for children with special health care needs. *Pediatrics, 105,* 760–766.

Nezu, A. M., Nezu, C. M., & Perri, M. G. (1989). *Problem-solving therapy for depression: Theory, research, and clinical guidelines.* New York: Wiley.

Noll, R. B., & Fischer, S. (2004). Commentary. Health and behavior CPT codes: An opportunity to revolutionize reimbursement in pediatric psychology. *Journal of Pediatric Psychology, 29,* 571–578.

Noll, R. B., & Kazak, A. E. (2004). Psychosocial care. In A. Atman (Ed.), *Supportive care of children with cancer: Current therapy and guidelines from the Children's Oncology Group* (3rd ed., pp. 337–353). Baltimore: Johns Hopkins University Press.

Noll, R. B., McKellop, J. M., Vannatta, K., & Kalinyak, K. (1998). Child-rearing practices of primary caregivers of children with sickle cell disease: The perspectives of professionals and caregivers. *Journal of Pediatric Psychology, 23,* 131–146.

Noll, R. B., Stith, L., Gertstein, M. A., Ris, M. D., Gruenich, R., Vannatta, K., & Kalinyak, K. (2001). Neuropsychological functioning of youths with sickle cell disease: Comparisons with non-chronically ill peers. *Journal of Pediatric Psychology, 26,* 69–78.

Noll, R. B., Vannatta, K., Koontz, K., Kalinyak, K., Bukowski, W. M., & Davies, W. H. (1996). Peer relationships and emotional well-being of youngsters with sickle cell disease. *Child Development, 67,* 423–436.

Norman, P., & Conner, M. (1996). The role of social cognition models in predicting health behaviors: Future directions. In M. Conner & P. Norman (Eds.), *Predicting health behaviors* (pp. 197–225). Philadelphia: Open University Press.

Norris, S. L., Nichols, P. J., Caspersen, C. J., Glasgow, R. E., Engelgau, M. M., Jack, L., et al. (2002). Increasing diabetes self-management education in community settings: A systematic review. *American Journal of Preventive Medicine, 22,* 30–66.

Oeffinger, K. C., & Hudson, M. M. (2004). Long-term complications following childhood and adolescent cancer: Foundations for providing risk-based health care for survivors. *CA Cancer Journal for Clinicians, 54,* 208–236.

Olness, K. (1981). Imagery (self-hypnosis) as adjunct therapy in childhood cancer: Clinical experience with 25 patients. *American Journal of Pediatric Hematology/ Oncology, 3,* 313–321.

Olsen, R., & Sutton, J. (1998). More hassle, more alone: Adolescents with diabetes and the role of formal and informal support. *Child: Care, Health and Development, 24,* 31–39.

Overholser, J. C., Spirito, A., & DiFilippo, J. M. (1999). Strategies for measurement and psychological assessment. In D. Drotar (Ed.), *Handbook of research in pediatric and clinical child psychology: Practical strategies and methods* (pp. 97–118). New York: Kluwer Academic/Plenum Publishers.

Pablos-Mendez, A., Barr, R. G., & Shea, S. (1998). Run-in periods in randomized trials: Implications for the application of results in clinical practice. *Journal of the American Medical Association, 279,* 222–225.

Padgett, D., Mumford, E., Hynes, M., & Carter, R. (1988). Meta-analysis of the effects of educational and psychosocial interventions on management of diabetes mellitus. *Journal of Clinical Epidemiology, 41,* 1007–1030.

Palermo, T. M. (2000). Impact of recurrent and chronic pain on child and family daily functioning: A critical review of the literature. *Journal of Developmental and Behavioral Pediatrics, 21,* 58–69.

Palermo, T. M., & Drotar, D. (1999). Coping with ambulatory surgery: Effectiveness of parent-implemented behavioral distraction strategies. *Behavior Therapy, 30,* 657–671.

Palermo, T. M., & Scher, M. S. (2001). Treatment of functional impairment in severe somatoform pain disorder: A case example. *Journal of Pediatric Psychology, 26,* 429–434.

Partridge, A., Avorn, J., Wang, P. S., & Winer, E. P. (2002). Adherence to therapy with oral antineoplastic agents. *Journal of the National Cancer Institute, 94,* 652–661.

Patenaude, A. F., & Kupst, M. J. (2005). Psychosocial functioning in pediatric cancer. *Journal of Pediatric Psychology, 30,* 9–27.

Paterson, B., & Thorne, S. (2000). Expert decision making in relation to unantici-pated blood glucose levels. *Research in Nursing and Health, 23,* 147–157.

Patterson, J. M. (1985). Critical factors affecting family compliance with cystic fibrosis. *Family Relations, 34,* 79–89.

Patterson, J. M. (1988). Families experiencing stress: I. The family adjustment and adaptation response model. II. Applying the FAAR model to health-related issues for intervention and research. *Family Systems Medicine, 6,* 202–237.

Patterson, J. M., Budd, J., Goetz, D., & Warwick, W. J. (1993). Family correlates of a 10-year pulmonary health trend in cystic fibrosis. *Pediatrics, 91,* 383–389.

Pegelow, C. H., Armstrong, F. D., Light, S., Toledano, S. R., & Davis, J. (1991). Experience with the use of prophylactic penicillin in children with sickle cell anemia. *Journal of Pediatrics, 118,* 736–738.

Perrin, J. M., MacLean, W. E., Gortmaker, S. L., & Asher, K. A. (1992). Improving the psychological status of children with asthma: A randomized controlled trial. *Journal of Developmental and Behavioral Pediatrics, 13,* 241–247.

Peterson, C. C., & Drotar, D. (in press). Family impact of neurodevelopmental late effects in survivors of pediatric cancer. *Clinical Child Psychology and Psychiatry.*

Peterson, C. C., & Palermo, T. M. (2004). Parental reinforcement of recurrent pain: The moderating impact of child depression and anxiety on functional disability. *Journal of Pediatric Psychology, 29,* 331–341.

Peterson, C. C., Palermo, T. M., Swift, E., Beebe, A., & Drotar, D. (2005). Assess-ment of psycho-educational needs in a clinical sample of children with sickle cell disease. *Children's Health Care, 133,* 227–239.

Peterson, L. S., Mason, T., Nelson, A. M., O'Fallon, W. M., & Gabriel, S. E. (1997). Psychosocial outcomes and health status of adults who have had juvenile rheumatoid arthritis. *Arthritis and Rheumatism, 40,* 2235–2240.

Peterson-Sweeney, K., McMullen, A., Yoos, H. L., & Kitzman, H. (2003). Parental perceptions of their child's asthma: Management and medication use. *Journal of Pediatric Health Care, 17,* 118–125.

Petitti, D. B. (1994). *Meta-analysis, decision analysis, and cost-effectiveness analysis: Methods for quantitative synthesis in medicine.* New York: Oxford University Press.

Peyrot, M. F. (1996). Causal modeling: Theories and applications. *Journal of Pediatric Psychology, 21,* 3–24.

Peyrot, M. F., & McMurry, J. F. (1985). Psychosocial factors in diabetes control: Adjustment of insulin-treated adults. *Psychosomatic Medicine, 47,* 542–557.

Phillips, D. F. (1996). Institutional review boards under stress: Will they explode or change? *Journal of the American Medical Association, 276,* 1623–1626.

Pichert, J., Snyder, G., Kinzer, C., & Boswell, E. (1994). Problem solving anchored instructing for diabetes-related nutritional knowledge skills and behavior. *Diabetes Education, 20,* 45–48.

Pieper, K. B., Rapoff, M. A., Purvical, M. R., & Lindsley, C. B. (1989). Improving compliance with prednisone therapy in pediatric patients with rheumatic disease. *Arthritis Care and Research, 2,* 132–135.

Pinkas-Hamiel, O., Solan, L. M., Daniels, S. R., Staniford, D., Khoury, P. R., & Zeitber, P. (1996). Increased incidence of non-insulin dependent diabetes mellitus in adolescents. *Journal of Pediatrics, 128*, 608–615.

Pless, I. B., Feeley, N., Gottlieb, L., Rowat, K., Dougherty, G., & Willard, B. (1994). A randomized trial of a nursing intervention to promote the adjustment of children with chronic physical disorders. *Pediatrics, 94*, 70–75.

Pless, I. B., & Nolan, T. N. (1991). Revision, replication and neglect: Research on maladjustment in chronic illness. *Journal of Child Psychology and Psychiatry, 32*, 347–365.

Pless, I. B., & Pinkerton, P. (1975). *Chronic childhood disorder: Promoting patterns of adjustment.* Chicago: Yearbook Medical.

Pless, I. B., & Stein, R. E. K. (1994). Intervention research: Lessons learned from research on children with chronic disorders. In R. J. Haggerty, L. R. Sherrod, N. Garmezy, & M. Rutter (Eds.), *Stress, risk, and resilience in children and adolescents: Processes, mechanisms and interventions* (pp. 317–354). New York: Cambridge University Press.

Powers, S. W. (1999). Empirically supported treatments in pediatric psychology: Procedure-related pain. *Journal of Pediatric Psychology, 24*, 131–145.

Powers, S. W., Byars, K. C., Mitchell, M. J., Patton, S. R., Schindler, T., & Zeller, M. H. (2003). A randomized pilot study of behavioral treatment to increase caloric intake in toddlers with cystic fibrosis. *Children's Health Care, 32*, 297–311.

Powers, S. W., Mitchell, M. J., Graumlich, S. E., Byars, K. C., & Kalinyak, K. A. (2002). Longitudinal assessment of pain, coping, and daily functioning in children with sickle cell disease receiving pain management skills training. *Journal of Clinical Psychology in Medical Settings, 9*, 109–119.

Powers, S. W., Vannatta, K., Noll, R. B., Cool, V. A., & Stehbens, J. A. (1995). Leukemia and other childhood cancers. In M. C. Roberts (Ed.), *Handbook of pediatric psychology* (2nd ed., pp. 310–326). New York: Guilford Press.

Pradel, F. G., Hartzema, A. G., & Bush, P. J. (2001). Asthma self-management: The perspective of children. *Patient Education and Counseling, 45*, 199–209.

Prochaska, J. O., & DiClemente, C. C. (1984). *The transtheoretical approach: Crossing traditional boundaries of change.* Homewood, IL: Dorsey.

Quittner, A. L. (2000). Improving assessment in child clinical and pediatric psychology: Establishing links to process and functional outcomes. In D. Drotar (Ed.), *Handbook of research in pediatric and clinical child psychology: Practical strategies and methods* (pp. 119–144). New York: Kluwer Academic.

Quittner, A. L., Drotar, D., Ievers-Landis, C., & De Lambo, K. (2004, August). *Changing adolescent adherence behaviors: The role of family relationships.* Paper presented at the 112th Annual Convention of the American Psychological Association, Honolulu, HI.

Quittner, A. L, Drotar, D., Ievers-Landis, C. E., Seidner, D., Slocum, N., & Jacobson, J. (2000). Adherence to medical treatments in adolescents with cystic fibrosis: Development and evaluation of family based interventions. In D. Drotar (Ed.), *Promoting adherence to medical treatment in childhood chronic illness: Concepts, methods, and interventions* (pp. 383–408). Mahwah, NJ: Erlbaum.

Quittner, A. L., Espelage, D. C., Ievers-Landis, C. E., & Drotar, D. (2000). Measuring adherence to medical treatments in childhood chronic illness: Considering multiple methods and sources of information. *Journal of Clinical Psychology in Medical Settings, 7*, 41–54.

Quittner, A. L., Opipari, L. C., Espelage, D. L., Carter, B., Eid, N., & Eigen, H. (1998). Role strain in couples with and without a child with a chronic illness: Associations with marital satisfaction, intimacy, and daily mood. *Health Psychology, 17*, 112–124.

Quittner, A. L., Opipari, L. C., Regoli, M. J., Jacobsen, J., & Eigen, H. (1992). The impact of caregiving and role strain on family life: Comparisons between mothers of children with cystic fibrosis and matched controls. *Rehabilitation Psychology, 37*, 289–304.

Quittner, A. L., Tolbert, V. E., Regoli, M. J., Orenstein, D. M., Hollingsworth, J. L., & Eigen, H. (1996). Development of the Role-Play Inventory of Situations and Coping Strategies for parents of children with cystic fibrosis. *Journal of Pediatric Psychology, 21*, 209–235.

Ramsey, B., Farrell, P., & Pencharz, P. (1992). Nutritional assessment and management in cystic fibrosis: Consensus conference. *American Journal of Clinical Nutrition, 55*, 108–116.

Rand, C. S., & Sevick, M. A. (2000). Ethics in adherence promotion and monitoring. *Controlled Clinical Trials, 21*, 241S–247S.

Range, L. M., & Cotton, C. R. (1995). Reports of assent and remission in research with children: Illustrations and suggestions. *Ethics and Behavior, 5*, 1–3.

Rapoff, M. A. (1999). *Adherence to pediatric medical regimens.* New York: Kluwer Academic/Plenum Publishers.

Rapoff, M. A. (2000). Facilitating adherence to medical regimens for pediatric rheumatic diseases: Primary, secondary, and tertiary prevention. In D. Drotar (Ed.), *Promoting adherence to medical treatment in chronic childhood illness: Concepts, methods, and intervention* (pp. 329–346). Mahwah, NJ: Erlbaum.

Rapoff, M. A., Belmot, J., Lindsley, C., Olson, N., Morris, J., & Padur, J. (2002). Prevention of nonadherence to nonsteroidal anti-inflammatory medications for newly diagnosed patients with juvenile rheumatoid arthritis. *Health Psychology, 21*, 620–623.

Rapoff, M. A., Lindsley, C. B., & Christophersen, E. R. (1984). Improving compliance with medical regimens: Case study with juvenile rheumatoid arthritis. *Archives of Physical Medicine and Rehabilitation, 65*, 267–269.

Rapoff, M. A., Lindsley, C. B., & Christophersen, E. R. (1985). Parent perceptions of problems experienced by their children in complying with treatments for juvenile rheumatoid arthritis. *Archives of Physical Medicine and Rehabilitation, 66*, 427–430.

Rapoff, M. A., McGrath, A. M., & Lindsley, C. B. (2003). Medical and psychosocial aspects of juvenile rheumatoid arthritis. In M. C. Roberts (Ed.), *Handbook of pediatric psychology* (3rd ed., pp. 392–408). New York: Guilford Press.

Rapoff, M. A., Purviance, M. R., & Lindsley, C. B. (1988a). Educational and behavioral strategies for improving medication compliance in juvenile rheumatoid arthritis. *Archives of Physical Medicine and Rehabilitation, 69,* 439–441.

Rapoff, M. A., Purviance, M. R., & Lindsley, C. B. (1988b). Improving medication compliance for juvenile rheumatoid arthritis and its effect on clinical outcome: A single subject analysis. *Arthritis Care and Research, 1,* 12–16.

Reisman, J. J., Rivington-Law, B., Corey, M., Marcotte, J., Wannamaker, E., Harcourt, D., & Levison, H. (1988). Role of conventional physiotherapy in cystic fibrosis. *Journal of Pediatrics, 113,* 632–636.

Reiter-Purtill, J., & Noll, R. B. (2003). Peer relationships in children with chronic illness. In M. C. Roberts (Ed.), *Handbook of pediatric psychology* (3rd ed., pp. 176–197). New York: Guilford Press.

Relling, M., Hancock, M., Boyett, J., Pui, C., & Evans, W. (1999). Prognostic importance of 6-mercaptopurine dose intensity in acute lymphoblastic leukemia. *Blood, 93,* 2817–2823.

Richardson, R. C., Nelson, M. B., & Meeske, K. (1999). Young adult survivors of childhood cancer: Attending to emerging medical and psychosocial needs. *Journal of Pediatric Oncology Nursing, 16,* 136–144.

Ricker, J. H., Delamater, A. M., & Hsu, J. (1998). Correlates of regimen adherence in cystic fibrosis. *Journal of Clinical Psychology in Medical Settings, 5,* 159–172.

Riekert, K. A., & Drotar, D. (1999). Who participates in research or adherence to treatment in insulin-dependent diabetes mellitus? Implications and recommendations for research. *Journal of Pediatric Psychology, 24,* 253–258.

Riekert, K. A., & Drotar, D. (2000). Adherence to medical treatment in pediatric chronic illness: Critical issues and unanswered questions. In D. Drotar (Ed.), *Promoting adherence to treatment in childhood chronic illness: Concepts, methods, and interventions* (pp. 201–236). Mahwah, NJ: Erlbaum.

Robin, A. L., & Foster, S. L. (1989). *Negotiating parent–adolescent conflict: A behavioral family systems approach.* New York: Guilford Press.

Rodriguez, M. A., Winkleby, M. A., Ahn, D., Sundquist, J., & Kraemer, H. C. (2002). Identification of population subgroups of children and adolescents with high asthma prevalence. *Archives of Pediatric and Adolescent Medicine, 156,* 269–275.

Rogosa, D., Brandt, D., & Zimonowski, M. A. (1982). A growth curve approach to the measurement of change. *Psychological Bulletin, 92,* 726–748.

Rolland, J. S. (1987). Chronic illness and the life cycle: A conceptual framework. *Family Process, 26,* 203–221.

Rose, B. M., Holmbeck, G. N., Coakley, R. M., & Franks, E. A. (2004). Mediator and moderator effects in developmental and behavioral pediatric research. *Developmental and Behavioral Pediatrics, 25,* 58–67.

Ross, J. A., Severson, R. K., Pollock, B. A., & Robinson, C. L. (1996). Childhood cancer in the United States. *Cancer, 77*, 201–207.

Rubin, R. R. (2002). Working with adolescents. In B. J. Anderson & R. R. Rubin (Eds.), *Practical psychology for diabetes clinicians* (pp. 139–147). Alexandria, VA: American Diabetes Association.

Rubin, R. R., & Peyrot, M. (1992). Psychosocial problems and interventions in diabetes: A review of the literature. *Diabetes Care, 15*, 1640–1657.

Rubin, R. R., & Peyrot, M. (2001). Psychological issues and treatments for people with diabetes. *Journal of Clinical Psychology, 57*, 457–478.

Ruggiero, L., & Prochaska, J. O. (1993). Readiness for change: Application of the transtheoretical model to diabetes. *Diabetes Spectrum, 6*, 21–60.

Rutter, M. E. (2000). Resilience reconsidered: Conceptual considerations, empirical findings and policy implications. In J. P. Shonkoff & S. Meisels (Eds.), *Handbook of early childhood intervention* (2nd ed., pp. 651–682). New York: Cambridge University Press.

Ryan, C. M. (1997). Effects of diabetes mellitus on neuropsychological function: A lifespan perspective. *Seminars in Clinical Neuropsychiatry, 2*, 4–14.

Sabbeth, B., & Stein, R. E. K. (1990). Mental health referral: A weak link in comprehensive care of children with chronic physical illness. *Journal of Developmental and Behavioral Pediatrics, 11*, 73–78.

Sahler, O. J., Fairclough, D. L., Phipps, S., Mulhern, R. K., Dolgin, M. J., Noll, R. B., et al. (2005). Using problem-solving skills training to reduce negative affectivity in mothers of children with newly diagnosed cancer: Report of a multisite randomized trial. *Journal of Consulting and Clinical Psychology, 73*, 272–283.

Sahler, O. J., Varni, J. W., Fairclough, D. L., Butler, R. W., Noll, R. B., Dolgin, M. J., et al. (2002). Problem-solving skills training for mothers of children with newly diagnosed cancer: A randomized trial. *Journal of Developmental and Behavioral Pediatrics, 23*, 77–85.

Satin, W., La Greca, A. M., Zigo, M. A., & Skyler, J. S. (1989). Diabetes in adolescence: Effects of multifamily group intervention and parent simulation of diabetes. *Journal of Pediatric Psychology, 14*, 259–276.

Sawyer, M., Antoniou, G., Toogood, I., & Rice, M. (1997). Childhood cancer: A two-year prospective study of the psychological adjustment of children and parents. *Journal of the American Academy of Child and Adolescent Psychiatry, 36*, 1736–1743.

Sawyer, M., Antoniou, G., Toogood, I., Rice, M., & Baghurst, P. (2000). Childhood cancer: A 4-year prospective study of the psychological adjustment of children and parents. *Journal of Pediatric Hematology/Oncology, 22*, 214–220.

Scarr, S. (1994). Ethical problems in research on risky behavior and risky populations. *Ethics and Behavior, 4*, 147–155.

Schafer, J. L., & Graham, J. W. (2002). Missing data: Our review of the state of the art. *Psychological Methods, 7*, 147–177.

Schatz, J., Brown, R. T., Pascaul, J. M., Hsu, L., & DeBaun, M. R. (2001). Poor school and cognitive functioning with silent cerebral infarcts and sickle cell disease. *Neurology, 56,* 1109–1111.

Schatz, J., Finke, R. L., Kellett, J. M., & Kramer, J. H. (2002). Cognitive functioning in children with sickle cell disease: A meta-analysis. *Journal of Pediatric Psychology, 27,* 739–748.

Schmidt, L. E., Klover, R. V., Arfken, C. L., Delamater, A. M., & Hobson, D. (1992). Compliance with dietary prescriptions in children and adolescents with insulin-dependent diabetes mellitus. *Journal of the American Dietetic Association, 92,* 567–570.

Schwartz, C. E., Chesney, M. A., Irvine, M. J., & Keefe, F. J. (1997). The control group dilemma in clinical research: Applications for psychosocial and behavioral medicine. *Psychosomatic Medicine, 59,* 362–371.

Schwartz, C. E., Feinberg, R. G., Jilinskaia, E., & Applegate, J. C. (1999). An evaluation of a psychosocial intervention for survivors of childhood cancer: Paradoxical effects of response shift over time. *Psycho-Oncology, 8,* 344–354.

Schwartz, L. (2004). *The relationship between self-identified goals and well being in young adults with a history of childhood chronic illness.* Unpublished doctoral dissertation, Case Western Reserve University, Cleveland, OH.

Schwartz, L., & Drotar, D. (2004). Effects of written disclosure on caregivers of children and adolescents with chronic illness. *Journal of Pediatric Psychology, 29,* 105–118.

Schwartz, L., & Drotar, D. (2005, April). *The impact of health on goal achievement and subjective well-being in young adults with various pediatric health histories.* Poster presented at the Great Lakes Conference on Child Health, Columbus, OH.

Seligman, M. E. P. (1990). *Learned optimism.* New York: Knopf.

Senturia, Y. D., McNiff-Mortimer, K., Baker, D., Gergen, P., Mitchell, H., Joseph, C., & Wedner, H. J. (1998). Successful techniques for retention of study participants in an inner-city population. *Controlled Clinical Trials,* 544–554.

Sharpe, D., & Rossiter, L. (2002). Siblings of children with a chronic illness: A meta-analysis. *Journal of Pediatric Psychology, 27,* 699–710.

Sheldon, K. M., & Elliot, A. J. (1999). Goal striving, need satisfaction, and longitudinal well being: The self-confidence model. *Journal of Personality and Social Psychology, 26,* 482–497.

Sindelar, H. A., Abrantes, A. M., Hart, C., Lewander, W., & Spirito, A. (2004). Motivational interviewing in pediatric practice. *Current Problems in Pediatric and Adolescent Health Care, 34,* 322–339.

Singer, L. T., Nofer, J., Benson-Szekely, M. S., & Brooks, L. J. (1991). Behavioral assessment and management of food refusal in children with cystic fibrosis. *Journal of Developmental and Behavioral Pediatrics, 12,* 115–120.

Smith, D. H., Malone, D. C., Lawson, K. A., Okamoto, L. J., Battista, C., & Saunders, W. B. (1997). A national estimate of the economic cost of asthma. *American Journal of Respiratory and Critical Care Medicine, 156,* 787–793.

Smith, N. A., Ley, P., Seale, J. P., & Shaw, J. (1987). Health beliefs, satisfaction, and compliance. *Patient Education and Counseling, 10,* 279–286.

Smith, N. A., Seale, J. P., Ley, P., Mellis, C. M., & Shaw, J. (1994). Better medication compliance is associated with improved control of childhood asthma. *Monaldi Archive of Chest Disease, 49,* 470–474.

Smith, N. A., Seale, J. P., Ley, P., Shaw, J., & Bracs, P. U. (1986). Effects of intervention on medication compliance in children with asthma. *Medical Journal of Australia, 144,* 119–122.

Smyth, J. M., Stone, A. A., Hurewitz, A., & Kaell, A. (1999). Effects of writing about stressful experiences on symptom reduction in patients with asthma or rheumatoid arthritis. *Journal of the American Medical Association, 281,* 1304–1309.

Spieth, L., Stark, L. J., Mitchell, M. J., Schiller, M., Cohen, L. L., Mulvihill, M. M., & Hovell, M. (2001). Observational assessment of family functioning at mealtime in preschool children with cystic fibrosis. *Journal of Pediatric Psychology, 26,* 215–224.

Spinetta, J. J., Masera, G., Eden, T., Oppenheim, D., Martins, A. G., van Dongen-Melman, J., et al. (2002). Refusal, non-compliance, and abandonment of treatment in children and adolescents with cancer: A report of the SIOP Working Committee on Psychosocial Issues in Pediatric Oncology. *Medical and Pediatric Oncology, 38,* 114–117.

Spirito, A., & Kazak, A. E. (2006). *Effective and emerging treatments in pediatric psychology.* New York: Oxford University Press.

Starbright Foundation. (2003). *Fitting cystic fibrosis into your life every day* [CD-ROM]. Los Angeles: Author.

Stark, L. J. (2000). Adherence to diet in chronic conditions: The example of cystic fibrosis. In D. Drotar (Ed.), *Promoting adherence to medical treatment in chronic childhood illness: Concepts, methods, and intervention* (pp. 409–428). Mahwah, NJ: Erlbaum.

Stark, L. J., Bowen, A. M., Tyc, V. L., Evans, S., & Passero, M. A. (1990). A behavioral approach to increasing calorie consumption in children with cystic fibrosis. *Journal of Pediatric Psychology, 15,* 309–326.

Stark, L. J., Janicke, D. M., McGrath, A. M., Mackner, L. M., Hommel, K. A., & Lovell, D. (2005). Prevention of osteoporosis: A randomized clinical trial to increase calcium intake in children with juvenile rheumatoid arthritis. *Journal of Pediatric Psychology, 30,* 377–386.

Stark, L. J., Jelalian, E., Janicke, D. M., Opipari, L. C., Powers, S. W., Mulvihill, M. M., & Hovell, M. F. (2005). Child behavior and parent management strategies at mealtimes in families with a school-age child with cystic fibrosis. *Health Psychology, 24,* 274–280.

Stark, L. J., Knapp, L. G., Bowen, A. M., Powers, S. W., Jelalian, E., & Evans, S. (1993). Increasing calorie consumption in children with cystic fibrosis: Replication with 2-year follow-up. *Journal of Applied Behavior Analysis, 26,* 435–450.

Stark, L. J., Mackner, L. M., Kessler, J. H., Opipari, L. C., & Quittner, A. L. (2002). Preliminary findings for calcium intake in children with cystic fibrosis following behavioral intervention for caloric intake. *Children's Health Care*, *31*, 107–118.

Stark, L. J., Mackner, L. M., Patton, S. R., & Acton, J. D. (2003). Cystic fibrosis. In M. C. Roberts (Ed.), *Handbook of pediatric psychology* (3rd ed., pp. 286–303). New York: Guilford Press

Stark, L. J., Miller, S. T., Plienes, A. J., & Drabman, R. S. (1987). Behavioral contracting to increase chest physiotherapy. *Behavior Modification*, *11*, 75–86.

Stark, L. J., Mulvihill, M. M., Powers, S. W., Jelalian, E., Keating, K., Creveling, S., et al. (1996). Behavioral intervention to improve caloric intake of children with cystic fibrosis: Treatment versus wait list control. *Journal of Pediatric Gastroenterology and Nutrition*, *22*, 240–253.

Stark, L. J., Opipari, L. C., Spieth, L. E., Jelalian, E., Quittner, A. L., Higgins, L., et al. (2003). Contribution of behavior therapy to dietary treatment in cystic fibrosis: A randomized controlled study within 2-year follow-up. *Behavior Therapy*, *34*, 237–258.

Stark, L. J., Powers, S. W., Jelalian, E., Rape, R., & Miller, D. L. (1994). Modifying problematic mealtime interactions of children with cystic fibrosis and their parents via behavioral parent training. *Journal of Pediatric Psychology*, *19*, 751–768.

Steele, R. G., Long, A., Reddy, K. A., Luhr, M., & Phipps, S. (2003). Changes in maternal distress and child-rearing strategies across treatment for pediatric cancer. *Journal of Pediatric Psychology*, *28*, 447–452.

Stefl, M. E., Shear, E. S., & Levinson, J. E. (1989). Summer camps for juveniles with rheumatic disease: Do they make a difference? *Arthritis Care and Research*, *2*, 10–15.

Stehbens, J. A. (1985). Childhood cancer. In D. K. Routh (Ed.), *Handbook of pediatric psychology* (pp. 155–161). New York: Guilford Press.

Stein, M. T. (1999). An adolescent who abruptly stops his medication for attention deficit hyperactivity disorder. *Journal of Developmental and Behavioral Pediatrics*, *20*, 106–110.

Stein, R. E. K. (2001). Home-based comprehensive care services for children with chronic conditions. *Children's Services: Social Policy Research and Practice*, *4*, 189–202.

Stein, R. E. K., Bauman, L. J., & Ireys, H. T. (1991). Who enrolls in prevention trials? Discordance in prevention of risk by professionals and participants. *American Journal of Community Psychology*, *19*, 603–627.

Stein, R. E. K., Bauman, L., Westbrook, L. E., Coupey, S. M., & Ireys, H. T. (1993). Framework for identifying children who have chronic conditions: The case for a new definition. *Journal of Pediatrics*, *122*, 342–347.

Stein, R. E. K., & Brooks, P. (Eds.). (1997). *Health care for children: What's right, what's wrong, what's next.* New York: United Hospital Fund.

Stein, R. E. K., & Jessop, D. J. (1982). A noncategorical approach to chronic childhood illness. *Public Health Reports, 97*, 354–362.

Stein, R. E. K., & Jessop, D. J. (1984). Does pediatric home care make a difference for children with chronic illness? Findings from the pediatric ambulatory care treatment study. *Pediatrics, 73*, 845–853.

Stein, R. E. K., & Jessop, D. J. (1991). Long term effects of a pediatric home care program. *Pediatrics, 88*, 490–496.

Stempel, D. A., Strum, L. L., Hedblom, E. C., & Durcanin-Roberts, J. F. (1995). Total cost of asthma care. *Journal of Allergy and Clinical Immunology, 95*, 217–222.

Stewart, J. L., & Mishel, M. H. (2000). Uncertainty in childhood illness: A synthesis of parent and child literature. *Scholarly Inquiry for Nursing Practice: An International Journal, 14*, 299–314.

Stinson, J. N., McGrath, P. J., & Yamada, J. T. (2003). Clinical trials in the *Journal of Pediatric Psychology*: Applying the CONSORT statement. *Journal of Pediatric Psychology, 28*, 159–167.

Stout, C., Kotses, H., & Creer, T. L. (1997). Improving perception of airflow obstruction in asthma patients. *Psychosomatic Medicine, 59*, 201–206.

Street, L. L., & Luoma, J. B. (2002). Control groups in psychosocial intervention research: Ethical and methodological issues. *Ethics & Behavior, 12*, 1–30.

Streisand, R., Rodrigue, J. R., Houck, C., Graham-Pole, J., & Berlant, N. (2000). Brief report: Parents of children undergoing bone marrow transplantation: Documenting stress and piloting a psychological intervention program. *Journal of Pediatric Psychology, 25*, 331–338.

Taitel, M. S., Allen, L., & Creer, T. L. (1998). *The impact of asthma on the patient, family, and society.* New York: Marcel Dekker.

Taylor, L. A., Wallander, J. L., Anderson, D., Beasley, P., & Brown, R. T. (2003). Improving health care utilization, improving chronic disease utilization, health status, and adjustment in adolescents and young adults with cystic fibrosis: A preliminary report. *Journal of Clinical Psychology in Medical Settings, 10*, 9–16.

Taylor, W. R., & Newacheck, P. W. (1992). Impact of childhood asthma on health. *Pediatrics, 90*, 657–662.

Teach, S. J., Lillis, K. A., & Grossi, M. (1998). Compliance with penicillin prophylaxis in patients with sickle cell disease. *Archives of Pediatric Adolescent Medicine, 152*, 274–278.

Tebbi, C. K., Cummings, M., Zevon, M. A., Smith, L., Richards, M., & Mallon, J. (1986). Compliance of pediatric and adolescent cancer patients. *Cancer, 58*, 1179–1184.

Tervo, R. C., Estrem, T. L., Bryson-Brockmann, W., & Symons, F. J. (2003). Single-case experimental designs: Applications in developmental–behavioral pediatrics. *Journal of Developmental and Behavioral Pediatrics, 24*, 438–448.

Thompson, R. J., Jr., Armstrong, F. D., Link, C. L., Pegelow, C. H., Moser, F., & Wang, W. C. (2003). A prospective study of the relationship over time of behavior problems, intellectual functioning, and family functioning in children with sickle cell disease: A report from the Cooperative Study of Sickle Cell Disease. *Journal of Pediatric Psychology, 28*, 59–65.

Thompson, R. J., Jr., Gil, K. M., Burbach, D. J., Keith, B. R., & Kinney, T. R. (1993). Psychological adjustment of mothers of children and adolescents with sickle cell disease: The role of stress, coping methods, and family functioning. *Journal of Pediatric Psychology, 18*, 549–559.

Thompson, R. J., Jr., & Gustafson, K. E. (1996). *Adaptation to chronic childhood illness.* Washington, DC: American Psychological Association.

Thompson, R. J., Jr., Gustafson, K. E., & Gil, K. M. (1995). Psychological adjustment of adolescents with cystic fibrosis or sickle cell disease and their mothers. In J. L. Wallander & L. J. Siegel (Eds.), *Adolescent health problems: Behavioral perspectives* (pp. 232–247). New York: Guilford Press.

Thompson, R. J., Jr., Gustafson, K. E., Gil, K. M., Godfrey, J., & Murphy, L. M. B. (1998). Illness specific patterns of psychological adjustment and cognitive adaptational processes in children with cystic fibrosis and sickle cell disease. *Journal of Clinical Psychology, 54*, 121–128.

Thompson, R. J., Jr., Gustafson, K. E., Gil, K. M., Kinney, T. R., & Spock, A. (1999). Change in the psychological adjustment of children with cystic fibrosis or sickle cell disease and their mothers. *Journal of Clinical Psychology in Medical Settings, 6*, 373–392.

Thompson, R. J., Jr., Gustafson, K. E., Hamlett, K. W., & Spock, A. (1992). Psychological adjustment of children with cystic fibrosis: The role of child cognitive processes and maternal adjustment. *Journal of Pediatric Psychology, 17*, 741–755.

Thompson, S. J., Leigh, L., Christensen, R., Xiong, D., Kun, L. E., Heideman, R. L., et al. (2001). Immediate neurocognitive effects of methylphenidate on learning-impaired survivors of childhood cancer. *Journal of Clinical Oncology, 19*, 1802–1808.

Tyc, V. L., Rai, S. N., Lensing, S., Klosky, J. L., Stewart, D. B., & Gattuso, J. (2003). Intervention to reduce intentions to use tobacco among pediatric cancer survivors. *Journal of Clinical Oncology, 21*, 1366–1372.

Vannatta, K., & Gerhardt, C. A. (2003). Pediatric oncology: Psychosocial outcomes for children. In M. C. Roberts (Ed.), *Handbook of pediatric psychology* (3rd ed., pp. 342–357). New York: Guilford Press

Varni, J. W., Blount, R. L., Waldron, S. A., & Smith, A. J. (1995). Management of pain and distress. In M. C. Roberts (Ed.), *Handbook of pediatric psychology* (2nd ed., pp. 105–123). New York: Guilford Press.

Varni, J. W., Gilbert, A., & Dietrich, S. L. (1981). Behavioral medicine in pain and analgesia management for the hemophilic child with factor VIII inhibitor. *Pain, 11*, 121–126.

Varni, J. W., Jacobs, J. R., & Seid, M. (2000). Treatment adherence as a predictor of health-related quality of life. In D. Drotar (Ed.), *Promoting adherence to* medical treatment in chronic childhood illness: Concepts, methods, and interventions (pp. 287–306). Mahwah, NJ: Erlbaum.

Varni, J. W., Katz, E. R., Colegrove, R., & Dolgin, M. (1993). The impact of social skills training on the adjustment of children with newly diagnosed cancer. *Journal Pediatric Psychology, 18,* 751–767.

Varni, J. W., Rapoff, M. A., Waldron, S. A., Gragg, R. A., Bernstein, B. H., & Lindsley, C. B. (1996). Chronic pain and emotional distress in children and adolescents. *Journal of Developmental and Behavioral Pediatrics, 17,* 154–161.

Varni, J. W., & Wallander, J. L. (1988). Pediatric chronic disabilities: Hemophilia and spina bifida, as examples. In D. K. Routh (Ed.), *Handbook of pediatric psychology* (pp. 190–221). New York: Guilford Press.

Vichinsky, E., Johnson, R., & Lubin, B. (1982). Multidisciplinary approach to pain management in sickle cell disease. *American Journal of Pediatric Hematology/ Oncology, 4,* 328–333.

Vinicor, F. (1998). Diabetes and asthma: Twin challenges for public health and managed care systems. *American Journal of Preventive Medicine, 14,* 87–92.

Wade, S. L. (2004). Commentary: Computer-based interventions in pediatric psychology. *Journal of Pediatric Psychology, 29,* 269–272.

Wade, S. L., Holden, G., Lynn, H., Mitchell, H., & Ewart, C. (2000). Cognitive–behavioral predictors of asthma morbidity in inner-city children. *Developmental and Behavioral Pediatrics, 21,* 340–346.

Walco, G. A., & Ilowite, N. T. (1992). Cognitive–behavioral intervention for juvenile primary fibromyalgia syndrome. *Journal of Rheumatology 19,* 1617–1619.

Walco, G. A., Sterling, C. N., Conte, F. M., & Engel, R. G. (1999). Empirically supported treatments in pediatric psychology: Disease-related pain. *Journal of Pediatric Psychology, 24,* 155–167.

Walco, G. A., Varni, J. W., & Ilowite, N. T. (1992). Cognitive–behavioral pain management in children with juvenile rheumatoid arthritis. *Pediatrics, 89,* 1075–1079.

Walders, N., & Drotar, D. (1999). Integrating mental health services in the care of children and adolescents with chronic health conditions: Assumptions, challenges, and opportunities. *Children's Services: Social Policy, Research, and Practice, 2,* 117–138.

Walders, N., & Drotar, D. (2000). Understanding cultural and ethnic influences in research with child clinical and pediatric psychology populations. In D. Drotar (Ed.), *Handbook of research methods in clinical child and pediatric psychology* (pp. 165–188). New York: Kluwer Academic/Plenum Publishers.

Walders, N., Drotar, D., & Kerscmar, C. (2000a). The allocation of family responsibility for asthma management tasks in African-American adolescents. *Journal of Asthma, 37,* 89–99.

Walders, N., Drotar, D., & Kercsmar, C. (2000b, April). *Family reports of barriers to adherence to asthma management in a pediatric intervention study: Assessment and goal setting.* Paper presented at the Southwest regional meeting of the Society of Pediatric Psychology, Oklahoma City, OK.

Walders, N., Kercsmar, C., Schluchter, M., Redline, S., Kirchner, H. L., Casey, T., et al. (in press). An interdisciplinary intervention for untreated pediatric asthma. *Chest.*

Wallander, J. L., Thompson, R. J., Jr., & Alriksson-Schmidt, A. (2003). Psychosocial adjustment of children with chronic physical conditions. In M. C. Roberts (Ed.), *Handbook of pediatric psychology* (3rd ed., pp. 141–158). New York: Guilford Press.

Wallander, J. L., Varni, J. W., Babani, L., Banis, H. T., DeHaan, C. B., & Wilcox, K. T. (1989). Disability parameters: Chronic strain and adaptation of physically handicapped children and their mothers. *Journal of Pediatric Psychology, 14,* 23–42.

Wallander, J. L., Varni, J. W., Babani, L., Banis, H. T., & Wilcox, K. T. (1988). Children with chronic physical disorders: Maternal reports of their psychological adjustment. *Journal of Pediatric Psychology, 13,* 197–212.

Warman, K. L., Silver, E. J., McCourt, M. P., & Stein, R. E. (1999). How does home management of asthma exacerbations by parents of inner-city children differ from NHLBI guideline recommendations? *Pediatrics, 103,* 422–427.

Weersina, V. R., & Weisz, J. R. (2002). Mechanisms of action in youth psychotherapy. *Journal of Child Psychology and Psychiatry, 43,* 3–29.

Weil, C. M., Wade, S. L., Bauman, L. J., Lynn, H., Mitchell, H., & Lavigne, J. (1999). The relationship between psychosocial factors and asthma morbidity in inner-city children with asthma. *Pediatrics, 104,* 1274–1280.

Weinberger, M., Oddone, E. Z., Henderson, W. G., Smith, D. M., Huey, J., Giobbie-Hinder, A., & Feussner, J. R. (2001). Multisite randomized controlled trials in health services research: Scientific challenges and operational issues. *Medical Care, 39,* 627–634.

Weinstein, A. G., & Cuskey, W. (1985). Theophylline compliance in asthmatic children. *Annals of Allergy, 54,* 19–24.

Weiss, C. (1998). *Collecting data: Evaluation methods for studying programs and policies* (2nd ed., pp. 152–179). Upper Saddle River, NJ: Prentice Hall.

Weiss, K. B., & Wagener, D. K. (1990). Changing patterns of asthma mortality: Identifying target populations at high risk. *Journal of the American Medical Association, 264,* 1683–1687.

Weisz, J. R. (2000). Lab–clinic differences and what we can do about them: The clinic based treatment development model. *Clinical Child Psychology Newsletter, 15,* 1–3.

Weisz, J. R., & Weiss, B. (1993). *Effects of psychotherapy with children and adolescents.* Newbury Park, CA: Sage.

Westbrook, L. E., Bauman, L. J., & Shinnar, S. (1992). Applying stigma theory to epilepsy: A test of a conceptual model. *Journal of Pediatric Psychology, 17,* 633–649.

Whitt, J. K. (1984). Children's adaptation to chronic illness related and handicapping conditions. In M. G. Eisenberg, L. C. Sutkin, & M. A. Jensen (Eds.), *Chronic illness and disability through the life span: Effects on self and family* (pp. 69–102). New York: Springer Publishing Company.

Wigal, J. K., Creer, T. L., Kotses, H., & Lewis, P. (1990). A critique of 19 self-management programs for childhood asthma: Part I. Development and evaluation of the programs. *Pediatric Asthma, Allergy & Immunology, 4,* 17–30.

Wild, M. R., & Espie, C. A. (2004). The efficacy of hypnosis in the reduction of procedural pain and distress in pediatric oncology: A systematic review. *Journal of Developmental and Behavioral Pediatrics, 25,* 207–213.

Williams, P. G., Holmbeck, G. N., & Greenley, R. N. (2002). Adolescent health psychology. *Journal of Consulting and Clinical Psychology, 70,* 828–842.

Wilson, J. J., & Gil, K. M. (1996). The efficacy of psychological and pharmacological interventions for the treatment of chronic disease-related and non-disease-related pain. *Clinical Psychology Review, 16,* 573–597.

Wolznick, L. A., & Goodheart, C. D. (2002). *Living with childhood cancer.* Washington, DC: American Psychological Association.

Wood, B. L. (1993). Beyond the "psychosomatic family": A biobehavioral family model of pediatric illness. *Family Process, 32,* 261–278.

Wood, P. R., Sadof, M. D., Kercsmar, C. M., & Kattan, M. (2004, May). *Research to implementation: The NCICAS asthma counselor model.* Paper presented at the annual meeting of the American Pediatric Society, San Francisco.

Woznick, L. A., & Goodheart, C. D. (2002). *Living with childhood cancer: A practical guide to help families cope.* Washington, DC: American Psychological Association.

Wysocki, T. (in press). Behavioral assessment and intervention in pediatric diabetes. *Behavioral Modification.*

Wysocki, T., Greco, P., & Buckloh, L. M. (2003). Childhood diabetes in psychological context. In M. C. Roberts (Ed.), *Handbook of pediatric psychology* (3rd ed., pp. 304–320). New York: Guilford Press.

Wysocki, T., Greco, P., Harris, M. A., Bubb, J., & White, N. H. (2001). Behavior therapy for families of adolescents with diabetes: Maintenance of treatment effects. *Diabetes Care, 24,* 441–446.

Wysocki, T., Greco, P., Harris, M. A., & White, N. H. (2000). Behavioral family systems therapy for adolescents with diabetes. In D. Drotar (Ed.), *Promoting adherence to medical treatment in chronic childhood illness: Concepts, methods, and intervention* (pp. 367–382). Mahwah, NJ: Erlbaum.

Wysocki, T., Harris, M., Greco, P., Bubb, J., Danda, C., Harvey, L., et al. (2000). Randomized, controlled trial of behavior therapy for families of adolescents with insulin-dependent diabetes mellitus. *Journal of Pediatric Psychology, 25,* 23–34.

Wysocki, T., Hough, B. S., Ward, K. M., Allen, A. A., & Murgai, N. (1992). Use of blood glucose data by families of children and adolescents with DM1. *Diabetes Care, 15,* 1041–1044.

Wysocki, T., Hough, B. S., Ward, K. M., & Green, L. B. (1992). Diabetes mellitus in the transition to adulthood: Adjustment, self-care and health status. *Journal of Developmental and Behavioral Pediatrics, 13*, 194–201.

Yoos, H. L., Kitzman, H., & McMullen, A. (2003). Barriers to anti-inflammatory medication use in childhood asthma. *Ambulatory Pediatrics, 3*, 181–190.

Young-Hyman, D. (2002). Identifying and treating youth at risk for Type 2 diabetes. In B. J. Anderson & R. R. Rubin (Eds.), *Practical psychology for diabetes clinicians* (pp. 171–180). Alexandria, VA: American Diabetes Association.

Zak, M., & Pederson, F. K. (2000). Juvenile chronic arthritis into adulthood: A long-term follow-up study. *Rheumatology, 39*, 198–204.

Zebracki, K., Drotar, D., Kirchner, H. L., Schluchter, M., Redline, S., Kercsmar, C., & Walders, N. (2003). Predicting attrition in a pediatric asthma intervention study. *Journal of Pediatric Psychology, 28*, 519–528.

Zimmerman, B. J., Bonner, S., Evans, D., & Mellins, R. B. (1999). Self-regulating childhood asthma: A developmental model of family change. *Health Education and Behavior, 26*, 55–71.

AUTHOR INDEX

Blew, A., 23, 159
Blount, R. L., 14, 24, 25
Boardway, R. H., 145
Boer, H., 43
Boland, E. A., 139, 145, 147, 151
Boles, S. M., 150
Bollen, K. A., 82
Bonar, L. K., 142
Bonin, D., 128
Bonner, M. J., 179, 180, 182, 190, 191
Bonners, S., 127, 131
Borduin, C. M., 236
Boswell, E., 151
Bowen, A. M., 217
Boyett, J., 162
Boyle, M., 13, 18
Brackett, J., 30, 41, 145
Bracs, P. U., 129
Bradshaw, B., 139
Branch, W. B., 182
Brandt, D., 82
Bratton, D. L., 137
Briery, B. C., 158, 168, 174, 177, 190
Bronfenbrenner, U., 48
Brooks, L. J., 216
Brooks, P., 246
Brooks-Gunn, J., 120
Broome, M. E., 184, 186
Brown, J. V., 131
Brown, M. B., 44
Brown, R. T., 4, 14, 17, 19, 41, 158, 159, 162, 163, 171, 173, 180, 182, 190, 217, 228, 248
Brownlee-Duffeck, M., 43, 44
Bryant, N. E., 125
Bryson-Brochmann, W., 68
Buckley, J., 161
Buckloh, L. M., 14, 139
Budd, J., 208
Bull, S. S., 231, 239
Burant, C., 111
Burbach, D. J., 37, 182
Burghen, G. A., 48, 143
Burkhart, M. T., 24
Bush, M., 15, 28
Bush, P. J., 128
Bussell, D. A., 116
Butler, R. W., 14, 158
Button, B. M., 208
Byars, K. C., 188, 207

Cadman, D., 13, 18, 19
Campbell, D. T., 73
Caplan, G., 65
Carden, F., 208
Carey, M. E., 158
Carson, J. W., 42, 184
Carter, R., 144
Caskey, J. D., 120
Cassidy, J. T., 192
Celano, M., 125, 127, 184
Centers for Disease Control and Prevention (CDC), 123
Chadwick, M. W., 24
Chalmers, T. C., 60, 128
Chambless, D. L., 70, 184
Charache, S., 181
Charette, C., 128
Charron-Prochownik, C., 44
Chasalow, F., 162
Chen, E., 184, 189, 190
Chen, H. T., 54
Chen, Y. Q., 130
Chernoff, R. G., 187, 188, 189, 211, 216, 231
Chesney, M. A., 74
Child Abuse Prevention and Treatment and Adoption Reform Act, 116
Chiofalo, N., 18
Chrisler, J. C., 142
Christian, B. J., 206
Christophersen, E. R., 194
Chung, N. B., 4, 15
Clark, N. M., 44, 129
Clarke, E., 101
Clarke, W., 42
Clay, D. L., 17, 19, 159
Clement, S., 151, 152, 153
Clingempeel, W. G., 80
Coakley, R. M., 54, 78–79, 229
Cohen, J., 4, 75, 82
Cohen, L. L., 14
Cohen, M. J., 182
Cohen, S. Y., 49
Cole, S. W., 184
Colegrove, R., 17
Collins, M., 183, 184, 189
Colton, P. A., 142
Conner, M., 43
Conrad, P. C., 43, 45
Conte, F. M., 4, 15, 194
Cook, T. D., 73

Gutai, J. P., 145
Gyato, K., 158

Haby, M. M., 129, 134
Hagglund, K. J., 195, 197
Hagopian, L. P., 212, 216
Hahlweg, K., 40
Hains, A. A., 213, 216, 217
Halfon, N., 10
Hallstand, T. S., 124
Halterman, J. S., 127
Hamlett, K. W., 37
Hampson, S. E., 145, 146, 150, 151
Hancock, J., 158
Hancock, M., 162
Hanson, C. L., 48, 143
Hardy, K. K., 182, 206
Harris, B. S., 148
Harris, M. A., 23, 42, 66, 145, 148, 231, 235
Hart, C., 47
Hartzema, A. G., 128
Hatton, C. L., 18
Hausenstein, E. J., 18
Hauser, S., 54
Hayford, J. R., 25, 194
Haynes, P., 206
Hazzard, A., 184, 185, 188
Health Insurance Portability and Accountability Act (HIPAA), 91, 109
Hedblom, E. C., 124
Henderson, Z. G., 206
Henggeler, S. W., 48, 80, 143, 236, 242
Henry, K. L., 120
Hermanns, J., 40
Hernandez-Reif, M., 208, 212, 216
Heuvel, F., 170
Hicks, D. A., 208
Hill, R., 37, 48
Hill-Briggs, F., 42
Hiss, R. G., 155
Ho, J., 30, 41, 145
Hoaglund, K. J., 81–82
Hoagwood, K., 115, 117, 118, 120
Hobbs, H., 21
Hobfoll, S. E., 29
Hobson, D., 143
Hoekstra-Weebers, W. E. H. M., 165, 170

Hoff, A. L., 46
Holden, G., 133
Hollon, S. D., 70, 184
Holmbeck, G. N., 30, 35, 54, 78, 80, 81, 83, 229
Holzheimer, L., 129
Houck, C., 170
Hough, B. S., 30, 31
Howard, R. I., 67
Howells, L., 147
Howite, N. T., 194
Hsu, J., 208
Hsu, L., 182
Hubert, N. C., 23, 159
Hudson, M. M., 166, 169, 175, 177
Hung, Y., 10
Hurewitz, A., 136
Hynes, M., 144

Ievers, C. E., 207
Ievers-Landis, C. E., 79, 136, 183, 218, 236
Individuals with Disabilities Education Act, 168
Ireys, H. T., 9, 18, 22, 76, 187, 188, 189, 197, 199, 211, 216, 231
Irvine, M. A., 74

Jacobs, J. R., 49
Jacobsen, J., 207
Jacobson, A., 241
Janicke, 199, 242
Janz, N. K., 43
Jarrett, L., 155
Jaspers, J. P. L., 170
Jay, S. M., 25, 163
Jelalian, E., 207, 209, 218
Jensen, P. S., 120
Jessop, D. J., 18, 22, 231
Jilinskaia, E., 169
Johnson, C. E., 25
Johnson, M., 183
Johnson, R., 191
Johnson, S. B., 16, 29, 117, 141, 142

Kaell, A., 136
Kalinyak, K. A., 183, 188
Kamps, J., 4, 15

Norman, P., 43
Norris, S. L., 149
Nowak, M., 60

Obrosky, D. S., 142
Oeffinger, K. C., 175, 177
Oesterle, A., 139
O'Fallon, W. M., 192
Offord, D. R., 13, 18
Ohene-Frempong, K., 183
Olfaway, N. J., 127
Olmsted, M. P., 142
Olness, K., 241
Olsen, R., 155
Olson, R. A., 25
O'Malley, J. E., 29, 159
Opipari, L. C., 207, 217, 219
Orr, D. P., 140
Overholser, J. C., 79, 105
Ozolins, M., 25

Pablos-Mendez, A., 100
Pachman, L. M., 25
Padgett, D., 144
Palermo, S. W., 14, 17
Palermo, T. M., 15, 68, 71, 174, 180,
    182, 191, 193, 244
Parks, P. C., 23
Partridge, A., 162
Pascual, J. M., 182
Passero, M. A., 217
Patenaude, A. F., 172, 175
Paterson, B., 42
Patterson, J. M., 36, 37, 38, 51, 54, 141,
    208
Patton, K. E., 236
Patton, S. R., 31, 203, 219
Pederson, F. K., 199
Pegelow, C. H., 183
Penati, B., 163
Pencharz, P., 205
Perri, M. G., 42
Perrin, E. C., 4, 20, 79
Perrin, J. M., 21, 130, 135
Peterson, C. C., 158, 172, 174, 175, 191,
    193
Peterson, L. S., 192
Peterson-Sweeney, K., 127
Petitti, D. B., 237

Petty, R. E., 192
Peyrot, M., 71, 141, 142, 143, 144, 145,
    149, 151, 153
Phillips, D. F., 109
Phillips, K. M., 127
Phillips, P. C., 158
Phipps, S., 160
Pichert, J., 151
Pieper, K. B., 194, 197
Piette, J. D., 155, 239
Piira, T., 14
Pinkas-Hamiel, O., 140
Pinkerton, P., 21, 36
Pless, I. B., 4, 13, 20, 21, 22, 36, 63, 66
Plienes, A. J., 216
Plumer, C., 168
Polin, I. S., 236
Pollock, B. A., 157
Porter, L., 42, 180, 181
Powers, S. W., 4, 5, 14, 24, 41, 42, 162,
    173, 180, 187, 188, 205, 207,
    208, 215, 217
Pradel, F. G., 128
Prochaska, J. O., 47, 53
Pruitt, S. D., 25
Pui, C., 162
Purviance, M. R., 194

Quittner, A. L., 29, 42, 79, 101, 118,
    136, 206, 207, 208, 209, 217,
    218, 236

Ramsey, B., 205
Ranalli, M. A., 180
Rand, C. S., 120
Randall, J., 242
Range, L. M., 120
Rapoff, M. A., 14, 16, 25, 28, 44, 47, 65,
    66, 72, 129, 192, 194, 195, 197,
    198, 199, 200, 201, 235, 249
Ratner, P., 129
Reaman, G. H., 102
Redd, W. H., 158, 161
Reddy, K. A., 160
Reeves, G., 24
Regoli, M. J., 207
Reisman, J. J., 208
Reiss, D., 171
Reissman, L. K., 18

Wang, P. S., 162
Ward, K. M., 30, 31
Ware, R., 182
Warman, K. L., 131
Warwick, W. J., 208
Waters, E., 129
Weil, C. M., 126
Weinberger, M., 74, 102
Weinstein, A. G., 129
Weiss, B., 75
Weiss, C., 238
Weiss, K. B., 123, 127
Weisz, J. R., 75, 234, 242
Weitzman, M., 13
West, S. G., 230
Westbrook, L. E., 9, 16
White, N. H., 23, 66
Wigal, J. K., 128
Wilcox, K. T., 37
Wild, M. R., 14
Wilder, J., 52
Wilkins, P. C., 101
Willard, V., 111
Williams, D. A., 181
Williams, J., 168
Williams, P. G., 30
Wilson, J. J., 15
Wilson, T. B., 80

Winer, E. P., 162
Winkleby, M. A., 123
Wolf, F. M., 24
Wolznick, L. A., 29
Wood, B. L., 39, 40
Wood, P. R., 132
Woods, G., 14
Woznick, L. A., 173
Wysocki, T., 23, 30, 31, 42, 66, 139, 141, 143, 145, 148, 154, 231, 235

Yamada, J. T., 228
Yang, M. C. K., 118
Yoos, H. L., 127
Young-Hyman, D., 140
Yu, C., 151

Zagorski, L., 247
Zak, M., 199
Zebracki, K., 76, 77, 95, 232
Zeltzer, L. K., 129
Zigo, M. A., 31
Zimen, R., 127
Zimmerman, B. J., 127
Zimonowski, M. A., 82

SUBJECT INDEX

Behavioral family systems therapy
        (BFST), 23
    for CF, 218, 236
    for diabetes, 148, 235
    home-based version of, 235
Behavioral interventions
    for CF, 209, 218
    for SCD, 184
Behavioral management approaches
    for CF, 217
    for diabetes, 147–148
Behavioral–psychopharmacological ap-
        proaches, in CD intervention,
        187, 188
Behavioral rehearsal, 25
Behavior modification, family-centered,
        for JRA, 200
Between-groups designs, 72–73
BFST. See Behavioral family systems
        therapy
Biobehavioral model, family-centered 39–
        40, 41
Biofeedback, frontallis electromyography,
        for asthma, 129
Biofeedback-assisted breathing and re-
        training control, 216
Bowel disease, in case example (Adam),
        17
Brain tumor, in case example (Joey), 17
Bundling of psychological services, 246
Bureau of Maternal and Child Health,
        247

Canada, home-care intervention in, 152
Cancer, 157
    case example of (Cassandra), 160
    cognitive–behavioral treatment for,
        25
    cognitive functioning affected by,
        158
    death of child from, 173
    imagery and hypnosis for, 241
    impact of on parents and family
        members, 160–161
    late effects of, 31, 158, 160, 174
    medical treatment for, 157–159
        adherence to, 161–162, 171
    and problem-solving theory, 42
    psychological impact of on children
        and adolescents, 159–160

psychological interventions for, 159,
        162–171
    in clinical settings, 172–177
    psychosocial interventions for, 166,
        173, 175–176, 177, 249
    recurrence of, 160
    research on interventions for, 171–
        172, 176
Care paths, for management of SCD
        pain, 191
Case studies and case series, 227–228
CDC, 132
CD-ROM-based educational approaches,
        for CF, 219
    *Fitting Cystic Fibrosis Into Your Life
        Every Day* (CD-ROM), 216
Cerebrovascular accidents, from SCD, 180
CF. See Cystic fibrosis
Change, five stages of, 47
Changes, in intervention protocols, 102
Change over time, analysis of, 81–82
Checklists, on families' behaviors during
        intervention, 100
Child (patient)
    and informed consent, 112–113
    as intervention target, 21
    responsibility for asthma manage-
        ment shifted to, 138
Child Abuse Prevention and Treatment
        and Adoption Reform Act, 116
Child Behavior Checklist, 79
Child (patient) centered models of psycho-
        logical intervention, 21, 24–26
Childhood chronic illness
    multifaceted psychological impact of,
        10–12
        child's psychological adjustment
            problems, 12–14
        distress associated with pain,
            14–15
        on family members, 18
        nonadherence to treatment,
            15–16
        in peer relationships, 16–17
        in school, 17
    prevalence of, 9–10
    varying success in coping with, 3
Child neglect or abuse, as ethical issue,
        116
Choice of research design, 62, 72–74
Chronic health condition, definition of, 9

Clinical care
    of asthma, 132–134, 138
    of cancer, 172–177
    for CF, 219
    of diabetes, 152–155
    of JRA, 200–201
    of SCD, 190–191
Clinical effectiveness, of diabetes interventions, 149–151
Clinical experiences with target sample, 61, 69
Clinical need and significance of target problem, 61, 68–69
Clinical settings and applications
    asthma interventions in, 135, 136
    diabetes interventions in, 145
    implementing of, 224
    as research stage, 226
    strategies to enhance, 224, 227, 234–240
    See also Practice settings
Clinical significance
    and intervention research, 227, 231–234
    of research and published reports, 240–245
    synthesizing of, 243
Cognitive approaches, for cancer patients, 173
Cognitive–behavioral approaches, 41–42, 55
    for asthma, 135, 136
    for cancer, 162–163, 166, 169, 171–172
    parents, 165, 166, 167, 169–170
    for CF, 213, 216–217, 218, 219
    for JRA, 195, 196, 197–198
    in pain management, 25
    for reasoned nonadherence, 69
    in SCD intervention, 184, 186, 189
Cognitive coping strategies, for SCD, 184
Cognitive deficits, interventions to remediate for cancer patients, 174–175
Cognitive restructuring
    for CF, 218
    for JRA, 200
Coinvestigators, 90
Collaboration
    in availability and success of intervention programs, 247

in providing optimal services, 246
    among researchers, 245
Collaborative context, for intervention research, 86, 87–92
Combined behavioral–psychopharmacological approaches, in SCD intervention, 187, 188
Combined educational and behavioral approaches, for CF, 217
Communication skills program, in cancer intervention, 164
Comorbidity, 12, 69, 232
Compensatory psychological and educational interventions, for cancer patients, 174
Comprehensive behavioral interventions, for CF, 218
Comprehensive care, 48–49, 55
    for asthma, 138
    evaluating and monitoring of, 238
    for survivors of pediatric cancer, 175
Comprehensive education and support program, for diabetes (costs vs. benefits), 151, 152
Comprehensive medical and psychological care, for SCD children and families, 190–191
Comprehensive and preventive psychological care, for cancer patients, 173
Computer-based interventions
    in cognitive rehabilitation, 174
    ethical issues in, 118
Computerized self-management approaches, for asthma treatment, 130–131
Confidentiality, and informed consent, 108, 116–117
Conflict resolution, in cancer intervention, 164
Consent, 112. *See also* Informed consent
Consolidated standards of reporting trials (CONSORT), 228
Contact information, for intervention studies, 97
Control group, 62, 72, 74–75
    clinical contact of, 99
Coping ability factors, 36
Coping behavior, 38
Coping skills training (CST), for diabetes, 145, 147

Coping strategies, for SCD, 181
Coping style, and parents of CF patients, 207
Cost-effectiveness, 236–237
Cost-offset, 237
Costs vs. benefits
    of comprehensive diabetes education and support program, 151–152
    of psychological interventions, 236–237
Course of chronic illnesses, individual differences in, 28–30
Critical reviews, of intervention research, 242–243
Crossover designs, 72
Cultural groups, generalizability of measures across, 81
Cystic fibrosis (CF), 30, 203
    age of diagnosis of, 28
    BFST for, 218, 236
    case example of (Alice), 12–13, 18
    case example of (Katelyn), 206
    CF-related diabetes, 204
    clinical care for, 219
    development of psychological intervention science for, 223
    future directions for intervention research on, 217–219
    medical treatment for, 203, 204–205
        adherence to, 207–208
    and problem-solving theory, 42
    psychological impact of on children, adolescents and young adults, 205–207
    psychological impact of on families, 207
    psychological interventions for, 208–217
    stressors faced by young adults with, 31
    in test of FAAR model, 38

Data-analytic plan, 63, 81–82
Database, for monitoring process and outcomes of services, 238
Data collection, settings for, 92–93
Data management, in psychological intervention studies, 101
Data safety and monitoring boards (DSMBs), 115

Death, of child from cancer, 173
Defining and measuring usual or standard care, 62, 78
Depression
    in case examples on diabetes, 16, 34
    as diabetes risk, 142
Design of intervention research, ethical issues in, 106–108
Design of psychological interventions, 59
    available resources for, 59–60
    decisions and considerations in selection of model
        clinical experiences with target sample, 61, 69
        clinical need and significance, 61, 68–69
        control group choice, 62, 74–75
        data-analytic plan development, 63, 81–82
        defining and measuring usual or standard care, 62, 78
        enhancing adherence to intervention protocol, 62, 78
        evaluating of available research, 61, 70–71
        impact of selective participation, 62, 76–77
        intensity and duration, 61, 66–67
        intervention fidelity, 62, 77–78
        and no-effect result, 63, 82–83
        operational definition of target problem and outcome, 61, 67–68
        outcome measures, 62, 78–81
        population and sample, 60, 61, 63
        and RCTs, 62, 73–74
        research design, 62, 72–74
        role of pilot and feasibility data, 61, 71
        role of theory, 62, 71–72
        sample methods, 62, 75–76
        sample size estimation, 62, 75
        scope of intervention, 61, 63–64
        standardizing of eligibility criteria, 62, 76
        target participants and behaviors, 61, 66
        timing and purpose, 61, 64–66
    and implementation, 83 (see also Implementing of psychological intervention research)

Developmental stage of child patient, individual differences in, 30–31

Developmental transitions, and psychological intervention, 30–31

Diabetes. *See* Type 1 diabetes; Type 2 diabetes

Diabetes, in adults
  CF-related, 204
  and problem-solving models, 42
  See also Type 1 diabetes; Type 2 diabetes

Diabetes Control and Complications Trial (DCCT), 113, 140

Diagnostic procedures, as painful, 14

Diagnostic and Statistical Manual of Mental Disorders, Fourth Edition (DSM–IV), 28, 176, 232, 233

Disability, stress, and coping model, 36–37

Distress associated with pain, 14–15

DM1. *See* Type 1 diabetes

DM2. *See* Type 2 diabetes

Documentation
  of adverse events (as ethical issue), 114–115
  of allocation and funding of intervention services, 247
  of changes in intervention protocols, 103
  of clinical significance, 234
    of diabetes interventions, 150
  on diabetes treatment in clinical settings, 145
  on impact of prevention interventions for JRA, 201
  of intervention fidelity, 98, 100
  for justification of interventions funding, 246

Double ABCX model of family behavior, 37–38

DSMBs (data safety and monitoring boards), 115

Duration of intervention, 61, 66–67

Eating disorders, as diabetes risk, 142

Economic level
  and access to care, 248
  and risk for severe chronic conditions, 10

Education
  of researchers in psychological interventions, 243–245
    on ethical issues, 120
  in self-management (diabetes), 152–153

Educational approaches, in SCD intervention, 185, 188

Educational-behavioral intervention
  in cancer intervention, 164
  for CF, 217, 219

Educational and support approaches, for JRA, 195, 197, 199

Education and support program for diabetes, costs vs. benefits of, 151–152

Efficacy or effectiveness, in RE-AIM model, 239

Electronic monitoring devices, 136

Eligibility criteria, standardizing of, 62, 76

Empathy, in cancer intervention, 164

End-stage renal failure, case example of (Johnny), 14

Equipoise, principle of, 107

Ethical issues
  anticipating risks in, 105–106
  child neglect or abuse, 116
  communicating with data safety and monitoring boards, 115
  communicating with Institutional Review Boards, 119
  in computer-based interventions, 118
  confidentiality, 116–117
  consultation on, 119–120
  in design of intervention research, 106–108
  documenting of adverse events, 114–115
  and domains of harm, 106
  education on, 120
  incentives and payments for expenses, 117–118
  informed consent, 108–114
    example on, 105
  managing participants with psychological problems, 115–116
  questions on, 119

Ethnic minority youths
  asthma prevalent among, 123
  See also African American children

Evaluation
    of asthma interventions, 136
    of available empirical research, 61,
        70–71
    of clinical significance of interven-
        tion change (four primary meth-
        ods of), 240
    of efficacy of tailored interventions,
        236
    of implementation of interventions
        in clinical settings, 239–240
    of intervention fidelity, 62, 77–78
Event congruence, 45
Exclusion criteria, 76, 94–95
Expectancies, outcome, 43–44

Factorial designs, 72
Family adjustment and adaptation re-
    sponse (FAAR) model, 37–38,
    39, 52
Family-based behavioral intervention pro-
    cedures, for diabetes manage-
    ment, 145
Family-based problem-solving, for
    asthma, 135
Family-based self-management training,
    for diabetes, 29
Family burden prevention program, for
    cancer, 172
Family-centered behavior modification,
    for JRA, 200
Family-centered biobehavioral model,
    39–40, 41
Family-centered psychological interven-
    tions
    for asthma, 126
    for diabetes, 148–149, 152
    for SCD, 190
Family conflict
    from miscarried helping, 40
    as risk factor, 50
    and stress, 40
Family Learning Program, for CF, 218
Family members
    asthma impact on, 125–126
    and barriers to interventions, 19
    cancer impact on, 160–161
    CF impact on, 207
    as intervention target, 21, 22–23

participation by and retention of,
    95–97
psychological impact of childhood
    chronic illness on, 18
SCD impact on, 182–183
See also Parents
Family processes, articulating role of, 51
Family systems models, 39–41, 52
Family therapy, for CF, 218
Feasibility and response burden, 80
Feasibility studies, 89
Fidelity of intervention, 62, 77–78, 97
    checking on, 98
Fitting Cystic Fibrosis Into Your Life Every
    Day (CD-ROM), 216
Flutter, the, 204
Foundations, research funds from, 89
Frameworks for intervention research. See
    Theoretical models and frame-
    works for intervention research
Frontallis electromyography biofeedback,
    for asthma, 129
Funding
    from National Institutes of Health,
        233
    for support of psychological interven-
        tion services, 246
    documentation of, 247

Generalizability of empirically supported
    interventions
    improvement of, 239–240, 243
    testing of, 235–236
Generalizability of intervention effects,
    231
    across multiple respondents, 80–81
Generalized or universal interventions,
    63, 175
Group family cognitive–behavioral inter-
    vention, in cancer intervention,
    164
Group therapy, multifamily, for diabetes,
    150

HbA$_{1c}$, and diabetes, 140
Health and Behavior CPT Codes, 20,
    233, 246
Health belief model, 43, 55
Health Buddy, 130–131

Health Insurance Portability and Accountability Act (HIPAA), 109–110, 119

Helping, miscarried, 40, 41, 52

High-frequency chest compression (HFCC) vest (ThAIRapy vest), 204

Home-based approaches, to asthma intervention, 131

Home-care intervention, for diabetes, 151–152

Home setting, for psychological interventions and data gathering, 93

Hypnosis, for cancer pain management, 241

Hypothesis testing, 81

Illness management, impact of chronic childhood illness on, 15–16

Illness uncertainty theory, 44–45

Imagery techniques
    for cancer pain management, 241
    for JRA, 200

Implementing of psychological intervention research, 85–86
    in clinical settings (evaluation of), 239–240
    developing collaborative context and resources, 86, 87–92
    managing of logistical challenges, 86, 92–101
    for multisite studies, 86, 94, 102 (see also Multisite intervention studies)
    in RE-AIM model, 239
    and unanticipated changes in protocols, 86, 102–103

Incentives
    as ethical issue, 117–118
    for family participation, 96, 100

Inclusion criteria, 76, 94–95

Individual behavioral management approaches, for diabetes, 147–148

Individual differences
    and manualized protocols, 106
    need for greater emphasis on, 53
    in response to psychological interventions, 26–31

Individual/family resource and risk factor models, 36–39

Individualized education plans, for SCD children, 191

Individuals With Disabilities Education Act (1997), 168

Informed consent, 108–114
    example on, 105

Institutional review board (IRB), 109, 118, 119

Insurance reimbursement
    and DSM–IV system, 233
    and managed care, 19

Intensity and duration of intervention, 61, 66–67

Interdisciplinary teams, 60, 90

International Society of Pediatric Oncology Working Committee on Psychosocial Issues, 162

Internet, research sharing on, 242

Internet interventions, privacy consideration in, 118

Intervention effects, testing mediation and moderation of, 82

Intervention efficacy, data needed for, 20

Intervention fidelity, 62, 77–78, 97
    checking on, 98

Interventionists, 90–91

Intrasubject replication designs, 72

IRB (institutional review board), 109, 118, 119

Journal articles, CONSORT guideline on, 228

Journal of Pediatric Psychology, 70, 144, 242, 242–243

JRA. See Juvenile rheumatoid arthritis

Juvenile rheumatoid arthritis (JRA), 191–192
    case example of (Tommy), 193
    educational and behavioral intervention for, 25
    medical treatment for, 192
        adherence to, 194
    psychological impact of on children and families, 192–193
    psychological interventions for, 194–199
        clinical applications of, 200–201
    research recommendations on, 199–200

JRA, *continued*
      social support interventions for, 22,
            197, 199

Ketoacidosis, 140, 153

Lance Armstrong Foundation, 89
Logistical challenges to study implementa-
      tion, 86, 92–101

Maintenance, in RE-AIM model, 239
Malignancies, pediatric, 157. *See also*
      Cancer
Managed care, and reimbursement for psy-
      chological intervention, 19
Management of acute episode, as self-
      management skill, 133
Manualized group behavioral interven-
      tion, for CF, 217
Manualized protocols, 106
Massage therapy
      for CF patients, 216
      for JRA, 195
Measurement of outcomes, for asthma in-
      terventions, 136
Mediation and moderation of interven-
      tion effects, testing of, 82
Mediators of intervention change, 35,
      52–53
Mediators of intervention effects, 229
"Medical home," 248
Medical neglect, 116
Medical treatment
      of asthma, 124–125
            adherence to, 127–128
      of cancer, 157–159
            adherence to, 161–162, 171
      of CF, 203, 204–205
            adherence to, 207–208
      of diabetes, 140–141
      for JRA, 192
            adherence to, 194
      for SCD, 180–181
            adherence to, 183, 189
Mental health disorders, and childhood
      chronic health conditions, 13

Meta-analyses
      of intervention research, 242–243,
            243
      of studies of psychological adjust-
            ment, 13
Minorities
      and access to care, 248
      asthma prevalent among, 123
      See also at African American
Minority parents, and asthma, 128
Miscarried helping model, 40, 41, 52
Models for intervention research. *See*
      Theoretical models and frame-
      works for intervention research
Moderation effects, analyses of, 82
Moderators of intervention change, 53–
      54, 230
Mothers
      in health belief model, 43
      See also Family members; Parents
Motivational interviewing, 47–48
MST. *See* Multisystemic therapy
Multidisciplinary care
      for asthma, 137
      for cancer, 277
      for SCD management, 191
Multifamily group therapy, for diabetes,
      150
Multiple baseline design, 72
Multiple informants, outcome data based
      on, 80–81
Multiple respondents, generalizability of
      intervention effects across, 80–81
Multisite intervention studies, 10, 86, 94,
      102, 245
      for CF, 218
      on SCD, 191
Multisystemic therapy (MST), 242
      for diabetes, 148–149, 237

National Cooperative Inner-City Asthma
      Study (NCICAS), 125–126, 132
National Cooperative Study of SCD, 191
National Institutes of Health, funds from,
      89, 233
National Institute of Mental Health, on
      mental disorder prevention, 64
National Institutes of Health (NIH)
      and access for minorities and eco-
            nomically disadvantaged, 248

career development training grants
sponsored by, 245
funds from, 89
National Jewish Hospital, 132
No-effect result of intervention, 63,
82–83
Nonadherence (noncompliance) to medical treatment, 15–16
for asthma treatment, 127–128
and treatment side effects, 125
for cancer treatment, 161–162
for CF treatment, 207–208
case example of (Brad), 208
for diabetes treatment (and MST),
237
discovery of as ethical issue, 117
and inconsistent parental reinforcement, 64–65
parents' vs. children's sensitivity to,
80
and tailored approach, 236
typology of problems in, 69
No-treatment control groups, ethical concerns over, 107
Nutritional education, for CF, 217
extension of, 219

Ontario Child Health Survey, 13
Open Airways program, 128
Operational definition of target problem
and outcome, 61, 67–68
Outcome evaluation, 238
quality control of, 101
Outcome expectancies, 43–44
Outcome measures, 62, 78–81
Outcomes, types of, 79
Outpatient management program, for dia-
betes, 152

Pain
competing models for response to,
35
distress associated with, 14–15
interventions for, 24–25
from JRA, 179, 192
from SCD, 179, 180, 191
in case example (Raymond),
181–182

Pain management
for cancer patients, 173
imagery and hypnosis in, 241
for JRA, 195, 196, 200
for SCD patients, 181, 189, 191
care paths for, 191
Pain reduction models, 41
Parents
of adolescent girls with diabetes, 141
cancer impact on, 160–161
and informed consent, 109–112
responsibility for asthma manage-
ment shifted to, 138
SCD impact on, 182–183
See also Family members
PAT (Psychosocial Assessment Tool),
176
Payments for expense, as ethical issue,
117–118
Pediatric Ambulatory Care Treatments
(PACT) program, 22
Pediatric asthma. See Asthma
Pediatric chronic illness. See Childhood
chronic illness
Pediatric diabetes. See Type 1 diabetes
(DM1); Type 2 diabetes (DM2)
Pediatric malignancies, 157. See also
Cancer
Peer-centered models of psychological in-
tervention, 21, 24
Peer relationships, 16–17
Personal meaning models, 45, 46
Pharmacological interventions, for can-
cer, 163
Pharmacotherapy, in cancer intervention,
171
Pilot studies, 89
of computerized interventions,
118
Policy applications, 224, 227, 245–249
Population-based systems approach, for di-
abetes care, 155
Posttest-only control group designs, 72
Posttraumatic stress disorder (PTSD)
among childhood cancer survivors,
160
among parents of pediatric cancer
survivors, 161
Posttraumatic stress symptoms (PTSS),
among parents of pediatric cancer
survivors, 161

Practice settings
    developing interventions in,
        234–235
    translation of psychological interven-
        tions to, 239, 243
    See also Clinical settings and
        applications
Practitioners
    in psychological intervention re-
        search, 91–92
    See also Primary caregiver
Prevention
    primary, secondary and tertiary,
        65–66
    as self-management skill, 133
Prevention and management of acute epi-
        sodes, as self-management skill,
        133
Preventive intervention approaches,
        248–249
    for cancer survivors and families,
        165, 166, 170–171
    cost-effectiveness of, 237
    for CF (young marrieds), 218
    for JRA patients, 200–201
Primary caregiver, as intervention target,
        21, 22
Primary outcomes, 79
Primary prevention, 65
Principal investigator (PI), 90
Privacy, in Internet interventions, 118
"Probably efficacious," 70
Problem-solving
    for asthma, 236
        family-based, 135
    for cancer, 164
        family-based, 167, 169–70, 190
    for CF, 218
    for SCD, 189, 190
Problem-solving theory, 42, 55
Process components, evaluation of, 238
Program evaluations, 238
Project coordinator, 90
Prospective research, 54
Psychoeducational interventions
    for CF, 209, 210, 216
    for diabetes, 145
Psychological adjustment problems, 12–14
Psychological interventions for childhood
        chronic illness
    barriers to, 18–20

    for asthma, 127–128, 131–132
    clinical applications for, 224,
        234–240
    costs–benefits and offset of, 236–237
    design of, 59 (*see also* Design of psy-
        chological interventions)
    different conditions at different stages
        of development of, 223, 225
    dissemination and development of,
        224, 241–242
    enhancing science of, 224, 226–231
    implementation of, 83 (*see also* Im-
        plementing of psychological inter-
        vention research)
    and individual differences, 26–31
    models of (target, method, out-
        come), 20–22
        child-centered, 21, 24–26
        family-centered, 21, 22–23
        peer-centered, 21, 24
        primary caregiver-centered, 21, 22
        school-based, 23–24
    need for examination of, 4–5
    need for greater access to, 248, 249
    number of participants available for
        study, 10
    and practice settings, 243–245
    recruitment of participants for,
        94–95
        HIPAA constraints on, 110
        resources needed for, 88
    research-based vs. clinical, 232–237
    researcher-practitioner interchange
        on, 241–242
    for specific illnesses
        asthma, 127, 128–132, 133
        cancer, 159, 162–177
        CF, 208–217
        diabetes, 143–146, 147–149,
            153–155
        JRA, 194–199, 200
        sickle cell disease, 183–184
    theoretical models and frameworks
        of, 33, 34 (*see also* Theoretical
        models and frameworks for inter-
        vention research)
    universal vs. selected vs. targeted,
        63–64, 175–176
Psychological intervention research. *See*
        Research on psychological inter-
        vention

Psychological problems, managing participants with, 115–116
Psychosocial Assessment Tool (PAT), 176
Psychosocial intervention, for cancer, 166, 173, 175–176, 177, 249
Psychosocial Therapies Research Group, 145
Psychosomatic family model, 39, 41
Psychotherapy, for CF, 218
PTSD. *See* Posttraumatic stress disorder
PTSS (posttraumatic stress symptoms), among parents of pediatric cancer survivors, 161
Published reports, enhancing clinical significance of, 240–245
Pulmonary events, from SCD, 180
Purpose of intervention, 61, 64–66

Quality control issues in psychological intervention studies, 97–101
   for outcome evaluation procedures, 101
Quasi-experimental designs, 72–73
Questionnaire data, 101

Randomization, parents' failure to understand, 111
Randomized assignment, 73
Randomized controlled trials of asthma management, 131–132
Randomized selection, 73
RCTs (randomized controlled trials), 62, 71, 73, 73–74
   and CONSORT, 228
   insufficient justification for, 235
   need for, 227
Reach, in RE-AIM model, 239
Readiness-to-learn model, for asthma intervention, 131
RE-AIM model, 239
Recommendations to enhance science, practice, and policy, 223–225
   and challenges to enhancing clinical significance of intervention research, 231–234
   conceptual framework for, 224–225
   on enhancing clinical applications, 224, 234–240

on enhancing clinical significance of intervention research, 231–234
on enhancing clinical significance of research and published reports, 240–245
on enhancing science of psychological interventions, 224, 226–231
on policy applications, 224, 245–249
Recruitment of participants in psychological intervention studies, 94–95
   HIPAA constraints on, 110
   resources needed for, 88
Relaxation techniques and training
   in anxiety and pain reduction models, 41
   for asthma, 129, 135
   for CF, 217
   and diabetes, 143
   for SCD, 181
Reliability, 79
Research assistants, 91
Research design, choice of, 62, 72–74
Research on psychological intervention
   access to services provided through, 20
   for asthma, 134–137
      future challenges to, 137–138
   for cancer, 171–172, 176
   challenges to, 31–32
   collaboration on, 245
   for CF, 217–219
   for diabetes, 149–152
   enhancing clinical applications of, 224, 234–240
   enhancing clinical significance of, 240–245
      critical reviews and meta-analyses of, 242–243
   for enhancing science of psychological intervention, 224, 226–231
   and family impact, 18, 19
   and identification of active ingredients, 229
   for JRA, 199–200
   new training methods and models for, 243–245
   participation rates for, 94
   policy applications of, 224, 245–249
   prospective, 54
   for SCD, 189–191
   stages of, 225–226

Social support approaches
    for CF, 211, 216
    for JRA (parents), 22, 197, 199
    in SCD intervention, 184, 187, 188
Specific intervention approach, 12
Specificity of models and frameworks,
    50–51
Stage of target problem, individual differ-
    ences in, 28
Stages of change models, 46–48
Standard care, defining and measuring,
    62, 78
Standardizing of eligibility criteria, 62, 76
Standards, for reviews of empirically sup-
    ported research, 70
STARBRIGHT world computer network,
    185
Statistical power, 81
Stress
    and acceptance of interventions, 29
    and diabetes, 143
    and family conflict, 40
    and parents of CF patients, 207
Stress management
    for asthma, 130, 135
    for diabetes, 145
    for cancer patient mothers, 167
Strokes, from SCD, 180, 181, 182
Surviving Cancer Competently Interven-
    tion Program (SCCIP), 171

Tailored intervention approaches, 63
to asthma intervention, 131
    evaluating efficacy of, 236
Tape recording
    ethical risks in, 106
    on fidelity of interventions, 77
Targeted approaches to psychological ser-
    vice allocation, 249
Targeted interventions, 63–64, 175–176
Target participants and model of interven-
    tion, 61, 66
Target problem, individual differences in,
    28–30
Tertiary prevention, 65–66
ThAIRapy vest, 204
Thank-you letters to participants, 97
Theoretical models and frameworks for in-
    tervention research, 33–36
    cognitive–behavioral theories, 41–42

comprehensive models, 48–49
family systems models, 39–41
individual/family resource and risk
    factor models, 36–39
and integration of theory, research
    and practice, 54–55
refining of, 49–50, 54
    articulating family processes role,
        51–52
    enhancing specificity, 50–51
    specifying mediators of interven-
        tion change, 52–53
    specifying moderators of interven-
        tion change, 53–54
social–cognitive models, 42–46
stages-of-change models, 46–48
Theory, in choice of intervention model,
    34–35, 62, 71–72
Tiered model of psychosocial care, 175–
    176, 200
Timing and purpose of intervention, 61,
    64–66
Trade-off, between clinical significance
    and statistical power, 68
Transactional stress and coping model, 37
Transitions, in life of cancer patient, 159
Transitions, developmental, and psycho-
    logical intervention, 30–31
Transtheoretical model, 47
Treatment adherence
    central characteristics of, 48–49
    See also Nonadherence to medical
        treatment
Treatment Options for Type 2 Diabetes
    in Adolescents and Youth (TO-
    DAY) study, 153
Triadic partnerships model, 49
Type 1 diabetes (DM1), 139, 140
    age of diagnosis of, 28–29
    and BFST, 23, 235
    case example on (Lisa), 34
    case example on (Sally), 16
    case example on (Sam), 142
    medical treatment regimen for,
        140–141
    MST for, 148–149, 237
    multifactorial interventions for, 31
    outpatient vs. inpatient model of
        care for, 237
    and problem-solving theory, 42
    psychological impact of, 141–143

ABOUT THE AUTHOR

Dennis Drotar, PhD, is professor of pediatrics at Case Western Reserve University School of Medicine, where he is director of the Division of Behavioral Pediatrics and Psychology. Over the course of his career, his research has focused on the psychosocial impact of physical chronic illness on children and families and interventions for these populations. His previous books include *Measuring Health-Related Quality of Life in Children and Adolescents: Implications for Research and Practice* (1998), *Handbook of Research Methods in Clinical Child and Pediatric Psychology* (2000), and *Promoting Adherence to Treatment in Chronic Childhood Illness* (2000). Dr. Drotar is actively involved in mentoring graduate students and fellows and directs the graduate research training program in pediatric psychology and the child health and behavior research fellowship at Case Western Reserve University.

He has served as president of the division of Child, Youth, and Family Services of the American Psychological Association (1995); president of the Society for Developmental and Behavioral Pediatrics (2001); and president of the Society of Pediatric Psychology (2005). He has received distinguished service awards for mentorship and significant research contributions from the Society of Pediatric Psychology.

His current research is focused on testing interventions to enhance informed consent to treatment in pediatric cancer, quality of life in pediatric chronic illness, and a randomized controlled trial of a problem-solving intervention to enhance adherence to treatment and illness management in children and adolescents with asthma and their families.